# Becoming a
# Master Counselor
## Introduction to the Profession

**Richard Hill Byrne**

University of Maryland
*Emeritus*

 I(T)P

**Brooks/Cole Publishing Company**
**An International Thomson Publishing Company**

Pacific Grove   Albany   Bonn   Boston   Cincinnati   Detroit   London   Madrid
Melbourne   Mexico City   New York   Paris   San Francisco   Singapore   Tokyo   Toronto   Washington

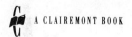

A CLAIREMONT BOOK

Sponsoring Editor: *Claire Verduin*
Editorial Associate: *Gay C. Bond*
Production Editor: *Penelope Sky*
Production Assistant: *Tessa A. McGlasson*
Manuscript Editor: *William Waller*
Permissions Editor: *Elaine Jones*
Interior Design: *Katherine Minerva*

Cover Design: *Laurie Hughes Design*
Interior Illustration: *Lisa Torri*
Art Coordinator: *Lisa Torri*
Marketing Team: *Connie Jirovsky and Margaret Parks*
Indexer: *Do Mi Stauber*
Typesetting: *Kachina Typesetting, Inc.*
Printing and Binding: *Arcata Graphics/Fairfield*

*For more information, contact:*

BROOKS/COLE PUBLISHING COMPANY
511 Forest Lodge Road
Pacific Grove, CA 93950
USA

International Thomson Editores
Campos Eliseos 385, Piso 7
Col. Polanco
11560 México D. F. México

International Thomson Publishing Europe
Berkshire House 168–173
High Holborn
London WC1V 7AA
England

International Thomson Publishing Gmbh
Königswinterer Strasse 418
53227 Bonn
Germany

Thomas Nelson Australia
102 Dodds Street
South Melbourne, 3205
Victoria, Australia

International Thomson Publishing Asia
221 Henderson Road
#05–10 Henderson Building
Singapore 0315

Nelson Canada
1120 Birchmount Road
Scarborough, Ontario
Canada M1K 5G4

International Thomson Publishing Japan
Hirakawacho Kyowa Building, 3F
2-2-1 Hirakawacho
Chiyoda-ku, 102 Tokyo
Japan

Printed in the United States of America

10 9 8 7 6 5 4 3 2 1

**Library of Congress Cataloging-in-Publication Data**
Byrne, Richard Hill.
    Becoming a master counselor: introduction to the profession /
Richard Hill Byrne.
        p.    cm.
    Includes bibliographical references and index.
    ISBN 0-534-25110-2
    1. Counselors.   2. Counselor and client.   3. Counseling.
I. Title.
BF637.C6B97   1994
158'.2.3'023—dc20                                    94-19530
                                                              CIP

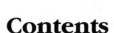

# Contents

**Part I
The Counselor
1**

# Chapter 6
## Affect in Clients' Lives
## 109

# Chapter 7
## Clients' Operant Behaviors
## 129

# Chapter 8
## Client Cognitions
## 149

# Part III
# Counseling Procedures and Techniques
# 163

## *Chapter 9*
## *Counseling Precepts and Practices*
## *165*

## *Chapter 10*
## *Counseling's Unique Communication Skills*
## *175*

# Chapter 11
## Other Counseling Issues
### 195

# Chapter 12
## Techniques for Helping Clients
### 209

# Chapter 13
## Counseling Procedures
### 237

## *Chapter 14*
## *Our Profession*
## *265*

# Preface

This book informs new students about counseling's cognitive content and technical practices, and it does so with a theoretical approach that differs sharply from other texts. It also shows that the essentials of counseling apply regardless of the agency or setting where they are offered (schools, colleges, rehabilitation agencies, marriage and family agencies), the specialized topics addressed (careers, sexuality, substance abuse), or the developmental concerns found in distinct subpopulations (different age groups, races, or genders).

The text is designed to be the first course in either a master's-level or doctor's-level program and to be informative for those experienced counselors who welcome learning about new conceptual approaches to counseling. It is also useful to anyone interested in learning what counseling is about and to those engaged in career exploration who may be considering counseling as a profession.

To aim at new students, I focus on main points, seeking to be comprehensive and coherent yet avoiding the extensive details characteristic of some other introductory texts. References too, featuring meta-analyses, have been kept to a minimum—enough to start students on a scholarly chase.

I find in some introductory counseling books an emphasis on technique with an insufficient treatment of the academic substance that must underlie practice. In this text I stress concepts. When concepts are mastered, counselors can create their own techniques.

## Unique Theoretical Content

The question of how people come to think, feel, and act as they do is central to all counseling topics. The concepts generated in response to that question give counseling its theory and the basis for its procedures and techniques.

Many introductory texts offer, without discrimination or critical judgment, a variety of counseling or therapy orientations or theories; students are to select one that satisfies them or create their own by melding several schools. Even if all the various theoretical options were defensible, that procedure would not be appropriate, because new students, not yet schooled in counseling, are unprepared to make that kind of scholarly judgment.

I take the position that a theory must agree with science—albeit postpositivist, or "new," science—a stand that reduces the tenability of some theories. I further demonstrate that current scientific reasoning and evidence eliminate the need for partial theories, even those that are somewhat compatible with scientific criteria. So often the schools of counseling described in introductory texts were formulated in counseling's early days. They were useful then, but now they deter counseling from achieving full professional status.

I see commitment to epistemic criteria as essential, so an early chapter addresses the topic of epistemology. One of the issues considered in that chapter centers on whether reality is "out there" or only in the "mind's eye." I believe that the best scientific thinking and evidence make clear that both the objective and subjective worlds are real. This position underlies the entire text.

I have applied that tenet and other criteria of nonpositivistic science to my examination of the theoretical and research literature. Consequently, I have rejected some theoretical propositions while finding portions of others tenable, even if seemingly contradictory, and have blended them into a new theoretical stance. I advance arguments that scientific reasoning and evidence give an explanation of why people think, feel, and act as they do that overarches prior theoretical offerings. This position is summed up in Chapter 9 in nine counseling precepts that constitute a theory, although I give that theory no label.

I am not saying that my theoretical stance is eclecticism, at least in the sense of piecing together of parts of seemingly discrete theories. Rather, it results from a fresh start by first committing to an epistemology and then seeking compatible ideas and practices. This results in a fusing of selected parts of past theories with new precepts, which produces a coherent single theory in which some parts of earlier theories can be recognized. For those committed to science and to the reality of both the objective and subjective worlds, this reworking precludes the need for the separate schools of thought that are usually found in counseling texts.

An important message emerges from that examination: in time, students should formulate their own epistemic commitment. Although this will be difficult for those who have not yet studied the issues, I nonetheless urge readers to adopt at least a tentative epistemic stand so that they can evaluate various proposals about counseling theory wherever they are found, including those offered in this book.

# Organization of the Text

## *Part I: The Counselor*

In Part I, I focus on counselors-to-be. Before students are led to see the need to make an epistemic commitment, they examine counseling as offered in a number of professions. This leads to a narrowing of the term to the type of counseling to which this text is devoted, which aims to resolve clients' psychological concerns.

I include the arguments made by those who have identified a shift in doctoral-level counseling toward clinical psychology and who accept that change. Those arguments are countered by those who think it is important to prevent counseling from sliding by default into an emphasis on the abnormal but to retain its adherence to enhancing the development of normal people, a purpose long synonymous with the word *counseling*. I favor the latter position. Most counselors will not be prepared beyond the master's level, so these arguments about doctoral-level practitioners do not apply to them. I therefore restructure the issue so that it also applies to the training of master's-level practitioners.

## Part II: The Client

In providing a comprehensive, coherent overview of counseling, I describe development of typical people. Development is examined at a depth that will let students see its relation to counseling and to prepare them for the advanced courses on development required in programs approved by the Council for Accreditation of Counseling and Related Educational Programs.

I include basic coverage of such biological factors as genes, the brain and neural system, and the endocrine system. Counselors who are aware of how biological factors influence mental processes, affect, and behaviors will better understand their clients.

## Part III: Counseling Procedures and Techniques

Through study of Parts I and II, students acquire the cognitive background they need to understand why counseling procedures and practices occur in the unique way they do—a "why" that is then summarized in the nine precepts upon which counseling practices are based. Readers go on to learn about the communication procedures that are unique to counseling, and they examine specific procedures for helping clients with concerns in the cognitive, emotional, and behavioral aspects of their lives. Then they are introduced to procedures and techniques that enhance healthy mental development and alleviate the nonpathological concerns of typical people. Finally, I examine such professional issues as approval of counselor-preparation programs and the certification or licensing of counselors.

## Other Philosophical Considerations

Chapters move in an increasingly advanced manner to explore how cognitions, feeling, and actions are formed and their significance for counseling. Because the fundamental commitment of this book is to a science that has moved beyond positivism, counseling is shown to be humanistic and existential. I clarify why these orientations are inescapable, how they are put into effect, and why counseling procedures that include them complement rather than compete with rigorous scientific evidence. Additionally, the writing is marked by these characteristics:

an emphasis on health and development, not cure or restoration
the view that people function as total entities and as systems in a variety of social contexts that are also systems
the idea that people are self-organizing, continuously striving to maintain and enhance their personal and social realities

## Counselor Formation Activities

I provide activities at the end of most chapters that are based on the assumption that to be a psychological counselor is to be more than just knowledgeable about counseling concepts, procedures, and practices. Counselors relate to other humans differently from laypeople; it is a function of a counselor-preparation program to facilitate the acquisition of those special characteristics. They cannot be acquired just through reading about them; deliberate effort to form them is needed. Some counselor-preparation programs devote course time to this end, but whether they do or not, the activities in this text can be performed by students on their own.

## Acknowledgments

Some of my interpretations and applications are based on the work of scholars of the past twenty years. I gratefully acknowledge my indebtedness to them. Colleagues at the University of Maryland and elsewhere, including those who disagree with my position, provided the intellectual anvils on which old concepts could be hammered into new professional shape. They have my gratitude, as do Audrey Newsome and John Rogers of Keele University (England), for professional responses that brought valued refinements to this text.

I am also thankful for the support of the staff at Brooks/Cole, especially Claire Verduin, Gay Bond, Penelope Sky, and William Waller, and to the following reviewers: Frank Asbury, Valdosta State College; David Lane, Columbus College; Arlene Lewis, Western Washington University; Anthony LoGiudice, Frostburg State University; Brent Mallinckrodt, University of Oregon; Janet L. Merrill, Southern Methodist University; Paul Power, University of Maryland; and Vince Peterson, Indiana University.

For editing that greatly helped me make the manuscript more readable, I remain beholden to special people: my wife Joy, and our firstborn, Chris.

*Richard Hill Byrne*

# 1
**PART**

# The Counselor

$$\boxed{1}$$

CHAPTER

# The Profession of Counselor

## Overview

This chapter clarifies what counseling is and what its practitioners do. It first points out that counseling is an activity found in a number of fields, such as health, law, finance, and religion. This breadth requires that the purposes and procedures characteristic of the counseling with which we are concerned be distinguished from the counseling offered in those other fields.

The counseling that interests us deals with the subjective (psychological) matters of clients' cognitions, emotions, and behaviors, which usually are present in a complicated mix. This chapter also introduces a related topic: the education and professional qualifications of counselors. Qualifications bear on whether counselors are professionals because professionalism depends on a degree of preparation that permits counseling to be a full-time occupation. Trained counselors are contrasted with those who help others with their cognitive, emotional, and behavioral development without having the formal preparation to do so.

For all history an individual who felt the need for help with a concern of the kind spoken of here as psychological would seek out a friend, family member, elder, neighbor, and so on. This historic form of counseling will always be provided, and by persons whose psychological knowledge and counseling experience are casual. This help offered by nonformally prepared persons is spoken of here as traditional counseling.

In contrast, the professional counselor, regardless of the field, is well educated and trained in that field and devotes full time to it. The professional psychological counselor is not only well prepared but also educated and trained in interpersonal relationships. In this and other chapters we see why this is so important a topic, how these relationships are developed, and how they function in counseling. We will see the role of communication skills in establishing and maintaining this relationship and in facilitating client growth and change. Those who provide traditional counseling typically lack awareness of what relationship should exist, and they lack training in communication skills.

Clarifying the role of the professional counselor is complicated by the fact that subjective (psychological) concerns are also the province of other professionals, such as social workers and clinical psychologists. Differences from other professionals, particularly clinical psychologists, are examined. In this chapter you will find both the general goals of counseling and three specific objectives of counselors. As part of the topic of objectives, counselors' life-views are defined, and the significance of these views for counseling is examined.

## Introduction: The Forms of Counseling

Phyllis is fortunate: she is 27 and has recently inherited over $200,000 from an aunt. Because she is inexperienced in financial matters, she looks for help in using her inheritance wisely. She calls upon an accountant who specializes in financial counseling. Alternatively, she might have asked a fellow employee who often brags about her financial wizardry.

Samantha, 36, has been experiencing a troubling lack of spiritual expression in her life. The daughter of nonreligious parents, she has come this far in life focusing only on the present. She had not mentioned her concerns to anyone but had been thinking that she would talk them over with her best friend, Jane. By chance, however, she met a female member of the clergy and has decided to engage in counseling with her.

Keith has had no concerns about spiritual matters and no need to discuss finances, even though he has accumulated a sizable fortune. But a cloud is looming: his former business partner has accused him of tampering with the books. Keith now has something to be worried about. At one time his brother, Bud, was similarly charged but wriggled out of it, so Keith first thought he had better have a chat with Bud. Today, however, he has decided to consult an attorney.

Betty has been married for seven years, since she was 16. The carefree euphoria of the first wedded years has long since withered, but she still wants to make something of her marriage with Carl, even though he has shown only lukewarm interest. She has frequently talked about her problems with Rose, who would have been Betty's bridesmaid had she not eloped to spite her parents. Talking with Rose did not help as much as she had expected; now she has gone to a marriage counselor.

Alan is a high school junior. Recent circumstances have made him eager to make serious plans for his occupational future. He has had some vague notions along that line but thinks they have been more fanciful than real. He now visits the school counselor and begins a series of interviews. He had occasionally discussed his future career with his father.

### *Traditional and Professional Counseling*

A choice faced all five: they could talk the problem over with a concerned friend or relative, or they could seek counseling with a professional. The counseling that Phyllis was seeking was financial, Samantha's was spiritual, and Keith's was legal. Shortly, we will look at the kinds of counseling that Betty and Alan wanted.

The label of counselor can be used, on the one hand, to describe anyone of goodwill and some experience who makes an effort to help another person solve a problem. On the other hand, it can be used to describe the trained professional who is committed to providing counseling assistance full time. Phyllis, Samantha, and Keith each chose the professional. Betty and Alan also chose the full-time practitioner over the untrained counselor. However, there is an important difference between the trained counselors with whom Phyllis and Keith conferred and the counselors consulted by Betty and Alan. The distinction lies in differences between the problems that these two pairs faced. (Samantha's concern is of a quite different order, to be inspected shortly.)

Phyllis's and Keith's concerns were primarily *objective,* involving financial and legal issues. The topics addressed by counselors in those fields involve clients' subjective states only peripherally. The prime topics of counseling in those instances are the objective realities of finance and the law.

Betty's and Alan's concerns, however, were *subjective.* They were concerned about how they felt about themselves, where they hoped to go in life, and how to get along with other people. Theirs are normal concerns in the psychological domain, so when they looked for professional help, they went to counselors whose interest and preparation are directed to enhancing the development of normal people with normal developmental needs. The topic of psychological counseling is the client, not an objective subject like law or finance. But what of Samantha? Were not her needs also subjective? They were, but psychological counselors are typically trained to handle concerns of this world, and Samantha also had otherworldly interests. She had the choice of counseling with a trusted friend or with someone well grounded in theology. A counselor prepared to deal with cognitions, emotions, and behavior would listen to Samantha, would help her define her concerns, and might provide some help. But her primary help will probably come from a person prepared to deal with matters of spiritual faith.

### Counseling about Psychological Development versus Other Counseling

Both trained and untrained people counsel, but there is a commonality in what happens. Whether or not the help being sought involves financial, legal, or health concerns, the person seeking help usually expects it to be in the form of advice. That will also be the case when someone seeks help about a developmental (psychological) matter from an untrained counselor. The difference between such an untrained helper and a professional lies in the professional's wealth of specialized knowledge and competence, which lets him or her know the uselessness of advice and the means to facilitate change without it. Dictionaries give the word *advice* as a synonym for counseling, and there can be no challenge to that when the topic of counseling is objective, as it is in law, health, or finance. In the practice of counselors trained to assist with the subjective (psychological) concerns of cognitions, emotions, and behavior, however, advice and counseling are not synonymous.

When giving advice, a professional practitioner in occupations that deal with the *objective* world is saying, in effect, "As an expert, I know what's best for you; take my advice." Advice provides clients with an immediate course of action for dealing with the objective world. On the other hand, the goal of a psychological counselor is to bring a permanent change in the way a client thinks, behaves, or experiences emotions—or all three together. This objective is not attained by giving advice.

When Betty talked about her marriage concerns with her friend Rose, she expected sympathy, of course, and advice. Rose's reactions were statements like "You ought to," "If I were you . . . ," or "You shouldn't let yourself get upset when that happens." That last bit of advice was particularly useless. If Betty was concerned because she got upset, just telling her not to be upset could not change her responses. The trained counselor, without using such phrases, would help her bring about permanent change in her cognitions, feelings, and behaviors. (These comments assume that Betty has come alone for marriage counseling.) As for her being upset about Carl's behaviors, the professional counselor would help her define and consciously experience her upset states, identify their causes, and learn to manage them and would engage in procedures to raise her self-esteem.

Advice, urging, and persuasion are feeble reeds for the professional to lean on. The effects of persuasion, Rehm and Rokke observe, "may be weak and temporary because [it] is not founded on [the client's] experience and may be quickly dismissed [by the client] in the face of experiential disconfirmation" (1988, p. 139). This is not to say that a trained counselor would never employ persuasion. As with advice and urging, it may occasionally be used, not as an impulsive technique but only deliberately after making a professional judgment of what may be best at the moment.

Let's summarize the ideas above:

1. To provide clarity to the public, the words *counselor* and *counseling* may need to be modified, depending on circumstances. There are full-time, trained counselors in a number of domains, such as finance, health, and law. Those counselors provide counseling under such titles as accountant and trust officer, nutritionist and physician, and paralegal and lawyer.
2. The concerns addressed by counselors in the financial, health, and legal fields are primarily objective ones; if these professionals deal with clients' subjective lives, it is only peripherally.
3. At any one time, large numbers of people will be experiencing concerns about their subjective (psychological) lives. These concerns are normal, some being the minor ones experienced by anyone at any time. Others, still in the normal range, may be of such proportion as to impede daily functioning.
4. The list of subjective concerns for which help is sought is lengthy; it includes unresolved early or recent traumas, senses of inadequacy or worthlessness, relationship problems (with friends, parents, spouse, children), job dissatisfaction, present or future career uncertainty, shyness, performance inadequacies, and insufficient control over emotions.
5. These and other psychological concerns occur in the normal development of typical people. The term *psychological counseling* will be employed here to

distinguish the processes treated in this book from counseling processes in other domains. Similarly, the term *psychological counselor* will often be used to emphasize the idea that the domain of counseling addressed is the psychological functioning of clients. At the same time, because the use of those two terms refers to developmental assistance to typical people, their connotations are not to be confused with what is meant by clinical psychology.

6. In any area of human concern, whether objective or subjective, counseling is more often sought from untrained people than from trained counseling specialists. Untrained counselors are handy, trusted, and respected, and their advice costs nothing. Additionally, many people see the seeking of help from a professional as a sign of weakness.

7. The seeking of help from untrained persons is more pronounced in subjective concerns partly because more people have more problems in the psychological domain than in others. Depending upon a number of variables, the help of untrained counselors may be not only ineffective but also harmful.

8. The verbal help given by *untrained* persons when they offer psychological counseling is similar to the assistance provided by both untrained and trained counselors who deal with objective matters like law, health, and finance. The help in these instances is primarily *advice,* perhaps coupled with persuasion, urging, or cajoling.

9. Professionally prepared psychological counselors relate to clients through procedures that are unknown to and unneeded by trained practitioners in the objectively focused professions. The task of the chapters that follow is to describe, in an introductory manner, the procedures unique to the practices of the psychological counselor.

## A Brief History of Counseling

The contemporary forms of providing psychological assistance have different points of origin. Everyone is familiar with the history of psychoanalytic psychology, starting with Freud. Another point of origin was clinical psychology, which developed in the early years of this century as an aid to physicians. Clinical psychologists at that time focused on psychological appraisal. Psychoanalytic psychology has retained its conceptual essentials, although in recent decades it has been generally replaced as a tenable accounting for the way people think, act, and feel. Clinical psychology has experienced evolutionary changes, due in part to the research orientation it has had from the start. Although the profession's title still retains its subservient adjective, "clinical," its practitioners often chose to function as independent professionals.

A quite different form of psychological help also appeared in the early part of this century. Some community-oriented people saw the need for children of immigrants and those who had finished eight grades of schooling to make a studied judgment about an occupation instead of just falling into some form of employment. This concern led to the establishment of vocational counseling. At the same time that vocational counseling for early adolescents was growing and changing along with other changes in public education, institutions of higher learning began to offer counseling for a considerably different population. It was in counseling for higher education that a new practitioner of psychology, the *counseling psychologist,* emerged about half a century ago.

Over the evolving years of this new profession, several forces led to the determination that counseling psychologists should be prepared at the doctoral level: it was natural to engage in research on counseling in university settings, university employment generally required a doctorate, and eventually an earned doctorate became a requirement for membership in the American Psychological Association (APA). This new occupation acquired its definition from the establishment of a Division of Counseling Psychology (Division 17) in the APA and from formal definitions of purposes set out by Division 17 in succeeding years. A major need for that definition was to differentiate counseling psychology from clinical psychology, to which it has a technical similarity. Shortly we will examine what those differences are.

Vocational (guidance) counseling in schools eventually lost its modifier to become just counseling, because counselors were expected to deal with all developmental concerns of students. A national association set up to define and sponsor research on a wide range of developmental concerns only slowly emerged from the single-interest association that started in 1913, the National Vocational Guidance Association. Today the American Counseling Association, which recently evolved from the American Association for Counseling and Development, provides definitional and research leadership for counselors whose specialty preparation is attained by a master's degree.

Counseling in public schools has developed over time to provide assistance (at least ideally) with an array of developmental concerns similar to those of counseling in higher education. Counselors in both settings attend to the psychological developmental competencies of their clients, in both immediate and long-term matters. To raise the effectiveness of school counselors to meet the newer professional needs, their training requirements have steadily increased to as much as 48 semester-hour credits, in contrast to the six courses prescribed by the U. S. Office of Education in the 1950s. As a body of counseling theory and skills emerged from the scholarly efforts of Division 17 along with some research from clinical psychology, professional psychological counseling spread out from educational settings to numerous specialties. Rehabilitation, mental health, and marriage and family are some examples. These require specialized training over and above a common foundation in counseling.

Given that history, it is no surprise that many of the defining terms of this profession originated with and were designed for those who will complete a doctor's degree. Scholars charged with examining the question would be expected to arrive at the broadest definitions and the maximum preparation required.

## *Psychological Counseling's Unique Characteristics*

The purposes and procedures of psychological counseling were first defined in the 1940s, fostered by people who eventually formed Division 17. The division issued reports recording alterations and additions to counseling concepts and practices as they developed. It would be harmful to believe that documents from an APA division defining counseling should apply only to doctoral-level counseling psychologists. Those preparing these thoughtful documents, which we will shortly be examining, included psychologists with a major interest in counseling as practiced anywhere, and particularly in schools. Two such men of historical note are Donald E. Super and C. Gilbert Wrenn.

This early history is examined by Jordaan, Meyers, Layton, and Morgan (1980), who offer as axiom the view that "all individuals can change, can lead satisfying lives, can be self-directing, and can find ways of using their resources" (p. 181). Commitment to that principle calls for interviewing procedures that set off those who help clients with normal psychological concerns from other practitioners. Those procedures require counselors to lead clients in "guided self-examination, self-discovery, and self-generated decisions [which] are more likely to lead to constructive actions and personal growth than *persuasion, exhortation, prescription, or advice*" (p. 182; emphasis added).

This early definition contrasted counseling with clinical psychology. In 1952 a Division 17 committee generated this statement:

> . . . we see . . . differences between clinical and counseling psychologists. One . . . is the amount of emphasis given [by counselors] to increasing individuals' resources for coping with their environments. [Counselors] spend more time in attaining comprehensive knowledge of the validities of psychological tests for predicting the outcomes of activities engaged in by clients during the normal course of their lives. . . . This is balanced by less preoccupation [by counselors] with the use of psychological tests for the analysis of the individual's inner life [Whiteley, 1980, p. 95].

A Division 17 gathering in 1964 (The Greystone Conference) produced five statements attributed to a group of leaders in counseling psychology—statements that distinguish counseling psychology from clinical psychology. They are paraphrased here, with core ideas emphasized.

1. The counseling psychologist works with *normal, convalescent, or recovered clients* who do not require long-term treatment because their problems are neither severe nor deep-seated.
2. The emphasis is on more typical (more normal) needs and problems that can be dealt with monthly on a *cognitive level*.
3. The focus is not on restructuring personalities [as it is with clinical psychology] but on drawing out and developing what is already there and on helping clients use their own resources.
4. Counseling psychologists attach importance to the roles of education and work in a client's life.
5. The counseling psychologist's role is essentially educational, developmental, and preventive rather than medical or remedial. This role calls not only for identifying, removing, or circumventing obstacles to *normal* development but also for helping individuals *achieve optimal development* [Whiteley, 1980, pp. 184–185].

It is noteworthy that this stance about the nature of counseling taken by Division 17 over 40 years ago remains unchanged. Promotional material issued by the division in 1992 to explain what counseling psychologists do informs readers that counseling focuses on the normal developmental needs and problems of adolescents and adults. This assistance is provided in diverse settings to meet a variety of needs.

Although the 1952 report describes the characteristics of counselors prepared at the doctoral level, those characteristics apply to all counselors. The concerns of human development are not affected by degree level. That is not to suggest that those prepared at the doctoral level are not more knowledgeable than those with less training. However, those with a master's degree are properly prepared for the level of service required of them. The intention here is not to examine differences in competency among practitioners at different levels of training but merely to record the leadership in defining counseling that originated with and continues to be provided by Division 17 of the APA.

## *The Struggle to Retain Counseling's Distinguishing Characteristics*

In ensuing years efforts to distinguish between counseling and clinical psychology continued. Super (cited by Pallone, 1980) in 1955 expressed the difference between the two psychologies by stating that "clinical psychology has typically been concerned with . . . *psychopathology,* with the abnormalities of even normal persons," whereas "*counseling psychology* concerns itself with *hygiology,* with the normalities of even abnormal persons" (p. 40; emphasis mine). Hahn did not see that distinction applying 25 years later but, rather, found the differences between the two rapidly diminishing (1980, p. 172). For example, he found listings in the "Positions Open" section of the APA *Monitor* stipulating that either clinical or counseling psychologists could apply. Such listings appeared more frequently than those asking for just counseling psychologists. At the doctoral level, given the extensive training, supervised practice, and experience of counseling psychologists, that may be a reasonable stipulation. However, for those positions held by the majority of psychological counselors—that is, those without a doctorate—the assumption is faulty: counselors with a master's degree cannot be compared to clinical psychologists.

A summary of the contrast between counseling and clinical psychologists is aptly provided by Super (1980a): "Clinical psychologists tend to look for what is wrong, and treat it, whereas counseling psychologists tend to look for what is right and how to help use it" (p. 15).

This profession may be defined either by principles emanating from representative bodies, or by practices that are not in line with those principles. Fitzgerald and Osipow (1986), for example, in writing about the long-standing emphasis on careers, find that attention to this heartland of the profession appears to be eroding. Indeed, empirical studies show little distinction between counseling and clinical psychologists.

Similarly, Watkins, Lopez, Campbell, and Himmel (1986) conclude that emerging trends in practice show the two specialties sharing several areas of convergence yet maintaining areas of distinctiveness: "It appears that clinical and counseling psychology have become increasingly similar over the years, and trends indicate that further convergence can be expected" (p. 582).

This convergence leads Levy (1984) to propose that the training of both specialties should be combined under the title human-services psychology. Steenbarger (1990) opposes that amalgamation. He summarizes research leading him to identify a theoretical basis for differentiating between the two professions. He sharpens the distinctions between a service that emphasizes *remediation* (clinical psychology) and one that emphasizes support of the *developmental* process (counseling). The latter may include some remediation, however. The theoretical term that Steenbarger employs is *developmentalism,* which he sees as a metatheory, "an overarching framework that guides the ways in which theories might be employed" (p. 435). A focus on developmentalism allows a wider base for examining differences than a focus on normal versus abnormal clients and problems. Historically, the counseling emphasis is on developmental and preventive processes. Steenbarger gives those historical ideas renewed viability with the concept of developmentalism.

Sprinthall (1990) offers several cautions to those who support a shift toward a common identity for clinical and counseling psychology. Should this drift be based on the lure of payments by insurance companies, this goal may be elusive; it can wither in the heat of economic realities that he examines. Clinical psychology as a field, furthermore, may come to resist infiltration by counseling psychologists. Be wary, he also cautions, of counseling-psychology programs being sent to the budget guillotine by the perennial campus cost-cutting prowlers who discover two programs preparing the same kind of practitioner, albeit under different names, and conclude that that is one program too many. Which program will be marked for extermination, he wonders: the long-established clinical program or the counseling program that has only recently moved into clinical preparation? The importance of this issue is grave for those counseling-psychology programs housed in colleges of education.

Beyond these political matters lie the critical professional ones, Sprinthall observes. In the matter of need:

> I fear that as we move in the direction of clinical treatment, we will move further away from behavioral science and from preventive practice. This may once again leave those with the greatest need for assistance out of the service loop [p. 460].

If there has been an insubstantial theoretical underpinning for preventive and developmental activities in the past, that is no longer the case, he contends, illustrating his argument with impressive recent developments in theory.

Counseling psychology, Sprinthall reminds us, has always sought to prepare a scientist-practitioner, one who provides the middle ground that bridges the understandable rift between the contending (and contentious) halves of the science and practice of psychology. The science element would be lost were the move to continue toward clinical practice away from counseling. He identifies the mission of counseling psychology (and, I add, of counseling practiced by whatever degree level of professional) as "educational and preventive and focused on promoting growth" (p. 461).

Steenbarger's developmentalism holds that psychological distress is not evidence of maladaptiveness or inappropriateness, which would require remediation. He holds that periods of disequilibrium are a normal by-product of natural change and, in fact, can be energizers leading to healthy growth: "Behaviors linked to distress often contain the kernel of new responses to developmental tasks, and as such are potentially adaptive" (1990, p. 453). Even though counseling and clinical psychologists may employ similar techniques, their views of client concerns are refracted by different theoretical and ontological prisms.

Stone and Archer (1990) take a developmentalist stand in their recommendations about university counseling centers in the 1990s. On the issue of normal versus abnormal behavior, they observe that:

> Given the evidence of problems related to pathological families and experiences, the definition of "normal" developmental issues becomes rather difficult. If 27% of the women in college have been raped since they were 14, is this becoming more of a "normal" developmental experience? [p. 546].

They comment that "it is clear that developmental issues for many of our students will include learning to overcome serious psychological problems" (p. 546).

## Counseling Defined

Combining the concepts cited above with ideas from other sources permits this definition of counseling, which represents a large degree of consensus: *Professional psychological counseling is provided by trained practitioners to cognitively competent clients of any age in order (1) to help them, by means of group activities and individual consultations, to work on common developmental tasks and (2) to assist most of them, usually in private consultations, to work through particular cognitive, affective, or behavioral obstacles impeding their development.* The primary developmental task is to attain and retain a sense of confident self-worth, paired with competence in forming and maintaining fulfilling and contributing relationships with others.

The most common socially specific developmental task, first appearing in adolescence and then anytime thereafter, is each individual's need to identify one or more appropriate, organized, consistent, and productive activities that will require a major investment of time and become part of his or her sense of personal significance and identity. These activities are an individual's occupation, whether paid or unpaid. Paid activities are easily thought of as occupations. It is not the pay that is of primary psychological importance, however, but the sense of personal meaning that those activities provide. In the 1960s and 1970s a noticeable number of youths were occupied full time being flower children and war protesters. In time they changed identities, and thus activities. These activities—these occupations—are now aimed at providing income and thus are occupations in the popular meaning of the word. The most common unremunerated occupation, which provides identity for many women today as it has in the past, is homemaker.

## *Diminished Concern with Career Development*

Despite this psychological centrality of occupations, some see a greatly diminished interest on the part of counselors in the role that occupations play in clients' mental health. Bishop (1990), in addressing this question, notes, however, that studies of college students show "some evidence that students are more inclined to participate in activities that assist them in career planning . . . than those that deal with more personal concerns" (p. 409). Career counseling, he further observes, is provided by 81% of university counseling centers.

Stone and Archer (1990) hold that "the need for psychologically oriented career counseling is great" (p. 552). In describing the opinions of directors of university counseling centers about the quality of preparation of counselors in career counseling and development, they report a score of 2.8 on a 5-point scale (5 = excellent). They conclude that college counseling centers should be concerned with career counseling and development because "career questions are inevitably connected to other psychological and developmental issues and someone trained in general counseling and developmental psychology theory can respond to career as a broad life-issue" (p. 552).

Bishop (1990) also supports the counseling center directors in their views about the poor quality of the training of counselors to deal with career questions. Perhaps that low quality is the reason for the reduced attention to career matters that Fitzgerald and Osipow report. Bishop writes that counseling students report the study of career psychology to be the least interesting course in their programs. Consequently, if study in that area is not required, few students select it as an option.

There may be a cyclical effect: doctoral students avoid studying career psychology or take only one course and find it unrewarding because it emphasizes dry-as-dust topics such as the *Dictionary of Occupational Titles,* career ladders, and occupational testing and interpretation. Anecdotal inquiry shows that students who take this sort of course fear that they must know these occupational data in order to serve as a career counselor. A course focusing on objective data lets students acquire the misunderstanding that career counseling is the brief sifting through of scads of information about the world of work and the client and then telling the client what is best for him or her.

What is sometimes peripheral or not even touched upon in such courses is that the term *career counseling* is mostly about the subjective nature of clients. Counseling examines important psychological issues of personal identity, such as self-concept and changes in it. It includes the imperatives of leading clients to their own decisions, which may indeed appear unrealistic to the counselor as unsupported romanticizing about an occupational future. Most clients, however, having sought out a counselor, can incorporate conclusions from this lengthy, intense psychological inquiry and make realistic decisions. It is the client's decision. These central topics of counseling are missed in some courses dealing with careers.

Some doctoral students eventually become counselor educators and thus influence the curriculum. If one course in career psychology survives, it is often assigned to a new faculty member as part of the rites of passage instead of to the most psychologically sophisticated instructor. This again reflects the common failure to see the centrality of occupations in humans' lives and in counseling about them. If the new instructor's view of careers was shaped by a deficient single course, the instructor looks forward to the day when he or she will have sufficient seniority to pass the course on to the next new member, thus being freed to teach a course in the "good stuff" in which lies the high status of working with the therapeutic needs in clients' lives.

If it is valid to be concerned that doctoral students are short-changed in their preparation for career counseling, the concern should be even greater when we recognize that master's students, the ones who will staff high school counseling centers, get little if any preparation in this area, which is of major concern to high school students. If the focus on careers in counselor preparation and practice is diminishing, the cause is not a declining interest on the part of clients.

### *Other Remedial Professions*

Psychological counseling includes remedial activities, but clinical psychology emphasizes the remedial function. In addition to clinical psychology, other professions have a remedial emphasis; they are mentioned here to complete the record.

Physicians who complete programs in clinical psychology become psychiatrists. Social workers who also study clinical psychology become psychiatric social workers; nurses who undertake similar studies become psychiatric nurses. Even though social workers are proficient in counseling, they are usually employed only in remedial agencies, in contrast to psychological counselors, who serve agencies concerned with prevention and development.

Clara E. Hill (1993), citing Gelso and Fretz (1992), observes that other helping professions, as well as counseling psychology, are concerned with remediation, prevention, and education/development. At the same time, the emphases of counseling psychology differ from those of other helping professions because counseling puts:

> (a) a focus on intact rather than severely disturbed people; (b) a focus on assets, strengths, and positive mental health regardless of the degree of disturbance; (c) an emphasis on relatively brief intervention; (d) an emphasis on person-environment interactions rather than an exclusive emphasis on the person or the environment; and (e) an emphasis on educational and career development [p. 252].

It must be pointed out that Hill is addressing the doctoral-level practitioner called a counseling psychologist. However, the characteristics she offers correctly describe all counseling that assists clients with cognitive, affective, and behavioral concerns (whether remedial, preventive, or educational/developmental), no matter the degree level of the practitioner or the specialty served.

## Relationship between Counselor and Client

Counseling on developmental matters differs from counseling in other professions in the nature of the relationship between counselor and client. Although an authoritative relationship is appropriate in professions in which the help given is advice, prescription, even urging (law, medicine), a notably different client/ counselor relationship is required in counseling on psychological matters. Counseling nurtures clients' self-examination, expects the process to result in their self-generated decisions, and teaches them how to manage their own lives—how to permanently alter cognitions, emotions, and actions to eliminate a current concern, prevent other concerns, and handle them satisfactorily if they do arise.

Those objectives are unique to counseling and require unique procedures to be employed within a unique relationship. This relationship is marked by communication devices that let clients know that the counselor is understanding their concerns. Such communication is characterized by those semiotic procedures (dealing with signs and symbols) that convey the counselor's esteem for and undivided interest in the client. These methods of communication establish the cooperative, nonauthoritarian tone that characterizes counseling. This relationship is sometimes called a working alliance, or therapeutic alliance, a concept that will receive detailed treatment later.

The initial period of counseling is marked by active listening, accompanied by clear signs that the counselor empathizes with the client (which does not mean that the counselor agrees with the client on issues). This relationship is sometimes a teaching/learning one, albeit not like the formal ones in structured education. The counselor at such times assumes the role of a caring tutor, or coach.

When a person employs the services of an attorney, accountant, or plumber— anyone who attends primarily to objective concerns—the person typically turns over to the practitioner the decisions about what work is to be done and how it is to be done, because the customer has no training or experience in making such decisions. The counselor, on the other hand, approaches clients from the stance (not the words, of course) that "we will work together, I sometimes as tutor and you as learner. I will create an atmosphere, an empathic relationship, that will help you along during any emotional states you may experience; these states may bring about needed personality restructuring. I will also help you acquire skills to manage your cognitions, emotions, and behaviors. Those coping skills will serve you through your lifetime and thus have a preventive function."

People who have not experienced professional counseling, upon meeting with a counselor for a first time, may expect the relationship to be similar to those experienced over the years with other professionals who deal with objective topics; that is, they may expect advice offered in an amiable but clearly authoritative tone. At the onset of counseling it may be necessary to clarify for some clients how the relationship and the approaches to be taken will differ from the client's prior experiences.

The client shares the counseling burden in terms of time spent during and outside interviews. In many instances the client will have to work far harder than the counselor. Clients learn early that they are not passive recipients of procedures applied to them by counselors, as may be acceptable in other professions where counseling occurs. In some instances, just experiencing a counselor for the kind of person she or he is, and being listened to by that person, may be sufficient for client needs. If there is a need for more specific changes in cognition, affect, or behavior, however, the counselor will initiate those procedures. Then the client will need to give considerable time to carrying out those procedures in the real world where the concerns lie. A coach spends some time training an athlete, but the athlete devotes more time to practice than was spent in the training session. So it is with some of the concerns addressed in counseling.

There are instances when a client requires extensive interviews. A client with a pronounced sense of inadequacy, for example, or one unable to ride through separation loss resulting from death, divorce, or other causes may become unable to function in most daily tasks. As noted earlier, however, maximum benefits occur for some clients solely from the counselor's attentive, active listening. Training to develop this skill is required for those counseling students whose accustomed manner of speaking when trying to help others is didactic, interruptive, or expressive of other communication impediments to professional counseling—all qualities difficult to change. Traditional counseling may offer this benefit of caring listening; a friend or relative of this kind is a valuable asset.

## Counselor of Individuals—Consultant to Agencies

From the beginning of the profession, counselors in institutions and agencies have consulted with their management and staff to study ways to enhance the social-psychological climate of the institution, thereby contributing to the development of its members. In these instances, a comparison of the counselor to the public health officer is useful. Public health officers treat patients (as counselors serve individuals) but also serve a variety of preventive functions in the community and supervise corrective measures if common health problems occur. Because counselors are mental hygenists, it is appropriate for them, too, to consult with employing institutions about mental-health matters among the population served.

Osipow (1980) sees counselors giving mental-health consultation in "environmental design, health (not sickness) settings, [and] legal settings . . . and [contributing] . . . to . . . social policy." Counselors "may continue to be the closest thing to a general practitioner that the mental health specialties provide" (p. 130).

Kagan and his colleagues (1988) elaborate on this theme in writing about university counseling centers. Services there fall into three categories: *prevention,* so as to forestall developmental difficulties, *enhancement* activities to facilitate student growth in coping skills, and *remediation* of psychologically debilitating life events. The resemblance is noticeable between these three services and the activities of the public health officer.

College counselors teach skills for effective living (Alschuler, Ivey, & Hatcher, 1977) and can contribute to broad mental-health goals (Krumboltz & Menefee, 1980). They do this by suggesting alterations in academic and social environments that have been "found to contribute to the problems in their client population." For example, "Counselors may advocate changes in the design of . . . residence halls . . ." (Krumboltz & Menefee, 1980, p. 197) to reduce problems in campus living. Whatever their consultation functions, counselors' activities encompass purposes reflected in Super's phrase, "community development and redevelopment" (1980b, p. 140).

# General Outcomes of Counseling

Psychological counselors carry out professional activities with individuals or with small groups of clients who have comparable concerns, and they also consult with institutions. They have common practices, regardless of specialty, and unique practices related to any specialized population they serve. What do counselors intend to accomplish by their consulting activities? To what outcomes do they put their professional skills? Some of these answers were given incidentally when other topics were covered, but the need now is for a more systematic inquiry. We begin by examining goals expressed by professional groups, because it can be assumed that these organizations speak for their members. They assert that counselors facilitate the psychological development of normal (typical) people by helping them make and carry out tenable plans for their future, by strengthening their resources, and by helping them remove obstacles to continued development.

Counseling objectives of the American Counseling Association (ACA) are specific to the different specialties that make up the ACA. On the other hand, the Division of Counseling Psychology of the APA was not only free to but also obligated to address fundamental issues about counseling as practiced by those who earned doctor's degrees, no matter the setting in which such professionals practiced. It is worth repeating that the positions published by Division 17 applied to all counselors regardless of degree level. It is a fact that Division 17 members, in the main, prepare counselors for all settings and are leaders within those settings. The division can speak knowledgeably about counseling no matter where it is practiced and at what degree level. Its prime concern, of course, is with the practice of counseling psychologists.*

## *Goals Set by Division 17*

Forty-some years ago Division 17 defined the scope of the doctoral-level psychological counselor. The bylaws then stated that the practitioner's purpose was "to extend the techniques of psychology to counseling and guidance activities in vocational, personal, educational and group adjustments including the disciplinary and behavioral problems encountered in educational institutions" (Whiteley, 1980, p. 29). Note the limitation of service to education, and the inclusion of the word "guidance." In 1954 new bylaws recognized additional emphases while dropping references to disciplinary and behavioral problems and the word "guidance." Newly included were industrial or business enterprises, government agencies, social agencies, and as a forerunner of an ever-increasing setting, private (independent) practice.

A report given in 1987 at the Georgia Conference, a national conference of counseling psychologists, stated that counseling was based on:

---

*In most states practitioners unlicensed by state boards may not identify themselves with the title counseling psychologist, psychological counselor, or any other title that uses the word *psychology* or a derivative word, without board sanction in those states. To identify themselves professionally, sub-doctoral counselors use a specialty's name, such as marriage and family, school, career, rehabilitation, and so on. These counselors, in actuality, address psychological concerns because they attend to cognitions, affect, and behavior.

1. a perspective that values the empowerment of individuals to gain mastery of their own lives and methods that focus on strengths, adaptive strategies, and strategies for change . . . and direct teaching of skills relevant to promoting the psychological health of individuals, groups, and systems
2. an understanding and appreciation of career development—the areas of work, work identity, leisure, and retirement—as related to human productivity, satisfaction with personal life-style, and socioorganizational health
3. a focus on development across the life span. . .
4. the importance of viewing people and their behavior in a contextual manner [to include the] variables of culture, ethnicity, gender, sexual orientation, age, and sociohistorical perspective
5. the value of programmatic research [Kagan et al., 1988, p. 351].

The mixed message of these several citations shows disagreement over whether counseling psychology overlaps with or even coincides with clinical psychology, a disagreement that resonates today in some training programs. Many hold that the difference between the purposes of clinical psychology and those of psychological counseling, defined by the five points above, is greater than the similarity. They contrast the developmental emphasis that marks counseling with the remedial focus of clinical psychology.

## *Goals Set by Institutions*

Goals stated by specialists within an organization are too broad to guide the individual counselor; they usually require further specification by employing institutions. Counselors in public schools, which employ more psychological counselors than any other institutions, are involved in students' critical years of development, marked by intense needs and unique concerns. This requires school counselors to determine objectives to meet those common needs and concerns. Additionally, schools gather up the entire population: able and disabled; genius, average, and below average; misanthrope and philanthrope. This mix of population and the commitment of schools to enhance the development of each student result in counseling goals or objectives unique to schools.

## *The Counselor's Objectives*

Whatever the goals stated by national, regional, or local associations and their divisions or by employing agencies or organizations, it is the individual counselor who provides the most specific set of objectives, partly in response to clients' concerns. One objective, set jointly with the client, is to reduce or eliminate the specific concern that produced the client's need for help. This specific aim is referred to here as an *intermediate* objective, given its stance between two other objectives, which will be explained below.

Even though these intermediate objectives are in some ways as varied as clients, in other ways client goals can be grouped into subclasses such as concerns with careers, with interpersonal relationships, with rehabilitation needs, with feelings or behaviors that impede effective coping, and so on. Some intermediate objectives are sharply defined: elimination of a phobia, choosing an occupation, or clearing up a difficulty in a relationship with a child or mate. On the other hand, a client saying, "I feel so worthless; can you help me?" is making a nonspecific plea but is staking an equally valid claim on a counselor's efforts.

When the client's goal becomes clear (it may take several interviews in complex cases), the intermediate objective has been set. No matter whether this objective is simple (to alter a study habit) or complex (to deal with and resolve antipathies about a long-dead parent, for example), the counselor will not reach it with the client by employing a single strategy. Attainment of intermediate objectives usually requires the client to reach several specific objectives. It is as if the counselor were to say, "First we'll have to do A, then make a start on B while you're still working on A, then get some closure on C," and so on. Some success with each of these specific objectives is required to accomplish the intermediate objective. Each of these small tasks, then, becomes for the counselor an *immediate* objective. An example: a client needs to resolve concern X, but to reach this objective, the counselor sees a need to reduce anxiety, to assist the client in changing some of his or her self-views, to reframe some cognitions, and to help the client acquire new coping behaviors.

What about broader objectives? Is there an objective beyond the removal of the concern that brought the client in for assistance? There is. It is an objective held out for clients by each counselor, who may be unaware that he or she is seeking to lead clients to this objective. It is called here the *ultimate* objective. Not only may the counselor be unaware of the operation of this objective, it is likely that the client is unaware, at least at first, of this further goal based on the counselor's views of what characterizes an ideally functioning person. Ultimate objectives are not only tenets about optimal mental health but can also be based on values. They are expressions of a counselor's *life-view*.*

Clients have life-views too, ones that may partly conflict with the counselor's life-views, and they require identification during counseling. In describing an interactional view of counseling, Claiborn and Lichtenberg (1989) note that a client's behavior is influenced simultaneously by the client's view of the world and the views held by others with whom the client interacts, an interaction that is an equally important phenomenon in counseling.

### *Ultimate Objectives, as Determined by Life-Views*

A recent profile in a popular periodical (Weschler, 1990) tells of a person who, as a graduate of MIT, became a renowned engineer in the space program. He then moved on to complete an MBA and became a successful executive in a financial institution. The article reports that he was ready for the next step in his career: to become a professional clown with a famous circus. Imagine him conferring separately with two counselors about the appropriateness of that action. One is enthusiastic about the decision ("I wish I had the courage to do that"); the other, weighing all past factors and measurement data, wonders about the abnormalities in this client's life ("What is he running away from?"). The first counselor sees this decision as a commendable step, showing the client's superb mental health; the other counselor may explicitly state disapproval or imply it with subtleties, also

---

*The phrase *world-view*, used by others, has somewhat the same connotations as *life-view*.

applying mental-health criteria. The second counselor may attach low value to the occupation of clown in contrast to the socially acceptable occupations of engineer and financier.

The issue here is not which counselor is correct. These hypothetical responses illustrate that counselors have views of the way humans function at their best—how they think, feel, and act when marked by good mental health and appropriate values—whether or not the counselors are aware of how these views impinge on counseling. These views, along with other perspectives, are part of a counselor's life-view. They become a variable during interviews, sometimes turning up in overt counselor responses but often in subtle ways of which even the counselor is unaware. In addition to voice tone and body posture that express disagreement or approval, facial expressions and counselor attention or inattention also convey reactions. These influences on counseling are undesirable when counselors are unaware of them, and perhaps unethical. When counselors are aware of these life-views, they are more likely to be able to control them.

Life-views include generalizations about philosophical issues. Some pairs of opposites show these contrasting assumptions and values that counselors (and clients) may hold:

1. Humans are completely free to act by rational choice when faced with decisions; or behavior is determined only slightly by reasoning, and more by internal and external stimuli not accessible to reasoning.
2. Morals are natural, apparent to everyone, and equally inborn to everyone (or required by a supreme being); or morals are learned, culturally determined social codes.
3. Humans are a higher order of animal life; or human existence has a transcendent or spiritual aspect that differentiates it from animal life.

Counselors' positions about those and other metaphysical questions will determine their ultimate objectives, the distant, long-range outcomes toward which they try to move the client, sometimes unknowingly, sometimes consciously and comfortably because "it is right." Counselors' life-views can be expected to be more potent than clients' because counselors are, by the very nature of counseling, the more potent persons in the dyad.

At the same time, on the basis of mental-health criteria counselors tend to agree about what are unacceptable client cognitions, feelings, or behaviors. For example, there would be almost no latitude among them about the undesirability of incest or suicide, or about the mentally unhealthy nature of feelings of racial or ethnic hate. There would be general agreement about what is undesirable by mental-health criteria (the narrow end of a figurative funnel) but disagreement about what thoughts and behaviors were *acceptable* by mental-health criteria (the wide end of the funnel).

Counselors apply their skills not only to help clients resolve current concerns but also to help them make general progress in life, either individually or in groups. Counselors must then be clear about how they would answer questions such as: What constitutes progress, What are the ultimate objectives of human existence, and What kind of person should this client become? In other professions where counseling occurs, such as law, finance, and health (but excepting the clergy), practitioners typically have little need to dwell on remote outcomes (on ultimate objectives). Practitioners' life-views are not an issue in those professions; their technical proficiency is all that matters. Those practitioners work solely toward the resolution of the client's concern, which, when removed, returns the help-seeker to the *status quo ante,* the outcome that the client also expects. In those other professions, counselors are not called upon to be professionally concerned about the psychological quality of clients' past, present, or future, whereas that is just what the psychological counselor is primarily concerned with. This kind of counseling differs from the others in that it has teleological objectives (ultimate ends) as well as ontological ones (the quality of being).

There is an opposing view: it proposes that counselors should keep from exercising any influence on a client's long-range existence. "Among the many things from which . . . clients need protection," says Kegan (1982), "is the practitioner's hopes for the client's future, however benign and sympathetic those hopes may be" (p. 296). Not that Kegan fails to have hopes for clients, "but they are *my* hopes. As much as I care about them, I care even more that people be protected from arbitrary influences upon them to shape up to someone else's favorite value" (p. 296). Whether or not a counselor considers it a counseling function to aim a client in the direction of a defined future, it remains an imperative for counselors to be aware of their ontological and teleogical values. We see the influence of these values as we look in on a hypothetical man just completing counselor training. His past experiences, including emotionally colored views expressed by his parents, others in his family, friends, and religious leaders, have equipped the student with values about women that were more common many decades ago among certain subcultures: men are superior and it is expected that they will dominate in any male/female relationship, particularly in marriage; men go out to work (and when home do no domestic tasks), but women by nature are home-oriented; men are rational (a highly valued trait), women emotional; and so on.

His counselor-preparation program (we hypothesize) regrettably provided no opportunity to raise these implicit elements of his life-view to an aware level, let alone evaluate them for their bearing on counseling. Now in his first job in a community counseling center, he is earnestly trying to help a woman resolve a complex relationship with a man. It is tenable to conjecture that his values about women will influence his counseling, maybe only subtly, and probably not to the client's benefit.

How would a counselor's relationship with a client be affected if the counselor held that the dominant drive in humans was economic, as in the old term *economic man?* Or what if the counselor held to the primacy of sexuality, or of power? What if the counselor's life-view orbited around tenets usually identified as fundamentalist Christian? A counselor so imbued might employ the same counseling techniques in a marriage problem as another would who carried the label of secular humanist. These two would attend to similar immediate and intermediate objectives, but there would be striking differences in their ultimate objectives.

In later chapters we will examine a number of distinctively labeled theories of counseling or therapy, each with distinctive practices and, perhaps, an espoused life-view. Collectively they are called here schools of counseling (or of therapy). Some schools differ little from some others. Other schools sharply differ in their ideas of how and why humans think and act as they do (theory) and in the approaches and techniques they employ to bring about desired changes. Some schools of counseling emphasize theory, and others emphasize techniques. In still others, a life-view may be a central feature; in other words, these schools emphasize the ultimate objective as much as or more than theory or technique. A feature of this text is that it eschews existing schools as integrated structures and bases its concepts and practices on the reasoning and findings of science. As such, it could not propose a life-view other than scientifically supported mental-health principles. Counselors have their own life-views, of which they should be aware, but this text will not propose what those should be beyond the position stated above.

From these arguments it follows that prospective counselors need training experiences that will bring to awareness any unconscious components of their life-view that are relevant to counseling. Some activities at the ends of the chapters of this book are designed for that purpose.

Professional associations provide statements of purpose broad enough to encompass a diverse membership. Divisions of those associations, as well as employing agencies, are even more specific in their goal statements. Ultimately, however, it is each counselor who makes any statement of objectives operational.

## Concluding Reflections

I have contrasted the counselor who helps clients work through normal psychological concerns with both trained and untrained counselors who serve clients in other fields. I have also emphasized the general purpose of psychological counseling as enhancement of the development of all clients, in contrast to the primary function of individual remediation engaged by clinical psychologists. Most times typical persons are able to take charge of their lives, brushing away obstacles that impede their progress or send them down inappropriate cognitive, emotional, or behavioral paths. At times these concerns can reach an intensity that moves them to seek some help in dealing with them. It is in the counseling of individuals that we find the maximum expression of professional skill, but because psychological counselors are oriented to development, ability to set up preventive, enhancing programs for all is also a prominent competence.

The programs that prepare people to be counselors are typically staffed by counseling psychologists (they have the earned doctorates required for teaching). If counseling psychologists on these faculties have been trained in programs that are distinctively in counseling psychology, they will have a development orientation and the knowledge needed to teach students how to initiate these development-enhancing programs. On the other hand, if the preparation of counseling psychologists is more and more melded with and takes on the characteristics of the training of clinical psychologists, it can be expected that counseling psychologists will be unable to teach students about these activities, and indeed may not even be sensitive to their need.

The increase in the number of psychological counselors who wish to be independent practitioners reduces the motivation of those counselors to study the developmental tasks central to those who will work in institutions. It contributes further to the shift toward identifying counseling as a therapeutic process, not a developmental one. If these trends continue, the time may come when psychological counseling will have to be reinvented at the doctoral level. The need for professionals to be concerned with facilitating normal development will not only remain but probably increase. This text is oriented to maintaining the historic development-enhancing thrust of counseling as defined at the start of the profession almost a half-century ago and continually restated by professional associations.

Most psychological counselors have not earned doctorates and thus cannot be counseling psychologists even though they do provide the bulk of psychological counseling. Because of a lack of training in abnormal states, their practice cannot resemble that of clinical psychologists, and thus their function will continue to emphasize development-enhancing activities. Increasing difficulties can be predicted for the counseling profession if the leaders and instructors available for the large group of subdoctoral practitioners are clinical psychologists or those who function as such even though under the title of counseling psychologist.

■                    **Points to Remember**                    ■

1. Counseling has been offered by family members, friends, and other untrained persons for all of history. Given its long history, this form of help is called here traditional counseling.
2. Professional counseling is relatively recent. It is oldest in the fields of law, accounting, and health and newest in the psychological areas dealing with cognitions, affect, and behavior. Professional counseling requires study in a unique body of knowledge and is a full-time occupation.
3. Unique knowledge is acquired in the preparation of the psychological counselor, including education and training in an area of study not needed in other fields: counseling relationships and the distinctive communication procedures that establish and maintain them.
4. To understand psychological counseling, it helps to contrast it with clinical psychology. The two fields differ in their major purposes. Clinical psychology, the older profession, is concerned with the diagnosis and remediation of major psychological problems. Psychological counseling, whatever the degree level of the practitioner, is designed to enhance the mentally healthy development of normal clients by helping them complete the developmental tasks common to all, and by helping individuals resolve cognitive, affective, and behavioral concerns.
5. This focus calls for counselors employed by institutions to organize programs to enhance the development of all members of the institution in addition to counseling individual members.
6. A master's degree is the minimum training required to practice psychological counseling. A psychological counselor who earns a doctor's degree in an approved program is a counseling psychologist.
7. Broad objectives for counselors have been established by Division 17 (the Division of Counseling Psychology) of the American Psychological Association. Although these objectives were set up in response to the needs of counseling

psychologists, they apply to all who practice psychological counseling. Divisions of the American Counseling Association have specified objectives for the clientele each division serves.

8. In serving individual clients, counselors have two objectives: the concern the client wants to alleviate, and the various subgoals to be reached in order to attain the client's objective. These subgoals have been labeled *immediate* objectives, while the client's goal is labeled the *intermediate* objective.

9. The intermediate objective is all that a client wishes to reach. The counselor, however, usually has one or more *ultimate* objectives of which she or he may not be fully aware. A counselor's ultimate objective reflects the counselor's view of what constitutes a mentally healthy person and also reflects his or her own subjective values and guiding principles. These beliefs are called here a counselor's life-view. The need is for counselors to be aware of these life-views and how they influence immediate and intermediate objectives.

# ■                    Counselor Formation Activities                    ■

Successful psychological counseling requires knowledge about cognitions, affect, and behaviors in order to be able to help those who become your clients. Academic knowledge is only one of a training program's outcomes; personal growth in ways that affect counseling is an equal imperative—growth that may be an extension of characteristics already present. In some instances, however, replacement of existing cognitions and behaviors with those appropriate for counseling may be required.

These end-of-chapter exercises give you the opportunity:

- to increase your knowledge of the chapter's academic content and the likelihood of your retaining knowledge
- to increase your self-awareness
- to evaluate and modify certain cognitions of yourself and the world—that is, to alter your life-views in ways that will remove obstacles to achieving counseling objectives
- to increase behaviors appropriate to counseling while eliminating undesired ones

Serious attention to these activities contributes to the formation of desirable counselor cognitions and behavior. Although some topics lead to growth in each student without discussion, other topics produce reactions of a greater personal intensity and so are more productive when discussed with a few other students with whom such thoughts will be regularly shared.

1. Recall brief events and longer periods of distress that occurred in your childhood, adolescence, and young adulthood that you judge to have caused developmental difficulties. Which of these did you talk about with an *informal* counselor (friend, neighbor, relative) to get some relief from your discomfort? For each of these, try also to recall:

   a. What was the relationship of that person to you?
   b. Why did you select that person instead of someone else?

   c. To which potential informal counselors would you *not* have gone to talk over that concern? Why not?

   d. Were the outcomes of those experiences good or bad?

   e. If the help was inadequate, what made it so?

2. Which developmental concerns have you had that you did not talk over with anyone, concerns that you identify as having kept you or as still keeping you from being the most functional and happy person possible? What deterred you from asking someone for help with these concerns?

3. Interview one or a few other adolescents or young adults about the questions raised in topic 1.

4. Interview one or a few counselors, clinical psychologists, social workers, or other professional helpers who are certified or licensed. Find out if they differentiate developmental difficulties that are typical of normal clients from those they classify as psychological abnormalities. On what basis do they make such a distinction? For those whose academic training is less than a doctorate, ask for examples of the kind of client concerns for which they have referred or would refer a client to a practitioner with more advanced training. What kind of practitioner would they select, what kind would they not select, and what are their reasons for selection or rejection?

5. Each of us has life-views—that is, comprehensive assumptions about humans. Refer to the life-view dilemmas posed in the latter part of this chapter. Consider in what ways your life-views would bear on each dilemma, such as your views of similarities and differences between genders. If you are male and were faced with assisting the female client who had relationship concerns, what assumptions about women and men would you be bringing to the interview? What views do you hold about adolescent privacy, punishment of children by parents, the appropriate relationship with certain ethnic groups and races, and the existence and function of free will? What was the origin of your original views on each topic, and how did your views change over the years? What were the causes of those changes?

■              **Complementary Reading**             ■

Graduate students, particularly at the doctoral level, are entrusted by society with the responsibility of increasing society's knowledge. Fulfillment of the role first requires students to know well the field of inquiry into which they have ventured, which means that to start graduate work is to embark on a never-ending literature pursuit. This text introduces you to the counseling-literature chase through the references cited in each chapter and gathered at the end of the book. The way to expand your knowledge is to peruse, or at least skim, references that have been emphasized.

A few references have been selected to round out your knowledge of each chapter's topic; these are given in the Complementary Reading section. Most of these works have their own cited references, so you will never be at a loss for published material to study. More likely, the converse will pertain: you will be overwhelmed by the plethora of journal articles and books, each of which may seem to be indispensable reading.

Chapter 1 takes a stand that distinguishes between helping normal people with normal developmental concerns and helping the minority whose coping problems are so intense and chronic that long-term therapy is required. By statistical definition, this latter group is made up of clients with abnormal difficulties who receive the kind of help for which clinical psychologists, and some counseling psychologists, are trained.

It is recommended that you regularly examine the *American Psychologist,* the *Journal of Counseling and Development,* and *The Counseling Psychologist* to look for articles that relate to topics treated in this text and to your eventual area of counseling expertise. The science on which counseling primarily rests is psychology—psychological thought and evidence as it applies to the development of normal people and to helping them maintain satisfactory development or, if need be, return to a mentally healthful state.

We recall that the shape and practices of counseling about psychological matters at any degree level owe much to the thinking and research of counseling psychologists. Therefore, I recommend:

WHITELEY, J. M., & FRETZ, B. R. (Eds.). (1980). *The Present and Future of Counseling Psychology.* Pacific Grove, CA: Brooks/Cole.

The help provided by doctoral-level practitioners is termed therapy or, most often, psychotherapy. The history of psychotherapy is also partially a history of counseling, so for a historical grounding of this profession I recommend:

FREIDMAN, D. K. (1992). *History of Psychotherapy: A Century of Change.* Washington, DC: American Psychological Association.

$$\boxed{2}$$

CHAPTER

# How Will I Know What to Do?

## Overview

The counselor-to-be may think: "I know generally what I'll be called on to do as counselor. I may plan and conduct programs to enhance the development of members of an institution. Whatever the setting, I'll help some individuals plan their future and help others eliminate developmental difficulties. But how will I know specifically what to do? What will my professional practices be?"

The answer begins in this chapter with the topic of epistemology—that is, the study of knowing, of what can be known, and of how it is learned. Some study of epistemology will improve your ability to determine which proposals about counseling to accept from among the numerous ones you will encounter. (You will also be better able to judge the proposals made in this text, because it differs from other such books in its epistemological emphasis.) The goal is to prepare you to make independent judgments about counseling, not to have you accept other people's statements.

The epistemic commitment of this text to "new" science, which will be explained below, requires an approach that overarches the variety of therapies or counseling systems commonly offered. The word *school,* used throughout to identify this variety, embodies two meanings. The first and more common is that of an organized institution of learning, such as Meadowville High School. At times even colleges are spoken of as schools. The other meaning, the one used here, is represented by the phrase *school of thought.* In this text, as we saw in Chapter 1, the term *counseling school* will mean a package of theory and practices offered under a distinctive name, such as person-centered therapy. Schools are examined by epistemic principles in this and other chapters. The results show that schools no longer serve an adequate explanatory function and therefore that counseling should be school-less, in the "school of thought" sense.

For years counseling's informing science, psychology, was almost exclusively objective and empirical—that is, positivist. The characteristics of positivism are examined in this chapter, as are those of once-excluded but now-acceptable subjectivism. That exclusion kept psychology from providing data needed by counselors who deal primarily with clients' subjective world—that is, with their cognitions and emotions, which are tied in with their behaviors.

This chapter examines the change in what is acceptable psychological science, a change which now makes acceptable the study of people's inner (subjective) worlds. This results in new information useful in counseling.


## Introduction

A counselor is interviewing Gail, who is 34 years old, married, and the mother of two children, age 9 and 5. Gail states her concerns as general unhappiness; vague dissatisfaction with her married life; and irritability, which she takes out on her children, who, she thinks, do not respect her. She thinks her husband loves her—at least he says he does. The counselor learns enough about her to be confident that there is no major personality disorganization and therefore that her concerns, psychological in nature, are appropriate for a counselor to address. The counselor is confident that through the unique relationship to be established and by helping Gail alter some cognitions about herself, some of her emotional responses, and some behaviors toward her children, she will be provided the relief she seeks. She needs to modify her views of herself and replace her inadequate coping skills.

The counselor begins procedures that will be based on what she knows of counseling's unique relationship, along with knowledge about how people acquire cognitions, emotions, and behaviors and how to help clients with difficulties like this one's. The critical question is: what *does* the counselor know about helping clients, and how did she acquire that knowledge?

To answer that question is to require some exploration of the fundamental topic of philosophy called epistemology, which is the study of how people know, what they can know, and how they learn it. Knowledge of this topic will enable you to evaluate what you hear and read about counseling during and after a program of counselor preparation.


## The Basic Source of Knowledge: Authority

Were we to inquire of most counselors what they know about counseling and how they came to know it, the answer might simply be that such knowledge was acquired during counselor training by reading texts, research reports, and articles and listening to lectures and other presentations. Inherent in that reply is the message that counselors acquire knowledge not by generating it but *by accepting as authoritative the written and oral statements of others.* This question then follows: how did those authorities come to know what they were reporting as the "truth" about counseling? Therein lies the dilemma of schools of counseling, those numerous, labeled packages of theory and practices that clamor for counselor allegiance.

## *The Problem with Schools of Counseling*

Most of what we know has been learned from others whose words we accepted on faith, starting with our parents. We were not far along in life before we ran into statements expressed by one authority, often about values, that conflicted with statements from other authorities. This required us to discriminate between these conflicting statements, perhaps by examining how each authority had acquired his or her knowledge. Disagreement about counseling theory and practices can be found among schools of counseling, with each school claiming to offer the correct explanation of how to meet clients' needs. Examination of counseling schools reveals differences among their epistemic bases. All methods of learning do not yield equally valid information, which requires us to persist in examination of this issue.

Instructors in some counselor-preparation programs generally agree on matters of theory and technique. Other programs pride themselves on being staffed by faculty members who hold diverse theories, and thus practice diverse techniques. Thirty-five years of teaching and advising have left me with memories of a common student complaint about these latter programs: "Professor M convinced me that counseling school A was correct, and I was an A-ian for a time. In Professor N's class, because he is a B-ian, we studied school B, and it made so much sense that I too became a B-ian. Professor O would not tell us what she was but made us study ten different schools and then told us to pick one of them as our own. My adviser is a hard-core C-ian, but I can't accept school C, and I can't change advisers. I'm soon to enter supervised practice, and I'm more confused than when I entered graduate study. I just don't see how I can be an effective counselor. Why is there such disagreement among counselor educators anyhow?!"

Students probably cannot wisely choose among counseling schools because their experience does not equip them with sufficient skill in reflective judgment (Brabeck & Werfel, 1985; King, Kitchener, Davidson, Parker, & Wood, 1983). Additionally, because many students are not grounded in epistemology, they will not have sorted out their own epistemic positions and thus will be unable to make even rudimentary evaluations based on epistemic criteria. Even with some prior study, one's epistemic commitments commonly require time to mesh into a comfortable whole. For some students, therefore, it is a matter of faith in authorities that leads to a commitment to one school or, on the other hand, to view that psychological counseling has arrived at a maturity that lets it now be school-less and, in fact, that the continued emphasis on schools may impede further maturation.

A central tenet of this text is that students, upon making some tentative commitment to a theory of learning, will not need to seek blindly for the surest explanations of human functioning and change from among the dozens of schools of counseling (therapy) that abound. Students' epistemic commitment will permit them to identify from what they read and hear those concepts that match their view of acquiring knowledge.

## An Alternative to Schools

Matarazzo (1987) finds support for the view that "[t]here is only one psychology, no specialties, but many applications" (p. 893). Translated to this text, the phrase might read, "one counseling, but a number of varied applications." The impropriety of students' studying counseling schools is asserted by Eysenck and Eysenck (1985). They observe that:

> [most] textbooks simply give a set of chapters [each] organized around one particular author, explaining his theory, quoting a few examples of empirical work more or less relevant to it: but they eschew the scientifically important and indeed essential job of judging the *adequacy* of the theory in terms of the experimental work devoted to it and thus fail to compare the adequacy of one theory along those lines with all the others. Thus what we have is not the evolution of a paradigm, but [an] *auction of ideas, alien to the spirit of science and conducive to arbitrary choice in terms of existing prejudices on the part of students* [p. 348; latter emphasis added].

Patterson (1980) puts it this way:

> Telling students to make their own choices is admitting that we have no basis for teaching, that counseling is not a profession. This is as if medical students were told that there is an infinite number of ways to perform an operation, and each must do it his or her own way [p. 349].

Krumboltz (1991) examined this issue by comparing theories to maps, which at best vary according to the information each is to convey and at worst may contain unintended errors based on limited information. In my version of this analogy, a map may be simply a schematic, a rough idea of reality, like a map of a subway system, which is accurate for a rider's needs but only approximates the system's actual routes. A school (theory) of counseling, like a map, may be "a distorted, inaccurate oversimplification of reality," Krumboltz asserts; "[t]he scientific ideal is to continue improving theoretical formulations to represent reality better" (p. 309).

# Nonscientific Sources of Knowledge

When we acquire knowledge from authorities, we in turn become authorities for that knowledge if we pass it on unmodified. The knowledge that was generated and passed on to others as authoritative in prescientific times had nonscientific origins: tradition, mysticism, and rationalism. Any one bit of knowledge can have contributions from several sources. As we seek to partially answer the question of how those who have become our authorities acquired their knowledge we must be aware that each way of acquiring knowledge operates in a less pure form than that presented here. The first two sources have little bearing on counseling knowledge but are offered nonetheless to widen the coverage of the topic.

## Tradition

When asked why a statement is true or how they came to know whatever it is that they have asserted, some people could respond: "All of us in this culture have always believed that. There never was a time when that was not one of our beliefs." In this context the source of knowledge is not just authority, it is also tradition. Such statements may not have a rational defense, but uncritical acceptance is expected of subordinates regardless.

Negative views of other races or ethnic societies and the long-held tenets of some theological systems come from this source. Indeed, in one Christian denomination tradition is seen as an authority equal to scripture. Tradition held in pre–World War II Japan that the emperor was a direct descendent of the sun god.

Tradition is powerful, as Galileo could no doubt testify, given the harm it caused him personally and in the suppression of scientific knowledge. People whose beliefs and actions originate in tradition, particularly those who are responsible for the preservation and transmittal of traditional knowledge, are typically hostile to any statements that counter the culture's beliefs, even if there is demonstrable evidence to the contrary: "If the facts do not agree with my beliefs, something must be wrong with the facts." It is to be expected that traditionalists will disagree with scientists. The proclivity of traditionalists to "roll back the clock" can be a threat to scientific advancement when they gain in numbers and political influence.

### Mysticism

Mysticism, once commonly relied upon as a source of knowledge, lost its potency as education spread, but it is regaining adherents even in the developed countries. Throughout history people have claimed that they acquired knowledge from dreams, from supernatural voices or visits, or from other esoteric sources. Astrology is put forth as a valid source of knowledge by a large number who apparently do not ever wonder how astrologers receive their knowledge. Faith does not require evidence, so such mysticism prevails in some advanced cultures where astrological omens weigh significantly in business, marriage, and statecraft matters. In the 1980s, astrology influenced significant political decisions, including the precise time of day at which the president was to be inaugurated (an apt word, incidentally; it originally showed dependence on omens mystically revealed by auguries).

One beneficial counseling procedure, meditation, has both mystical and nonmystical connotations. It is the latter connotation that justifies including meditation in the counselor's armamentarium. The intention of mystical meditation is to journey inward to find knowledge at a higher plane. This goal is based on the premise that at one time humans had superior knowledge from a divine source but that this knowledge has become hidden under worldly debris. Mystical meditation seeks to tap into that lost knowledge.

### Rationalism

This classical epistemology, exemplified by scholasticism, centers on reason. It appears at first glance to be the thinking person's source of knowledge, but it too is at fault because it holds that knowledge can be obtained by reasoning alone—that there is no need to seek empirical confirmation. Rationalism is often illustrated by an apochryphal anecdote about monks of centuries ago who had gathered to discuss how many teeth horses have. They did not go to the barn to count them, an empirical action that would have been untenable because it is contrary to rationalism.

There is a difference between rationalism as a source of knowledge and reasoning as a process. This text is committed to a theory of science in which reasoning is central but in which empirical data are acquired when possible.

## Two Cautions

Epistemology is a complex scholarly inquiry. These few pages do little more than recall that complexity to some who have studied the topic and provide a few terms to those who have not. You are urged to pursue the topic far enough to gain a functional grasp of it.

The other caution is generated by the fact that tradition, mysticism, and rationalism, being inappropriate as sources of knowledge for counseling, must not be viewed as nonproductive in other aspects of living. Much social good can be attributed in ancient and present cultures to knowledge based on tradition and mysticism, and conversely all can see the social harm, as in environmental damage, that has come about by applying technologies based on scientific thinking. Knowledge based on any source can result in both social good and harm. Our interest here is to ask what source or sources of knowledge will be defensible for counselors whose ethical practice is assumed. The answer for this text is scientific thought.

# Science: Counseling's Primary Source of Knowledge

It is safe to say that most people look on experiments as the defining activity of science. Although controlled empiricism is a powerful source of knowledge, the counseling student requires a more refined understanding than that of the typical person. To increase that understanding, we start with a brief look at the major characteristics of scientists and science.

## Scientists and Science

To some extent science is defined by what people do in its name. Scientists are usually intellectually gifted, curious, skeptical, objective, and educated to the highest level available in their respective specialties. The quality "curious" connotes a must-know urge, a compulsion for "emotionally satisfying intelligibility" (Rosenberg, 1983). Scientists identify a gap in knowledge that must be filled because, like the mountain, "it is there."

In a number of sciences the equation *science = experimentation* has been axiomatic. The position that reflects that equation is called *positivism,* which is the technical theory in epistemology that the world is objective and thus that the seeking of knowledge must be only in the objective realm. It is positivism's tenet that knowledge, although processed necessarily by reason, must come through the senses—that is, through observations. Those observations must be controlled, and that requires experimentation.

## Revolution in the Science of Psychology

Among the philosphers of science, the publications of Kuhn (e.g., 1970) are regarded as benchmarks of change. Kuhn musters arguments to demonstrate that scientific progress comes not primarily as a result of accumulating experimental evidence but, in fact, occurs only when scholars in a scientific area periodically redefine the area in a radical manner. He labels these changes revolutions, a shift into a new paradigm from one that had been dominating the science.

Kuhn defines a paradigm as a matrix of distinctive elements: (1) the assumptions, theories, and problems studied: (2) the specifics of those problems and how they are studied; and (3) the instrumentation typical of that science. These characteristics make up the disciplinary matrix common to the science at a certain period of its development. When one or more creative scholars come to think differently about the science's questions, assumptions, and techniques, a "shift of conceptual web" occurs (Kuhn, 1970, p. 194). This leads to the appearance of a new paradigm in that science that will borrow from the old but will employ those old elements in new ways. These new proposals may draw people from the established paradigm, especially students, and in time the new paradigm is established, destined for a while to be a concurrent alternative within that science. Over time, if the new paradigm produces greater success than its predecessor in solving the science's questions, it will increase in status as the matrix within which scholarly activity in that science should occur.

The paradigm shift in psychology has been the result of a variety of interacting changes that effect a number of practices. One cause of the shift is the increasing acceptance of the idea that some important psychological questions lie more outside the objective world than in it, and therefore are not observable solely through experiments of a positivist nature. Excluding attention to the objective world, many now contend, is no more intellectually defensible than the opposing stand—that only subjective (phenomenological) experience is real.

Pribram (1985) identifies the decade between 1955–1965 as the primary period of paradigm shift in psychology. He attributes the shift to a "convergence of technological innovation, mathematical invention, and a host of innovations in the neurosciences" (p. 5). Among these, he notes, have been remarkable accomplishments in:

> information measurement in communication; servomechanism in control systems; computers and programming techniques to analyze problem-solving; studies of natural language grammars . . . ; and the analysis of learning from the vantage of sampling and decision theories (p. 5).

Pribram believes that psychology will be made whole when its ruling paradigm reflects "the totality of subjective behaviorism" (p. 6). He therefore submits the term *holistic* as the one appropriate to "this next turn in the development of scientific and professional psychology" (p. 6).

The change in many sciences, including psychology, has seen the displacement of the epistemically exclusive stand of positivism by a more relativistic stand. Doppelt (1983) sees this change as an appropriate abandonment of rigid positivism in favor of a theory of scientific rationality that incorporates the insights of historicism (the theory that historical forces cause events to occur) while not accepting historicism's complete relativism.

## Realism and Idealism

Psychology's paradigm shift has given the concepts of realism and idealism a new importance, reflected by the question "Is it better to speak of realism versus idealism or realism *and* idealism?"

A classic philosophical question is "Is there a real world out there—objective and knowable—or are my *perceptions* of whatever is out there the only reality?" If my position is that there is a knowable real world and I consider it to be of primary importance, I am a realist. If I hold that my perceptions and those of each individual are the only reality, I am a phenomenologist, or idealist. (In this usage the word *idealist* differs from its common meaning of one who strives for or subscribes to only the best.)

Although the arguments concerning this issue fill volumes, this text takes the approach that neither realism nor idealism is correct by itself; both are correct. Pribram (1986) puts the issue this way, in paraphrase: Are my perceptions (my phenomenal experiences) the "real," or does the content of those perceptions make up the "real" world? My phenomenal experiences are mental; the world as it appears to me is material. I can give primacy to my experience and become a phenomenologist, or I can give primacy to the contents of the experience and become a materialist (realist). But I can also give primacy to neither and attest to the dual nature of reality. Materialism and phenomenology run into difficulty only when each attempts to deny the other (p. 510).

It is acceptance of both the objective and subjective that constitutes the "cognitive revolution" in psychology, a revolution in the Kuhnian sense—that is, a paradigmatic shift of major importance. The details of this revolution are still to be resolved, but there can be no doubt that it will permanently affect psychological inquiry, whether under the labels of radical constructivism (Von Glaserfeld, 1984), constructivism (Pribram, 1986), structural realism (Manicas & Second, 1983), or others.

If a paradigm shift from positivism had to occur in any science, it was psychology. By definition there is no subjectivism in the content of the material, or "hard" sciences. On the other hand, in psychology (a probabilistic science—it deals with probabilities, not absolutes) the subjective world is also real, and its study is as imperative as study of the objective world.

## Science and Medicine

An examination of science allows us to weigh psychological counseling on science's scales. We can best do that by first considering the role of science in an analogous profession, medicine.

In past centuries there was only a tiny base of substantiated knowledge on which medical practice could be based; in consequence, the sources of knowledge underlying healing practices were assumptions, folklore, and conjectures passed on by authorities. One such conjecture: diarrhea is a natural process for ridding the body of evils, a theory that called for the practice of administering physics or laxatives, as one approach to treating patients, the practice of which led to calling medical practitioners physicians.

The Renaissance promoted scientific inquiry into a number of dormant and new scholarly areas and thus improved the quality of medicine. The oldest science of medical value, predating the Renaissance by millennia, was anatomy; bones were easy to see without supplemental vision, and a knowledge of anatomy was valuable in sculpting and painting, highly prized activities during this period. Eventually, biology and chemistry emerged, with biology providing more useful knowledge as instruments to improve the senses were developed. Later, biology was wedded to other sciences with further benefit to medicine's purposes, as in the cases of biochemistry and biophysics. Sciences did not emerge primarily to serve medicine's needs but evolved as individual scientists were compelled to climb intellectual peaks because they were "there."

The gist of this review is that medicine is artful practice based on knowledge provided by several areas of scientific inquiry. It is artful because the physician has to create a concept of a patient's physical state and then create a course of medicine that addresses the specifics of that patient's condition.

## Counseling and the Science of Psychology

To what sciences could counselors in the early 1950s refer to support their artful practice? Because the concerns of clients were psychological, it followed that psychology would be the informing science. But that was not so.

Psychology moved out of the domain of philosophy in 1879 when Wilhelm Wundt established the first psychology laboratory in Leipzig. For the next 30 years psychologists studied individuals' conscious states—they were phenomenologists. By about 1920 a paradigmatic shift was under way, one that called for psychologists to reject the study of inner states and experiment only with observable behavior, the positivist epistemology that characterized "respectable" sciences at that time. This trend led to experimental treatment of objectively acquired data from the real world, an approach to psychological study called behaviorism. This was the general tone of psychological inquiry in the early 1950s.

As appropriate as this research direction was for psychology as an emerging science, it did not provide information useful for counseling because it did not address counseling's problems, which are subjective as well as objective and therefore require an emphasis on inner states. Behaviorists did not deny the existence of inner states, they just considered them outside the purview of scientific inquiry in psychology, a position congruent with the realism they espoused.

### Early Psychology and Counseling

In the 1950s, given the shortage of psychological theory and practices on which counseling could be based, most counselor-preparation programs trained students in C. R. Rogers's client-centered therapy, which was rooted in idealism. Whatever else may have caused commitment to this particular school, the two alternatives appeared less acceptable. Psychoanalysis, the first alternative, was rejected for three reasons, any one of which was sufficient: (1) The problems it addressed were not ones that counselors faced, (2) the length of time and expense required for training were both unrealistic for counselors, and (3) the likelihood was that counselors would not be admitted to a training program because of lack of qualifications, even if neither of the other factors pertained. Today an additional reason would deter some students: the fact that psychoanalysis has little scientific support for explaining thoughts, feelings, and behaviors. In those days there were programs in clinical psychology, of course, but these too were usually analytically oriented. In addition to the other impediments, psychoanalytic programs of study and their adjunct, clinical psychology, were applicable primarily to "patients" classified as abnormal, whereas client-centered practice employed no such labels and primarily attended to the concerns that any client brought.

Another counseling orientation was available, but it was not theory-based. It was developed by E. G. Williamson (1939, 1950) at the University of Minnesota as a rational, problem-solving model and assumed that counselors were authorities about how the world operated. Counseling was conducted within an expert/novice relationship similar to that of physician/patient because counselors were considered to be knowing people to whom the less knowledgeable came for help. The Williamson model originated with and was directed toward a university student population. For that reason there was a pronounced career-oriented facet to this model, one easily duplicated in any educational institution.

By midcentury, the psychoanalytic model was rejected for the reasons given, and the Williamson model was viewed as too restrictive. This left only the client-centered model for consideration.

### *Client-Centered Therapy*

The theoretical heart of client-centered therapy is phenomenology, which maintains, as we have seen, that reality lies only in each person's perceptions of the world. It is on this epistemic tenet that the details of this school's counseling procedures are constructed. It is a view that constitutes the school's major deficiency when judged by the standards of science, because reasoning and evidence do not support the conclusion that the inner world of a person is the only reality. Both the inner and the objective worlds are real, a position that requires moving beyond the precepts (but not all of the practices) of client-centered therapy (now titled person-centered) *as a system,* just as positivism must be rejected for its one-sided position.

To reject person-centered therapy, however, is to put oneself in the prejudicial error of rejecting everything about it and thus to overlook any valuable contribution it can make to science-oriented counseling. There is no need to throw out the baby with the bathwater. It is a defensible conjecture that most counselors today, whether aware of it or not, are sensitive to clients' phenomenological world owing at least partly to Rogers's emphasis on that point. And they use communication procedures that he partly identified and developed to deal with that subjective world.

For an illustration of the baby-with-the-bathwater issue, consider Anton Mesmer's contributions to the improvement of the human lot. All bathwater, no baby? Mesmer proposed mystical procedures to corral magnetic forces that flowed from cosmic bodies. His followers were coached in procedures to trap these forces, procedures that included a form of meditation that resulted in a trance. Although this was not a new technique, it became well known through Mesmer's work, and he was immortalized when it became known as mesmerism. The technique's name today is hypnotism. Although still occasionally employed as parlor entertainment, it is a significantly useful tool among some counselors and many clinical psychologists and psychiatrists. It is a baby that needed saving when throwing out the bathwater of Mesmer's theory.

## Three Other Counseling Schools

From time to time other schools of counseling will be briefly reviewed in this text to encourage applying epistemic criteria, and also to seek out any "babies" that may lurk in their "bathwaters" as we pursue the idea of school-less counseling. Three schools among many are selected somewhat arbitrarily for this purpose.

***Gestalt therapy.***   Gestalt therapy, founded by Frederick and Laura Perls, is also a phenomenological school and is thus not defensible under the criterion that reality is both internal *and* objective. "[Gestalt therapy's] goal is awareness and only awareness" (Simkin & Yontef, 1984, p. 279), and although there is agreement with the imperative need for awareness, there can be no epistemic justification for maintaining a school with that purpose alone when there is need to address other cognitive realities as well. But be wary of committing the baby-with-the-bathwater error with this school; useful counseling techniques come from it.

***Reality therapy.***   Like other schools that originated decades ago when science-based knowledge about human conduct was scarce, reality therapy is a product of one person's observations and ideas. As with person-centered therapy, its origina-tor was not a scholar/researcher but a pragmatist who was dissatisfied with the primary choices of counseling systems, which were psychoanalysis in its original form and several mutations. William Glasser (1984) writes that reality therapy attempts "to teach people better ways or better behaviors to deal with the world" (p. 324), a claim made by most counseling schools. He contends that people choose their own behavior and must be held responsible for it, a desirable value statement appropriate in anyone's life-view and also in accord with social science. Reality therapy does not attend to a number of client concerns, does not employ a number of tested procedures available to counselors, and does not contribute any new ideas or techniques to the pool of scientific knowledge.

***Rational-emotive therapy.***   In the 1950s the founder of rational-emotive ther-apy, Albert Ellis, began to reflect in his clinical-psychology practice the paradigm shift occurring in psychological science. As mentioned, this shift was from positiv-ism to a less restrictive epistemology that provided scientific credibility to the study of cognitive processes, and to clinical practice that reflected that study. Ellis, like others, found that the psychoanalytic model in which he had been trained did not contribute concepts and practices useful with typical clients. Although others had previously found that clients' views of themselves and conflicts between their values and actions and those of others were causes of distress, Ellis's persistent emphasis on these phenomena helped in establishing the validity of this subjectiv-

ism. He focused on clients' cognitions and vigorously espoused the scientific
legitimacy of attending to these inner states.

One characteristic of this school is its life-view, which is seen by some as
essential but considered by others as unacceptable. Probably no other counseling
school has so clearly explicated the values to which counselors should subscribe.
This school, says Ellis (1984), is "humanistic, existentialist, and hedonistic" (p. 234).
The latter attribute is central in this school's tenets because humans are seen as
biologically and culturally predisposed to seek pleasure but are thwarted in that
goal by learning to conform to other values. From the start Ellis has challenged
clients who say that they "must" behave in certain ways, such as that they must forgo
a desirable activity because of parents' preferences. The need to challenge remains
central in this school and is reflected in a word Ellis coined that regularly appears
in his writing, *must*urbation (his emphasis). That characteristic is to be eliminated,
or at least minimized, along with perfectionism, grandiosity, and intolerance. This
minimizing "was also attempted by religious leaders such as Buddha, Jesus, and St.
Francis of Assisi; but because they refused to stay with logico-empiric methods, they
strayed into irrational pathways" (p. 212). "[People's] inborn and acquired person-
downing, antihumanistic, god-and-devil inventing philosophy encourages them to
have . . . foolish thoughts . . . and inappropriate feelings that drive them to whine
and rant and live less joyously" (p. 235).

This emphatic, sharply delineated life-view provides immediate, intermediate, and ultimate goals for counselors who adhere to this school. The
importance attached to these values is demonstrated by the creation of an institute
to propagate rational living according to the principles maintained by this school.

The school's original and primary technique, confrontation of clients using a
vigorously argumentative approach, apparently reflects the founder's personal
style. Recent statements suggest that there are now additional approaches to clients,
with techniques described as explicatory and didactic.

## The Contribution of Schools Today

Schools were useful during the early days of psychology. They provided some
systematic bases from which counselors could assist clients, even though the
choice of a school to which to be committed was, in the expression of the Eysencks,
a choice that did not express any scientific reflection but only the existing prejudices of students (Eysenck & Eysenck, 1985).

Four schools, most with large followings, have been given cursory inspection
in this chapter. Three of these schools were established by individual practitioners,
not researchers, a characteristic of other schools not reviewed here. The other
school, behavior therapy, is the outcome of the continuing research of many
persons. The significance of the one-practitioner origin is that those schools
express one person's it-seems-to-me empiricism, which is uncontrolled and thus
not scientific. Although changes have to start in just that way, when a scientist
develops a hypothesis—"It seems to me" or "I am led to think"—it is necessary to
involve the scientific community to perform critical evaluation, a central principle
of science. The proposer is expected to experiment and present hypotheses and

early findings to others. If sufficient merit is found, other scientists may join in the inquiry by conducting their own investigations. Such careful, critical study has not characterized schools of counseling, with the exceptions of early client-centered therapy, behavior therapy, and cognitive-behavioral therapy. Most other schools' tenets are based on uncontrolled empiricism but are offered by their originators as if they were substantiated findings.

It is appropriate to refer to most counseling schools as sects, because like the blind persons seeking to describe an elephant, each describes some portion of the full array of extant knowledge about human conduct and its change. Some schools may also be classified as cults, because the sect's founder has become an essential element in the definition of the school. That is epitomized by the adulation directed at Rogers by his followers although not sought by him.

One characteristic common to a number of schools is the claim by each that its concepts are more accurate and its procedures more effective than the ideas and procedures of others. Research into these claims has consistently failed to prove the greater effectiveness of one approach (except behavioral) over others. Recent research repeats these findings: "Despite clear demonstrations . . . of systematic differences in therapists' techniques, most reviews of psychotherapy outcome research show little or no differential effectiveness of different psychotherapies" (Stiles, Shapiro, & Elliot, 1986, p. 165). Some change occurs simply from a client's having taken the initiative to seek help; 50% of the change sought by clients is the figure some use (but not necessarily accurately). Another source of change independent of counselor assistance is called spontaneous remission* by medical practitioners. The possibility of the operation of other, unknown variables must also be acknowledged.

Neophyte counselors may be justifiably skeptical of the claims of school X that it produces a high rate of change, particularly in contrast to school Y. When you have mastered research and statistical procedures, you will be able to appraise those claims by evaluating the treatment given to their dependent and independent variables. Indeed, you may find that those variables were not systematically investigated.

For example, much is known today about the genetic determiners of cognitions, actions, and feelings, yet examination of the teachings of counseling sects shows little or no attention given to that vital information. This may be because those schools were originated by one person at a time when such biological information was not available. But why not incorporate that knowledge now? Schools were established and are maintained today with little change; otherwise they would not be schools. Person-centered therapy would not be that if it were to accept as valid the proposition that reality can also be objective. If schools were modified to incorporate the current scientific knowledge and techniques and to forgo any unsubstantiated precepts and procedures that characterize them, a large part of their tenets and practices would become identical. Their major distinguishing attribute would be their title.

*This is a potentially misleading phrase, because for some people spontaneous remission or reversal often connotes a *sudden* and *unexplainable* change. "Unexplained reversal with no external intervention" is a better description of such events, which usually are not sudden. Science assumes that the causes of these rare reversals can be explained and will be in time.

There are no schools (theories) of engineering among which students must chose. There are specialties, of course, but each of these is informed by the same disciplines, just as counseling can be informed by science as its single source of knowledge, regardless of the institution or specialty in which counselors practice.

It is important to note that a fallacy may occur in comparing the conceptual integrity of engineering to the practice of counseling. Engineering is based on absolute (or "hard") sciences because it deals only with the objective world. Additionally, it is a relatively closed system in its practices; that is, the variables that impinge on engineering projects are relatively few and stable. On the other hand, numerous variables impinge on clients, and they occur in patterns unique to each client, particularly in clients' phenomenological world. In addition, the pattern of variables present in this week's interview may differ from that of last week's, because humans are open systems and are subject to changes in environments and to changes originating within the person. It is defensible to assert that the typical engineer is called upon for less ingenuity and creativeness than a counselor is.

## Eclecticism

Eclecticism is the practice of selecting and amalgamating what appear to be the best portions of various doctrines, methods, or styles. Eclecticism provides both undesirable and valuable outcomes when applied to counseling, depending on whether it is theoretical or technical eclecticism.

**Theoretical eclecticism.**   I have previously expressed the undesirability of a student's studying a number of counseling schools and then selecting one of them as the basis of his or her counseling practice because it conforms with personal prejudices. It would be every bit as undesirable for a student to study the theoretical tenets of a number of counseling schools and select some principles from two or more schools for his or her own theory *without having an epistemic justification* that would give coherence to this mix. Eclecticism without epistemic criteria— that is, choosing bits and pieces from the buffet of theoretical concepts without reference to an epistemology—is theoretical eclecticism, and is undesirable.

The error in the following statement is apparent (the statement is not fictional; it epitomizes those made by counselors from time to time): "I am a person-centered counselor, although with certain clients I am a behaviorist." These are incompatible theoretical positions, and thus the speaker is demonstrating a lack of grounding in epistemology rather than the even-handedness or objectivity (or mastery of skills) he intends to demonstrate.

**Technical eclecticism.**   If theoretical (epistemic) eclecticism can be undesirable, technical eclecticism, on the contrary, is not only desirable but also imperative for a person who is committed to the scientific epistemology. Had the counselor's statement cited above been, "I use proven techniques from both person-centered and behavioral theories when I find them useful," the counselor would have been attesting to the wise practice of technical eclecticism.

Among science's characteristics is its pragmatism, and thus a counselor will employ any technique no matter where it originated as long as its efficacy has been demonstrated and as long as it is in accord with the values of the counselor's life-views. This position about pragmatism does not favor an approach to counseling technology that is based solely on "what works," however; that stance would result only in pragmatists, in technicians, and mark those practitioners as theoretically sterile.

Some years ago a team of physicians from the United States examined the healing practices of nontechnological, nonliterate peoples to search for techniques and materials to add to the Western medical armamentarium. This is praiseworthy technical eclecticism. That team, however, could not have accepted as valid the statement that certain forest demons had caused the diseases treated by those effective procedures and materials and then have incorporated that "fact" in their findings. To have done so would have shown theoretical eclecticism without epistemic justification in addition to technical eclecticism. To have done so would have been scientifically untenable.

## Counseling: Theory, Technology, and Art

This text proposes that the time has come for psychological counseling to be school-less. Most schools are faulted for being too narrow in scope and therefore providing inadequate explanations both of how people come to think, behave, and feel as they do and of what are appropriate counseling procedures. This text seeks to offer as complete a picture as possible of principles and techniques that originate from the epistemology of science. The resulting product exemplifies what a theory is: a tenable explanation for observed phenomena. It follows that without an acceptable explanation (theory), there can be no counseling. Traditional counselors also operate from theory—from an explanation of the world that is agreeable to each. These theories, however, are not based on extensive study of human cognition, affect, and behavior. For those providing nontraditional counseling, the theories incorporating those three areas have been informed by only their personal experience. Most of these "home-grown" theories would be found unacceptable by professionally trained counselors.

Counseling cannot be just an array of techniques, either. As noted earlier, should counseling courses teach only "what works," graduates would be technicians, not professionals. While it may be better to have technicians giving help than no one, counseling is more than theory-validated technology. It is also an art, and an art requires a theory to inform it. The theory that informs counseling practice is not primarily *counseling* theory, although that position is more a matter of academic hair-splitting than a practical one. Theory originates in the sciences from which the technology is derived. Psychology is the major science that supplies the theory on which the technology of counseling is based, to which are added some findings from the social sciences.

Medicine is a technology and an art also: a technology when the diagnosis is absolute and the cure is patent and an art when the diagnosis and cure are obscure. A broken bone provides a simple illustration. The physician does not heal the fracture but does create the best conditions for it to heal itself, and may provide analgesia for the pain experienced immediately after the break. Is this only technology? Perhaps; enough so that a medical technician can carry out the procedures.

The physician, however, rooted in theory, may see conditions related to the break and the patient's general health that the technician does not see. The physician may have to create healing circumstances beyond simple technical procedures when a puzzling medical problem turns up, one for which there is no one-to-one correlation between the diagnosis and the procedures required for cure. The physician creates medical procedures unique to this patient and thus is practicing artfully. These creative procedures are not based on medical theory, it is argued, just as the counselor is not practicing from a basis of counseling theory. The theories that undergird a physician's artful practice grow out of the disciplines on which medical practice is based: chemistry, biochemistry, neurology, anatomy, and biophysics, as examples.

Each authority who originated a school of counseling in years past sought to convince counselors that he or she offered an accurate portrayal of human concerns and how to deal with them. Each, in fact, offered partial knowledge acquired from varying sources. A goal for all students, therefore, is to assess their own present epistemic convictions and to advance them through further study, thereby becoming able to evaluate the propositions of those authorities for themselves.

## Concluding Reflections

At times counselors must challenge a client's assertions about what he or she knows. Whatever the specific reason at the moment, such a challenge is justified because the client's developmental growth requires an increased knowledge of self.

It is equally valuable for counselors to understand the origins of their own knowledge. When it comes to professional practices, it is imperative that counselors be able to justify the tenets to which they subscribe. Doing that requires some understanding of epistemology and some consciously made epistemic commitment after reasoned deliberation. This chapter provides a brief excursion into that imperative.

Intellectually, as well as physically, the cosmos is fluid—marked by continuing change (which creates a difficulty in maintaining one's values). We lessen our effectiveness as counselors if we never challenge the tenets we hold, never question our counseling practices. Some counselors may hesitate to conduct a regular examination of their ideas because that may seem to be a weakening of value judgments that are essential or may threaten the comfortable professional stands they adopted in the past. Alertness to epistemic issues and the application of epistemic criteria to professional matters can let us be professionally progressive yet retain essential values.

## ■ Points to Remember ■

1. Counselors will be faced with claims by individual schools of counseling theory and practice that seek their loyalties. Some knowledge of epistemology is required to enable counselors to judge whether any school earns that loyalty or whether some alternative to schools, such as is proposed here, is defensible by epistemic criteria.

2. The topic of epistemology, the study of knowing, is complex, but the starting benchmark is authority, the source of knowledge for most of what each of us knows.

3. There are several prescientific sources of knowledge, of which three deserve some thought: tradition, mysticism, and rationalism.

4. The primary body of knowledge that informs counseling is psychology—"new" psychology.

5. The science that dominated psychology for over a half-century is called positivism. This science attends only to objective reality. A recent paradigm shift has brought a different kind of science of psychology to the forefront. This "new" science recognizes the need to incorporate clients' subjective realities, such as cognitions. Recent findings in the field of psychology are highly applicable to counseling.

6. In the past, before psychological science had progressed to the point where it could offer comprehensive knowledge about how and why people think and feel as they do and how to produce desired changes in thoughts, feelings, and behavior, some practitioners developed techniques and published them as separate therapies, or schools of counseling. Schools still dominate in most preparation programs but are held here as anachronisms. Schools were explanations for thought and action that served useful purposes in counseling's early days. They have been made redundant by recent scientific findings and reasonings.

8. In its theory and procedures one counseling school emphasizes clients' subjective world, a phenomenological epistemology. Another emphasizes only clients' objective world. Neither subscribing to the exclusive objectivism of positivistic science nor the subjectivism of phenomenology is defensible. Both realism and idealism, to employ other terms from epistemology, are correct.

9. It is questionable eclecticism to select portions of theories and be committed to them solely because they have surface appeal. Such choices must be made on defensible epistemic grounds.

10. As in some other professions, such as medicine, the technical practices employed in counseling are based on scientifically supported theories and bodies of knowledge. There is not a one-to-one match between technique and changes sought, however. Counselors are educated and trained both to reason out and experiment with techniques from the pool of proven ones and to invent new techniques. Counseling is an art because its practitioners creatively employ techniques adapted to each client.

## ■   **Counselor Formation Activities**   ■

1. This activity is intended to cause you to ponder how you know what you know. Through a Chapter 1 activity you became more aware of assumptions that determine your behaviors and feelings, parts of your life-view. Over the years you have acquired numerous beliefs, general knowledge, and facts. Has there been a single source of knowledge on which their acquisition has been based? Do you describe yourself as one whose knowledge and beliefs are fundamentally rooted in

science, mysticism, rationalism, tradition, or another source? In thinking about yourself, you will probably find that you are committed to differing sources of knowledge depending upon the area of learning, such as religion, health, or the nature of the physical world. Regardless of the epistemic underpinnings of these commitments, with respect to counseling it is the specific life-views stemming from it that are significant. What those life-views are now may not be what they were years ago. Give studied thought to the origins or reasons for any changes in epistemic commitments you identify that have resulted in life-view changes.

2. Interview one or more counselors or other providers of psychological services to learn by what theory or school of counseling (therapy) their professional practice is governed. Ask the practitioners about the source of knowledge on which that theory is based. Make an effort to determine the relative emphasis of uncontrolled empiricism, controlled empiricism, reasoning, other sources of knowledge, or mixes of them that informed their authorities. Also inquire about their stand on the phenomenology/reality issue. Do they stand clearly in one or the other camp, take a stand in the middle, or remain vague about where they stand? The purpose of these inquiries is to assist you in identifying your own positions and to increase your appreciation of the counseling significance of whatever epistemic positions a practitioner takes.

3. Do you enter this counselor-preparation program with a preference for a named counseling school (person-centered, reality, Gestalt) or even a commitment to it? If so, can you identify the epistemic principles on which this school is based?

■                           **Complementary Reading**                           ■

Psychology's recent shift from a pronounced positivism to a more inclusive paradigm is not to be read as the appearance of a new movement in psychology. It is a newer emphasis of a model that has a long history, one that should be known beyond the introductory coverage in this chapter. I urge study of this essay:

CAHAN, E. D., & WHITE, S. H. (1992). "Proposals for a Second Psychology." *American Psychologist, 47*(2), 224–235.

The study of epistemology can be daunting for newcomers to the topic. The best starting place is any standard encyclopedia.

A major tenet of this text is that schools of counseling have outlived any usefulness as unique explanations for human covert and overt behaviors. For that reason, schools are not systematically examined here. To be more fully informed about schools or theories, you can read the full statements made by schools' founders or heirs or by acknowledged leaders in *Current Psychotherapies* (Corsini, 1984). Selectively compare material offered there with that found in:

COREY, G. (1991). *Theory and Practice of Counseling and Psychotherapy,* 4th ed. Pacific Grove, CA: Brooks/Cole.

Corey not only provides analysis and interpretation of schools but also covers other topics related to counseling.

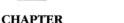

# Experiments:
# An Epistemological Imperative

## Overview

This chapter is related to Chapter 2 because it extends the theme of epistemology with a detailed look at controlled empiricism, in the form of experiments. Experiments have been the hallmark of positivist psychological science, but because of the "new" science in psychology—the new paradigm—some people may be led to think that experimentation has lost its importance. To the contrary, experimentation remains essential in the new paradigm. The change from the exclusive empiricism of positivism does not mean that empiricism no longer has a place; it does mean that psychology is moving away from the idea that empiricism is *exclusively* important. Because the epistemology of this text is science—albeit the science of the new paradigm—the examination of the major defining activity of science, the experiment, is necessary.

There are other reasons for this focus on experimentation. One is that by providing you with a better understanding of the empirical side of science, you will better be able to understand science as a major source of knowledge. This can result in clarifying why parts or entire schools of counseling (therapy) are judged to be no longer appropriate. The other purpose is to inform prospective writers of theses and dissertations of the essentials of experimentation in case they choose that route of empirical research or it is required of them.

## Introduction

As noted in Chapter 2, science is defined by more than experimentation—that is, by more than empiricism. "Psychology has been the most aggressively empiricist of all academic disciplines," Kukla observes, but now philosophers of science seem "to agree that the role of empirical research in scientific progress was vastly overestimated by the logical positivists of the previous generation" (1989, p. 785). He endorses the proposition that science is more than empiricism, illustrating his point with scientific activities that are nonempirical. One example is the scientific reasoning that occurs in theory construction, including the investigation of the logical coherence of a theory and the construction of new conceptual schemes. The reasoning in scientific thinking is informed by the study of logic, and its conclusions will be shaped by the hard-nosed evaluation of fellow scientists.

Because the controlled experiment will always be a feature of most sciences (it cannot be fully so in astronomy and geology, for example), its desiderata need to be understood.

## Characteristics of Experiments

Experimentation is controlled empiricism. Because *uncontrolled* empiricism has been spoken of negatively, we will examine that topic first to see why it is a dubious source of knowledge and to provide a contrast that lets us better understand controlled empiricism. Another reason to investigate this process is that prospective counselors need to be aware of its shortcomings, because some counseling schools are based on it.

### *Uncontrolled Empiricism: A Risky Epistemology*

Uncontrolled empiricism is the receipt of knowledge through the senses but with no test of that knowledge's validity. For millennia, people's knowledge about the movement of the sun around the earth was empirical, received through the sense of sight with no reason to question what was seen—a historical example of this epistemology. This common knowledge, whose validity was unimportant in daily life but was important to those interested in the truth about the cosmos, could not be contested, let alone tested, until several conditions converged. First a paradigm shift had to occur. Copernicus stimulated that shift at a time when another need was satisfied: a device to enhance vision of distant objects, called the telescope. Then came a burgeoning interest in astronomy that led to the controlled observations necessary to test beliefs about the nature and movement of heavenly bodies. The knowledge provided by uncontrolled empiricism was thus proved false.

The earth's rotation around the sun also provides an illustration of authority as a knowledge source. Each of us sees the sun appear to move around the earth, yet we all deny the validity of that empirical datum. Is that because each of us has established the fact through her or his own study in astronomy? No; yet we adamantly persist in our view that the earth rotates around the sun. We hold to that view because those whom we accept as authorities have told us that our observation is an illusion contrary to the fact. We accept their statements as authoritative despite what our sense of sight tells us, even if these authorities do not support their explanations with evidence.

### *Controlled Empiricism*

Experimental methods, unlike theory development, concept evaluation, and other logic-demanding aspects of science, are easy to understand because they are definable techniques. No matter how intellectually competent typical scientists are in manipulating the logic of science, they also need to know the role of experimentation in their science and to be competent in conducting experiments.

Experiments are carried out to test whether some assumption, guess, or conjecture about the real world can be verified. Such assumptions, labeled *hypotheses,* are subjected to controlled observations in laboratory or nonlaboratory conditions. Operational definitions of the hypothesis permit the results of those observations to be numerical, which in turn permits statistical treatment and generalization.

## *The Hypothesis*

Individuals differ in their responses to phenomena they experience. Some of them show no curiosity about causes. Others *are* curious but accept any plausible explanation without regard to the authority's qualifications. Some arrive at answers that are not based on earlier findings and seek no empirical proof of their conclusions. Others set up hypotheses about the causes and pursue knowledge about them tenaciously and carefully through controlled observation; these people are scientists.

The originator of the scientific method in the Western world, Thales, observed the same phenomena that his fellow Ionians did over 2000 years ago. All Ionians had equal opportunity to see the solid and liquid components of the earth, observe the effects of air, and peer at the cosmos day and night. Others may have systematically observed and conjectured about what they saw, but it was Thales who wrote about his observations and conclusions and became known as history's first scientist.

When a scientist notices a phenomenon for the first time, he or she wonders "Why?" "How did that happen?" "What caused that?" These questions lead to conjectures, or informed guesses, that are formally termed *hypotheses*. A hypothesis, clearly stating what is to be observed and measured, leads to experiments that provide either support or rejection of the scientist's conjectures about the "what," "how," and "why" questions. Upon observation of the phenomenon, a scientist may start by engaging in scientific activities other than experiments, such as theory building, but at some point will conduct experiments.

**Refutability of hypotheses.**    Let us assume that a scientist observes phenomenon P and, after studying P's concomitants, hypothesizes that a variable, V, has an effect on or is in some way associated with P. The scientist cannot directly validate this hypothesis but instead will carry out observations to show that the hypothesis is false. For this purpose a hypothesis must be stated negatively: it is a *null hypothesis.* Any idea about the real world that someone wishes to check for accuracy, therefore, must be a statement (hypothesis) that can be proven false. Hypotheses can be eventually accepted only when observation after observation, carried out by a number of scientists, have not proved them to be false. These observations are carried out by trying to prove the validity of a *null hypothesis,* as we will shortly see.

Some rural folks a century ago "knew" that thunder was the cause of milk turning sour. If that view were stated as a hypothesis, it would meet the criterion of falsifiability. The refutation did occur when it was experimentally demonstrated that the hypothesis was not valid and that the cause of milk's souring was the rapid multiplication of bacteria, not thunder. Thunder occurred incidentally because the same heat that resulted in the reproduction of bacteria also caused electrical storms.

Some folk beliefs are not refutable and therefore cannot be validated. When a group is told by someone accepted as an authority that an affliction, such as an earthquake or a flood, was divinely sent because of the sins of the group, no hypothesis can be forwarded because the assertion that sins caused the affliction cannot be refuted by controlled experimentation. It is the absence of refutability that denies use of the label *hypothesis.* We are reminded that some testing of hypotheses can be carried out rationally—that is, without collecting new data through experimentation. The use of existing data may suffice. More commonly, however, new testing is carried out experimentally for each hypothesis proposed.

***Null hypothesis.***    The technical act of refutation is to state the hypothesis so that it contradicts the conjecture held by the researcher; it is stated and tested in the null form, as "There is *no* relationship between P and V." If the null hypothesis is not supported by statistical treatment of the data—that is, if the data the researcher gathers and submits to statistical testing do *not* require the rejection of the statement that P and V are not related—it does not thereby follow that the positive statement (the research hypothesis, "P and V are related") is valid. There can be increasing confidence that the research hypothesis is true only after repeated research continues to show no support for the null hypothesis and after no competing hypothesis is supported. Additionally, confidence in the validity of the research hypothesis can be maintained only if control over observations was sufficient to account for all variables that might affect the results. If the null hypothesis is supported after a number of observations, the researcher who developed the hypothesis may be disappointed, but the cause of knowledge will have been served.

When scientists propose a hypothesis, it is assumed that they will conduct some research to verify it and eventually, through conference reports and publications, will explain the reason for the hypothesis and the research findings to date. It was noted earlier that some counseling practitioners develop a conjecture or hypothesis and then state it as if it is a postulate, a discovered truth, even if their conclusion is supported only anecdotally and not by controlled observation. The result of forgoing controlled observation may be yet another counseling school.

After a scientist reports his or her ideas and the first research findings, other scientists may become interested in the topic and conduct further research, a step necessary to validate any hypothesis.

## A Research Essential: Tedious, Controlled, Accurate Observation

Experimentation is defined by the process of controlled observation. Both scientific and nonscientific methods begin with casual observation of some phenomenon, which is uncontrolled empiricism. When experimentation is possible, this casual observation will be followed by formal, controlled observation, beginning with a description of the variables related to the phenomenon. Scientists may also study problems that are not directly accessible either to observation through the senses or to experimentation. In either case science-oriented reasoning dominates. The early study of atoms and quantum mechanics illustrates the impossibility of direct observation. The study of cognitions in the field of human conduct is another illustration, because cognitions cannot be directly sensed.

Experimentation is an advanced form of observation, to be carried out when possible, but inquiry may nonetheless be scientific even if control of major variables is not possible. The validity of scientific inquiry without direct experimentation is demonstrated by cosmic research. Cosmic phenomena have had to be studied without manipulation of major variables, but all alternative procedures are carried out in a controlled manner. That we have extensive knowledge of the cosmos despite the impossibility of the manipulation of major variables is demonstrated by interplanetary spacecraft. Experimentation cannot be performed on some of the major variables of meteorology and geology either, but these sciences are not to be faulted as resting on uncontrolled empiricism. Nor can studies like anthropology, sociology, or archaeology. In these studies, unlike counseling schools founded by one person on the strength of his or her experience without carrying out controlled studies, investigators pool their observations and reasoned conclusions. Most counseling schools' founders are practitioners, not researchers.

Observations of a phenomenon permit one or more hypotheses to be generated as explanations of the phenomenon. Adequate testing of hypotheses calls for numerous observations of a quality that probably requires training in experimental observation. The scientist differs from the nonscientist also in observing elements of a phenomenon that would probably be missed by the nonscientist because the scientist is sensitized to them by experience and research methods. Additionally, the scientist will carry out observations over a long period, in minute detail. Sample after carefully chosen sample needs to be observed, experimentally when possible.

***Instruments.***    To carry out those observations, a scholar may need to create one or more instruments. These could be a cyclotron costing hundreds of millions of dollars or a new personality inventory costing but a few hundred dollars. The use of both established and new instruments additionally distinguishes a scientist from a nonscientist who may notice the same phenomenon. A layperson observes with unaugmented senses, whereas the scientist supplements his or her senses with a variety of instruments (Morrison & Morrison, 1987). The discovery of Jupiter's satellites serves as example. The casual observer of the night sky in the mid-17th century could see Jupiter, as had casual observers for millennia, but could not see its satellites. The astronomers' vision, when eventually augmented by telescopes, showed those satellites, and being scientists, not naturalists, astronomers were eager to account for the satellites' motions. That required detailed, tedious observation, which Galileo, among others, provided. "It's quite remarkable that he could follow the four satellites well enough to be able to make fair predictions *after only two or three years of watching*" (Morrison & Morrison, 1987, pp. 34–35; emphasis added).

## Reliance on Quantification

The attempt to refute a hypothesis calls not only for controlled observation but also for mathematical observation of the data collected, which is why the components of the hypothesis must be quantifiable. To illustrate, let it be hypothesized that regular and frequent pledging of allegiance to the flag results in patriotic citizens. Reciting can be quantified; patriotism cannot. But, one might ask, cannot citizenship be indirectly measured? After all, neither gravity nor magnetism occupies space, nor can they be seen or felt, but their effects can be measured. The effects of gravity and magnetism, however, are relatively consistent and can be defined mathematically. But how can one define patriotic citizenship to the satisfaction of all observers? It is assumed that it cannot be defined, and therefore its effects cannot be measured. The outcomes of allegiance-pledging must necessarily remain in the domain of faith.

***Quantifying intelligence.***   The scientific process sometimes requires that gaps in a theory be filled in by creating ideas that refer to things that do not actually exist but are used in the theory as if they did. These creations are called hypothetical constructs. The most prominent of these constructs in counseling are mind, intelligence, and the unconscious. No method has been devised to quantify the concepts of mind and the unconscious (understandably), and thus no scientific measures are possible. There are numerous measures of intelligence, but at the same time there is wide disagreement about what they are measuring. The hypothetical construct called gravity, on the other hand, is mathematically defined and thus readily, consistently, and accurately measurable. In consequence, the effects of gravity can be predicted, and thus controlled, as demonstrated by space flights.

The range of definitions of intelligence precludes agreement on what is to be observed, which in any case cannot be observed directly, only its effect. In consequence, prediction and control based on data said to measure intelligence are rare outcomes. The inconsistencies related to this construct exemplify why the probabilistic science of behavior is also called an inexact one ("less exact" is a better term). Those sciences spoken of as absolute, or exact, are able to address components that occupy space, or have agreed-upon constructs when constructs are required to explain a phenomenon, and have agreed-upon scales, measurements, and instruments for observing (for collecting data about) the phenomenon.

Were observation controlled in the P and V study used above for illustration, P would have to be observed under a variety of values of V. That is, V would have to be altered a number of times in quantity and frequency, with measures of effects on P made for each change in V. In addition, other variables that could possibly influence P would have to be observed along with V.

## Assumption of Lawfulness and Determination

In Chapter 1 we noted the importance of assumptions for counseling. The assumptions referred to were those macrocosmic tenets about human existence called life views. Whatever the sweep of large assumptions that constitute our life views, each of us also subscribes to assumptions about the more specific and detailed aspects of daily life. Our thoughts and actions are dominated by these countless microcosmic assumptions as well as by the global ones.

This phenomenon can be observed operating in daily life. Select a brief period of any day, and recall the actions you took during that time. For each action, ask what you assumed before taking that action. You will find that some assumptions are accounted for as extrapolations of experience. When you mail a letter, you make numerous assumptions, one of which is that it will be delivered. A young child causes damage while doing some prohibited act. Hearing a parent approach, the child assumes from her past experience that a painful event is to ensue. Easily managing the wiles of childhood, she speedily works up tears accompanied by protestations of love for the parent and sorrow for the action. The relatively unaware assumption behind this accomplished acting is that it will result in parental guilt about any planned punishment and will produce, if not a full pardon, at least a less painful consequence. Driving in traffic would be impossible were we not able to make assumptions about others' driving behaviors.

Some assumptions are based not on experience but on assertions by those viewed as authorities. When a person is told by an authority that if X is done (sex), undesirable Y will result (blindness, hell), the person may abstain from doing X solely on that basis, assuming entirely on faith that the pronouncement corresponds to reality.

Scientists have to be skeptical about, if not reject, unverified assumptions about phenomena. If the theological statement that the cosmos is about 5000 years old is assumed to be accurate by a youth who later develops aspirations to become a geologist or astronomer, either the assumption or the career goal will need to be abandoned.

Just as counselors are influenced professionally by life views they hold, so too are scientists' professional behaviors affected by assumptions characteristic of the philosophy of science. One such assumption is that *phenomena are lawful* (based on laws of nature, such as gravity) *and thus determined,* with the scientific enterprise directed to uncovering lawfulness where it may exist. This is relatively easy to do when the phenomena studied are interactions among material things and agreed-upon forces, as is common in the more exact (absolute) sciences, which are relatively closed systems. It is far less easy to uncover lawfulness in sciences that examine open systems, such as human behavior. It is difficult or even impossible to hold behavioral variables steady; in an open system, variables can "leak out," or other variables can intrude—a potentially harmful condition when those unwelcomed variables are not noticed during an experiment.

This lawfulness, this orderliness as it may apply to humans in general, is what the researcher of cognitions, affect, and behavior hopes to identify. It will be described in quantifiable terms when possible and will include the antecedents (conditions that precede), concomitants (conditions that occur at the same time), and prospective results of the phenomenon studied because those are variables in the occurrence of thoughts, feelings, or actions. Antecedents, concomitants, and expected results are major determiners of those events.

The view that human thoughts, feelings, and actions are determined by forces not under an individual's control is repellent to some, but this tenet is not as harsh and "mechanical" as it may seem. It is valid to say that at any moment a person's behavior *is* determined by antecedents, concomitants, and prospective results, but that does not imply forces found only outside the person. A large number of those determiners are internal—that is, are part of the person's consistent ways of thought, life views, and feelings associated with them. In any case, if some determiners cannot be changed, whether of internal or external origin, the *effect* of those determiners can often be altered, an activity for which counseling is a helpful resource.

People usually wish to understand what causes events. When verifiable causes are not immediately forthcoming, those recognized as authorities sometimes create plausible reasons, which then become assumed knowledge, part of tradition and folklore. During the Middle Ages, medicine was practiced on the basis of epistemologies other than science. The affliction now called epilepsy was assumed in certain cultures to result from possession by a demon, a conclusion based on mysticism and rationalism, preserved by tradition, and passed on over generations by authority. The cure dictated by this theory was exorcism, the ritual driving out of demons. The natural and normal subsidence of symptoms was available as "proof" that the theory and its technique were valid.

In the Western world science has replaced mysticism in most applied fields. When medical problems arise for which there are no science-based explanations (theories) and cures, prescientific explanations are not assumed. "We don't know about that yet," is the typical stance, a statement that shows faith in the eventual discovery of a science-based cure.

Should that not also be the stance in the case of the knowledge on which counseling is based? Behavior is complex, in part because it is a component of an open system, and is therefore subject to change. It is an area that yields its laws reluctantly, yet the scientific search must go on. Where there is no knowledge of substance, there is no justification for filling in the gaps with fictional explanations from nonscientific domains, no matter how rational they appear. In the absence of empirical evidence, the counselor, informed by theory, performs as an artist, creating a procedure that adheres as closely as possible to confirmed scientific evidence or reasoning but does not go beyond that.

# Concluding Reflections: Part 1

A text on psychological counseling for new students must necessarily cover only highlights or major themes and is forced to examine those aspects in only an overview fashion. While this limitation may be regrettable, it is not necessarily a handicap. Getting to know a new city to which one has moved serves as analogy. The positions of certain tall landmarks are fixed, and the appearance and routes of major streets are learned. That done, the newcomer can comfortably get around the city without being expected to claim complete knowledge of it; those features serve only as starting points for that knowledge. In like fashion, this text provides you with a few landmarks, which have been simplified in some cases. Continuing study will permit you to expand and complete this basic knowledge.

The topic of epistemology, for example, cited here as important knowledge for the counselor-to-be, has been treated in a cursory manner. It is hoped, however, that the coverage has been sufficient for those encountering the topic for the first time to understand its importance and some of its essentials so that further study can be pursued.

One of the essentials is the realism/idealism issue. Because it is complex, you may have to engage in considerable reading and discussion before arriving at a position on the issue that is reasonably comfortable. The epistemologically competent student or counselor will not need to look for an authority to serve as a mediator between the scholars who write about counseling, on the one hand, and an evaluation of what is written, on the other. The ability to judge for oneself will be there.

Any profession has its sinners as well as its saints, a way of saying that counselors are as diverse in morality and ethics as those in all other areas of endeavor. While the positive is emphasized here, students should be aware of the potency of human frailties occasionally found in the sciences underlying counseling or among its practitioners. "Subjectivity, personal prejudice, and pet notions have not been vanquished . . . in psychotherapy," Kazdin and Wilson (1978, p. 8) observe, nor will they ever be. Despite a diligent effort to make the theoretical and technical portions of this text objective, you are likely to find instances of the three sins that Kazdin and Wilson identify. As you gain sophistication in counseling, you will be readier to note the scholarly vices or inadequacies of your authorities and be sufficiently able to ignore those vices and inadequacies so you can absorb the products of the virtues.

Illustrations in this chapter and Chapter 2 show counseling primarily as a problem-solving activity—the elimination of obstacles to normal client development. Recall that a major function of the psychological counselor is the enhancement of good development, a facilitation of ongoingness, through instructional activities with groups and through consultation with agency management. Counseling of individuals, however, is the most professionally demanding activity, and the one over which more disagreement is found among schools of counseling. It requires most of our current attention; programmed activities for enhancement are to be explored later.

When life is going well, we humans form bonds, attachments, and affiliations with a variety of people playing a variety of roles. These affiliations provide assurance of our well-being, fill the need for belongingness, give living its purpose, and enable our development to progress along satisfying lines. Bonds and affiliations enhance the likelihood of our coping with anxieties, and they nurture an essential for effective living: accurate self-awareness. They can also result in a centering, in achieving a life focus, and in supporting continuing movement toward idiosyncratic purposefulness. When all goes well (it often does not), lives will be marked by a surging, reciprocated love of some others, a caring for many, comfort with spirituality (or its absence), and deeply rooted self-confidence.

Where is science in this portrayal of the ideal human existence? It is not there—we cannot expect science to contribute to the fundamental definition of humanness. Here we are in the domain of values, of what it is for each person that describes the optimally living human in terms that are not amenable to operational definition or quantification. These terms will include soaring, ongoing, constructive, and self-actualized. Such imprecise concepts describe persons who are existentially marked by self-realization and have the capacity to live with conflicts that are beyond personal resolution.

Can most people achieve these outcomes on their own? Is a person to shrug off the presence of an obstacle that naiveté or circumstance has dropped in his or her developmental path as just one of life's irreparable misfortunes? No, psychological counseling can ameliorate, if not remove, these deterrents. Counseling holds that individual purposefulness can be enhanced and can be aimed to the achievement of life goals such as those cited above, although they may be only partially attained. "Life" is not a science, but counseling, an aid in maximizing the quality of life, *is* based on science. A client may need love, acceptance, a sense of unshakable affiliations, and an increased sense of existential worth and direction, but the counselor does not enter the client's life as others might to provide for those needs. The counselor cares about and encourages emotional bonds with clients but does not love them—does not intentionally substitute for friend, lover, parent, or sibling. The counselor is fully aware that these and other affiliations are imperative to maintain mental-health-oriented goals but also knows that the affiliation between counselor and client is unlike those others, knows it is not intended to, nor can it, provide clients with the quality of life those other affiliations provide.

Counselors also know the techniques that permit them to let a client find out why these essential affiliations have not been achieved, and how to go about attaining them. The scientific thrust of this chapter (which, to reiterate, is not equated with positivism) is offered not with the view that it is to be extrapolated to the value and existential aspects of living but solely as the epistemology that is to inform counseling practice.

The counselor artfully applies science-based techniques to help others attain the life-view objectives mentioned above. Away from the counseling setting, counselors are but humans who may be struggling to maximize themselves through affiliations that are falling apart. They may face anxiety-producing developmental problems or may have a brooding sense of decreasing worth, of loss of purpose, and of being. In short, counselors also may have developmental concerns that motivate them to seek help from a psychological counselor.

# ■                      **Points to Remember**                      ■

1. The epistemology of science includes more than conducting experiments. At the same time, fundamental to science is the imperative to study any phenomenon that deserves study, when possible, by means of *controlled* observations, or empiricism. Uncontrolled empiricism is a daily experience of all, but it frequently leads to erroneous conclusions.

2. In experimentation, variables associated with a phenomenon are manipulated in a controlled manner over time so as to increase knowledge about it.

3. Not all science is experimentation. For example, some natural phenomena cannot be studied through direct manipulation of them. Nonetheless, study in such fields (geology is an example) is as solidly scientific as that in any field in which elements of the phenomenon can be experimentally manipulated.

4. The basis for experimentation is a conjecture that if variables are manipulated in a certain way, a precisely defined and measurable outcome will result. That conjecture is labeled a hypothesis.

5. An experiment's hypotheses cannot be proved true; they can only be proved not false. Hypotheses, therefore, are tested in null form. This negative statement says that the experiment will be conducted in an effort to sustain the null hypothesis. If this negative hypothesis (the opposite of what the researcher believes) is rejected, the conclusion can be only that the hypothesis is not false.

6. The epistemology of science, including one of its major distinguishing features, experimentation, provides criteria for examining the numerous schools of counseling. People committed to this epistemology will find the origins and propositions of some schools unacceptable. This text is committed to counseling theory and procedures based on scientific findings, scientific thinking, and the concurring thoughts of reputable scientists in psychology and the practice of counseling.

■   **Counselor Formation Activities**   ■

Obviously, numerous areas of knowledge are treated experimentally, psychology being one of them. Within psychology there are specialties, each with its own focus and some with unique experimental methods. Because your specialty is counseling, you should quickly develop a sense of the experiments conducted in this specialty. Even though it may be assumed that you do not yet have the technical knowledge to understand, let alone evaluate, those reports, choose an area of specialization in counseling, and examine recent issues of the *Journal of Counseling Psychology*, published by the American Psychological Association, and the *Journal of Counseling and Development*, published by the American Counseling Association, to look for one or more research reports related to that interest. Of course, this is not normally how you will go about carrying out a systematic study of a topic. That is not your intention at this time. The purpose is to become familiar with some of the research literature in counseling.

The outcome of this activity, as for most in this formation series, will be enhanced by discussing what you have found with others in your small training group. In the group, describe the topic you researched and the researcher's interpretation of the findings. Additionally, discuss how the findings of this research might affect your theoretical knowledge or technical skills.

■   **Complementary Reading**   ■

In time you will systematically study research methods, but meanwhile, to acquire some familiarity with how research in counseling is systematically carried out, you can consult:

HEPPNER, P. P. (1992). *Research Design in Counseling.* Pacific Grove, CA: Brooks/Cole.

One advantage of this volume is its focus on counseling, in contrast to more widely focused texts.

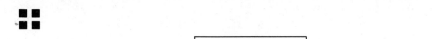

# 2
**PART**

# Clients

**CHAPTER**

# Effect on Clients of Biological and Other Variables

## Overview

What people think, feel, and do is partly biologically determined, and there-fore counselors need to know more than the average person about body organs that affect thoughts, emotions, and behaviors. This does not mean that psycholog-ical counselors are expected to modify those physiological determiners; changes of that nature cannot be made by any kind of professional at present. Counselors can help clients, however, by enabling them to modify the ways in which those physiologically determined thoughts, feelings, and actions are expressed.

In the section "Biological Elements," some of the influences of *genes* on behavior are examined, followed by a description of the role of the *brain* on clients' concerns. These two physiological variables establish the boundaries within which specific cognitions, affect,* and behaviors will develop as the person trans-acts with social systems.

The topic of personality development, which is influenced by one's genetic inheritance, is examined under two titles: "Temperaments and Their Traits" and "Cognition and Abilities."

Under the heading of "The Environmental Variable" the relationship between a person's biological inheritance and the numerous environments in which that person interacts is examined. Individuals function as systems, as entireties, and are locked into unique environments in symbiotic relationships with others. The term *transaction* is preferred to *interaction* as the better label for many of those relationships. Interactions can be observed, whereas a transaction is an invisible physiological interlocking with one or a few persons in a particular environment.

Interactional and transactional relationships, influenced by one's biological inheritance and modifed by experience, produce the unique pattern of thinking,

---

*The word *affect* subsumes both emotion and mood. *Feeling* is a synonym for affect.

feeling, and action that characterizes each individual. That experience is called learning. There is a brief examination of three learning modalities: modeling; classical, or respondent, conditioning; and operant, or instrumental, conditioning.

Selected developmental steps and changes that occur through the life span are also briefly examined.

## Introduction

A counselor who had only an average person's knowledge about how the feelings, actions, and mental processes of people in general were formed would be professionally handicapped. A counselor must not only know the effect of the environment on how one thinks, feels, and behaves but more basically must also be apprised of the function of biological factors. Counselors will be able to assist a client if they have some understanding about how these three facets of life originate. Such knowledge will let them account for the amazing diversity among people's affect and behaviors, particularly among those with the same parents and apparently similar environments.

The complexity of human functioning is emphasized for us through awareness that humans' cognitions, feelings, and behaviors, originally formed and maintained by biological and environmental factors, have been compounded over time into a unity. To further this thought, we consider the making of a cake. A cake recipe includes a list of ingredients (the content), and directions (the process). A cake is more than just the sum of the ingredients; the processes of mixing and heating cause the ingredients to combine and create a new product. The consumer is interested in the final product, but the baker must be concerned with the role of each ingredient, with how too much or too little of each can result in a defective product, and with the process that blends and changes those ingredients.

The major weakness of this analogy is that cake ingredients are relatively inert and that baking processes are elementary when compared with the complex and changing variables and processes of human development. The essential analogy holds, however: any client is more than a sum of the "ingredients" of that person's existence and the processes affecting them. These ingredients, if exogenous (entering from the environment), are introduced into a system that was already functioning at birth, to interact with some endogenous (genetic) ingredients.

## People as Systems

To comprehend the individual as a system, it is necessary to identify both internal and external variables that affect personality attributes. Systems theory holds that a person functions as an entirety but in a selective manner, typically incorporating at any one time only those new elements that are compatible with the existing system and, conversely, rejecting elements that do not fit in with the total system. Individuals as systems will change over time, the result of internal and external variables acting on personality attributes. Sometimes this change is rapid, as during adolescence, when relatively seismic changes may occur.

The significance of the systems concept is summarized by Caple (1985). He notes that the self-organization paradigm shows that mind and body function as an entirety and that the human organism is a system that "organizes and reorganizes itself throughout the entire life span" (p. 177). Learning about humans is easier when we know something about the ingredients, the "building blocks," which are the elements of any personality. When we seek to serve a client, however, we meet a person in whom these elements have interacted to produce a whole. A counselor does not need to know every client as an entirety but, with the client's help, assesses which element is performing in a faulty manner and then plans with the client to induce a change in that element, or at least to control its effects. Giving attention to changing only one element of a system is based on the evidence that change in one can change the entire system. A powerful emotional experience, for example, might change all other elements of a system. The emotion following the tragic death of a child or young friend can change thought patterns or behaviors, as can the emotional experience of imprisonment, which has been shown to reform cognitions and behaviors. Cognitive restructuring can alter emotions and behavior, and directed behavior change can affect cognitions and feelings. Counselors' successes are partly dependent on their ability to identify the elements that make up the whole person and to identify the processes that combine those ingredients into the whole person—into a living system.

Despite the fact that psychology provides some precise knowledge about people in general, about "the complex mechanisms that . . . underlie performances by individuals acting in the world," we cannot expect it to explain everyday behavior because "the acts of persons in life settings are open-system events that involve an enormous range of codetermining structures and systems" (Manicas & Secord, 1983, p. 407). Because people as systems are "open"—that is, the system is amenable to change from either internal or external sources—the explanation of human functioning is "a multidisciplinary effort and, though based on the behavioral sciences, necessarily transcends them to involve both biology and the social sciences" (p. 405). Because there is some science in the counselor's approach to clients and considerable art, it can be said that the counselor seeks to create a science of each client and is thereby "engaged in understanding the concrete person and his or her life history and particular patterns of behavior, including . . . self understanding" (p. 411).

Each person functions psychobiologically as a system within his or her cocoon of skin. At the same time, each has a place in temporary or fixed social environments, which also function as systems. It is the social systems in which people live that provide dimension to an individual and are the source of life's rewarding moments and problems. This text emphasizes the importance of social systems, while retaining an awareness that each individual in those systems is also a self-contained psychobiological system.

How can a counselor account for the differences in the mental processes, feelings, and behaviors of individuals? This chapter seeks to provide some useful answers by addressing selected biological and social variables that affect development and result in the distinctive person that each individual is. If some of these biological and social variables are not accessible for direct change through counseling, their *outcomes* can often be changed. Development cannot be reversed, but some outcomes can be modified, or otherwise counseling would be purposeless.

# The Biological Variable

Among variables beyond the direct reach of counselors are the genetic ones, although the particular ways in which genetic variables appear in thoughts, feelings, and actions are open to some counselor intervention. Even if genes cannot be directly altered, "[it] doesn't follow that counselors . . . cannot do a tremendous amount to help [the client] live a more effective and satisfactory life" (Skovholt, 1990).

Counselors can help move behaviors away from being antisocial, for example. The violent behavior of hundreds of people in one study showed evidence of brain dysfunction and neurological defects, Elliott (1988) reports, while other evidence (Eron, 1988) shows the contribution of the environment to these harmful behaviors. Antisocial or criminal behavior is rooted in the genes, thus making certain people biologically predisposed to these behaviors, Raine and Duncan (1990) assert. But they also write that when further research permits identification of children so genetically disposed, "[it] would then be possible to concentrate intervention on developing skills, interests, and aptitudes that those individuals clearly possess" (p. 642).

## *Transactions and Biological Interactions*

Frequent reference will be made to people transacting with others in social systems. Because the concept of transaction may be unfamiliar, some explanation follows.

There are two ways in which the relationship between an individual and others or the environment is commonly described. One, and the less acceptable, is to speak of an individual *and* his or her environment. The separateness of an individual from other people is conveyed by that phrase. This may be appropriate at times, such as when an individual is in a randomly assembled group of people but is interacting with none. It is not an appropriate term when considering counseling issues.

"An individual *in* his or her environment," meaning other people in that environment, is a better formulation, but it still does not convey the condition of being "locked" into a social system.

Transaction conveys the idea that the interactions among two or more persons in a specific environment have a depth or degree of bonding that results in indistinct psychological boundaries between an individual and others in that environment, a partial melding of personalities. This idea will be expanded upon in Chapter 5. The individuals who are in transaction can be observed as separate entities, but the transaction itself, the dynamics of this subjective, partial union of personalities, can be known only through a lengthy observation.

An individual's biological inheritance, as it becomes modified through transactions in many environments, provides the framework for that person's unique cognitive processes and content, for the degree of sensitivity to situations that will affect moods and arouse emotions, and for how she or he acts. These biological determiners are primarily in the chromosomes and genes, in the brain, and in the endocrine systems, and they have different effects associated with different developmental periods (Papalia & Wendkos Olds, 1988).

## Consequences of Transactions

Transactions with other persons in given contexts can have positive or negative consequences for an individual, and often both. These consequences are customarily called pleasant or painful, but psychologically they mean more than just physical pleasure or pain. A mentally healthy person may engage in actions that further that person's sense of purpose but at the same time result in physical discomfort. A polar explorer or a researcher studying wildlife in conditions some others would call trying is psychologically enhanced by that activity even though there are consequences of physical discomfort. Astronauts spending many days, even months, in a cramped space vehicle experience physical discomfort, but the positive psychological consequences outweigh the negative physical ones.

A consequence that is more positive than negative (whether or not an individual is conscious of it) increases the probability that the pattern of thoughts, feelings, and actions that produced that consequence will be repeated, assuming the individual's control over events. If the outcome is more negative—more punishing—than positive (a psychologically punishing consequence is often more potent than a physical one), the probability is increased that the pattern that resulted in the consequence will not be repeated. A 14-year-old boy, eager to show off before his peers, takes the family car during his parents' absence, intending only to drive around the block. His driving competence is less than he assumed, with a neighbor's destroyed mailbox as evidence. The exhilaration from the driving is promptly outweighed by the sharp negative consequences he experiences from his parents. These, in fact, may not include any physical punishment; shame and guilt can be far more potent deterers. The probability is greatly increased that the youth will not repeat that or a similar act.

## Biological Elements

### Genes

If the Declaration of Independence were being written today, it might read, "All people are born equal before the law" and might even make some reference to social equality. To be even more accurate, however, the document would have to add, "But all people are not born biologically equal, and therefore are not born psychologically equal." It is axiomatic that genetic inheritance, determined at the moment of conception, will result in temperaments (a component of personality) and traits, including individuals' proclivities for feeling emotion and how emotion is expressed. These general dispositions are shaped over time through interactions that result in the awesome variability found among individuals.

Genetically determined characteristics acquire their specific and idiosyncratic manner of expression as a result of people's experiences, but these experience-shaped responses lie within the boundaries of expression that are gene-determined for each person. The fact that some degree of change can be made within these genetically determined limits authenticates counseling.

Facts concerning the genetic basis of the unique behavior patterns shown by individuals are the result of a long history of scientific inquiry. Gregor Mendel initiated research in the field of genetics in 1857. His findings, published in 1860, were overlooked for 40 years,

> . . . which is unfortunate, since Mendel's laws neatly fit a major gap in Darwin's theory. Darwin knew that variation occurred, but he did not know how it was inherited. Mendel's laws described [that] mechanism [Hellmans & Bunch, 1988, p. 396].

Fleming reported the discovery of chromosomes in 1882, but their control over hereditary traits through the genes located on them became clear only in the first half of the 20th century. Knowledge concerning the significance of genetics has been enormously enhanced by the technological advances of the past few decades, such as the identification of the DNA double helix. Genetic engineering and gene transplanting, unthinkable a few decades ago, are now taken for granted as subjects of research.

Specific pairs of chromosomes have been linked with specific body dysfunctions, such as cystic fibrosis (pair 7), and Alzheimer's disease (pair 21). The absence of a single gene can result in a disorder, such as phenylketonuria (an inherited metabolic disease), whereas undesirable behavior patterns, such as aggression and excessive alcohol consumption, are determined by a pattern of genes (Groves & Rebec, 1988). Genetic research, recently begun and of stunning potential, will result in the mapping of each gene's spot on the chromosome where it is located. The project's purpose is "to identify the genes related to human disease" (Hall, 1990, p. 45). Although the purpose is limited, it leads us to expect that in time the genetic basis of behavioral characteristics will also be identified. This further demystification of life may cause distress to some people, but later generations will accept that knowledge as commonplace. In any case, it is behavior, intertwined with cognitions and affect, that is the concern of counselors, not the physical dysfunctions from which it originates.

Gatz (1990) proposes that "personality is genetically influenced," with traits found to have "inheritabilities in the range of 30% to 50%" (p. 601). It is experiences *unique to each person* that interact with that individual's unique genetic inheritance to produce personality traits, accounting thereby for the remaining variability. Shared experiences, Gatz finds, such as those of siblings are not the source of personality traits.

Rowe (1990) supports this idea, which counters conventional belief. He notes that a "common dose of family environment" has little effect on most personality traits, contrary to common belief. Studies of monozygotic (identical) twins permit not only that conclusion but a surprising general one: *family environment, including specific child-rearing techniques, has little effect on personality.* "The major environmental influences on personality may well be accidental factors and extrafamilial influences" (p. 609).

Not only are shared family experiences of minimal significance, conclude Baker and Clark (1990), but "parenting styles and traditional family variables may be relatively unimportant in understanding problem behavior" (p. 598).

The fact that genes affect observable body characteristics is axiomatic, not just in such broad indexes as racial characteristics but also in specific ways, such as a child's facial features resembling those of a parent in impressive detail. Far more than surface similarities are genetically determined. Even people who are not familiar with the specific results of genetic research have learned from popular publications, from television, and from personal experience that some health traits are common to a genetic line and that genes influence internal body structure and function. One of the organs that is genetically influenced is the brain. Because the brain is a major determiner of behavior, affect, and mental processes, we can expect the accumulating research data to increasingly reveal the degree of that influence.

The proliferation of studies carried out over long periods of monozygotic twins' lives provides the primary source of data about genetic influences. Only identical twins have identical genes, which accounts for their greatly similar appearance, thinking, feeling, and behavior. (See Segal's 1990 summary of twin research with its significance for counseling.) This similarity persists even in identical twins who are separated and who thus experience cultural and child-rearing differences during formative and later years.

Dissimilarity between two siblings who are not identical twins does not mean that they therefore have inherited completely dissimilar genes; that is impossible when each child has the same parents. Genes may give a general direction to behavior patterns, but the specific nature of those patterns is the product of the *unique experiences of each person.* Genes determine that males will be aggressive and competitive but do not determine how those characteristics will be expressed. Other genes, and the person's unique experiences, provide the specifics. Competition may be expressed in a consuming interest in chess, in wrestling, in medical research (which is competitive), or in working in a car dealership.

## *The Brain*

Our interest is not with the brain in general so much as with specific sections that serve specific functions, such as the halves into which it is divided.

***The hemispheres.***    Although the structure of the two halves is similar, their functions differ noticeably between genders and less so among persons of the same gender. In general, the right half processes stimuli so that people "see" wholes, or entireties, whereas the left hemisphere "looks for" details. The right hemisphere sees a room; the left, the furniture in that room. The right hemisphere transduces (translating the coding of one system into the coding of another) the metaphorical and analogical information characteristic of emotions.

The two halves have independent capabilities for consciousness, memory storage, communication, and control of motor activities. In these matters, however, the two hemispheres operate cooperatively through the *corpus callosum,* which joins the two halves, while emotional responses between the two sides are unified through the *anterior commisure.*

Certain portions of each hemisphere dominate when one action or cognitive response is required, such as verbal activity, which originates in the left hemisphere. In women, this occurs mostly in the front of that hemisphere; in men, in both the front and back. For vocabulary, on the other hand, both halves of the female brain are employed, and both the front and back portions of each, whereas word defining in men is predominantly processed in the left hemisphere, both front and back.

To repeat, these are dominations, not exclusives; the whole brain functions in these activities. Even though both hemispheres function in the formation of ideas, the fact that the left half dominates in ideation is partly a function of its larger size at birth (Guyton, 1986, p. 654). As the larger hemisphere, it is more likely to receive stimulation as the infant interacts with its surroundings, and consequently it grows even more dominant.

***Brain systems and behavior.*** Portions of the brain function together as systems, such as the limbic system. Parts of this system, particularly the *hypothalamus,* provide sensations of pleasure or rage when the *periventricular* portion is excited. Hormones secreted by the brain also play an important role. Psychological counselors who serve large populations, such as those in secondary schools and colleges, may expect 1 in 20 persons to show symptoms of clinical depression. Those counselors will not be called on to intervene in any but the milder forms because the more severe instances require the help of clinicians trained in abnormalities. Nonetheless, it behooves counselors in those settings to be able to identify the symptoms of depression, particularly because more severely afflicted clients may be suicidal. Those severely affected report or demonstrate long periods of otherwise unexplained despair, misery, insomnia, loss of sex drive, and withdrawal. The giving away of possessions may point to a depressive person inclined to suicide.

The individual afflicted with a true mood disorder (formerly called affective disorder) will probably demonstrate inappropriate and excessive emotional responses. The psychological counselor who works with adolescents will be called upon to distinguish between the occasional high and low peaks of emotional responses and mood swings that are common to everyone, but particularly to adolescents, on the one hand, and the pervasive and extreme mood swings that mark a true manic/depressive disorder, on the other.

Students may be reported to the counselor for their unusual excitability, a sense that they can "lick the world," or an exaggerated euphoria not attributable to illicit drugs. People so identified may be in a manic state, a mood that may either cycle with depression or occur without cycling. These mood swings baffle, even terrify, the afflicted person as much as they puzzle and concern others.

It is currently hypothesized that such mood disorders result from faulty secretion of chemical transmitters in the brain's hormonal system—that is, of abnormal amounts of norepinephrine in the brain's *reticular formation,* of serotonin in the *midline raphe nuclei,* or both. Too much, the conjecture is, yields mania; too little, depression. The normal secretion of these two hormones results in the potentiality for happiness, contentment, normal appetite, appropriate sex drive, psychomotor balance, emotional stability, and other normalities.

## Nerve and Endocrine Systems

It is common to think of the brain as the receiver of sensory stimuli, as indeed it is, but it also originates stimuli as an organ of cognitive processes. Additionally it operates as a biochemical drug factory, as we saw in the discussion of mood disorders. All humans are born with the same organs, or are identical in biological structure. It is the difference in biochemical functioning, modified by experiences, that produces differences in cognitions, affective states, and behaviors.

There is evidence, Thompson (1988) reports, to show that the differences in biochemical secretions "may represent genetic variability, . . . a variety of transient biological factors (diet, drug use, health, menstrual cycle, sleep-wake cycle etc.), . . . environmental history, [or] individual differences in cognitive coping strategies" (p. 331). Some secretions or their effect can be modified by cognitive procedures (see Beck, Rush, Shaw, & Emery, 1979, regarding treatment of depression). But most of the undesired behaviors resulting from endocrine imbalances have to be modified by chemicals. Although these drugs must be prescribed by a physician, lobbying to permit clinical psychologists to prescribe or administer them has been under way for a few years.

Nerve systems operate integrally with the brain and endocrine system. Not only is the brain a drug factory, but "hormones [are] circulating extensions of the nervous system" (Reiser & Reiser, 1985, p. 1167). The quality of endocrine operation as it transacts with the nervous system (a condition of no direct concern to counselors) affects brain function and therefore affects the reasoning processes and overt behaviors, which are conditions with which counselors do deal. Endorphins, which have strong analgesic properties, and opiates occur naturally in the brain. Endorphins regulate the pain/pleasure continuum, as well as alertness/ anxiety. It is clear that doing, thinking, and feeling are a product of genetics, biochemistry, and environment. Although we are aware that social experiences affect the nature of social interactions, the great effect of hormonal quality and quantity, particularly on sexual and aggressive dispositions, is sometimes overlooked.

The function of the complete endocrine system is beyond the scope of this text. This brief look is intended to reinforce your awareness that thoughts, feelings, and actions are not casual, chance occurrences, as capricious as the wind, nor are we in full control of them. However, the fact that there can be some control over thoughts, feelings, and actions is important because if people had no ability to develop such control, there would be no reason for counseling.

## Intrauterine Influences

Counselors in their consultative role may be called upon to educate a clientele about prenatal influences on the fetus. Some negative influences have been known for years: the high probability that alcohol, nicotine, and the mother's improper nourishment will result in birth defects, for example. Now there are "crack babies" to be concerned about, those whose development has been severely damaged by the mother's use of crack cocaine during pregnancy. Scans show the crack-killed spots on the brain of these babies, which explains the children's rages and aggressiveness, which some expect will translate into violent, felonious behaviors when they reach adulthood. Other postnatal difficulties suspected to be of prenatal origin, such as hyperactivity, may result from deficiencies in prenatal cortex growth.

It is reasonable to expect counselors to better understand the behaviors of adults if they know about fetal development, such as the preliminary finding that prenatal hormones may be a variable in sexual orientation. If further evidence accumulates, same-sex erotic attraction will be better understood. The present psychiatric conclusion is that:

> there appears to be no definitive action of hormonal or other biological factors on sexual identity or object choice. Rather, there appears to be a complex interaction between biological, environmental, and mental factors that affect the expression of sexually dimorphic behaviors [Meyer, 1985, p. 1058].

Meyer's observation is of interest because he includes the biological variable among the interactions that may determine sexual orientation; consultation with parents, teachers, and others ought to reflect the evidence that sexual orientation may not be solely the result of the environment or of rational choice. The widely held view that an individual's sexuality is solely a matter of choice may not be justified in light of the evidence that brain and prenatal hormonal factors, along with environment, may also determine sexual orientation.

### Mind, Intelligence, Consciousness, and the Unconscious

To complete this brief examination of biological variables, we consider in more depth the terms *mind, intelligence, consciousness,* and the *unconscious,* which were introduced in Chapter 3. They are often misunderstood or are otherwise sources of disagreement. No text on anatomy or physiology reports any physical structure connected with those names or even assumes their existence, for the obvious reason that they have no material existence. But are they, as reductionists would contend, merely convenient ways to talk about the functioning of a material thing, the brain? Because the question's answer is mixed, we use the analogy of speech for some understanding.

No physiology text reports the existence of an organ named speech, either, only the existence of lungs, larynx, and mouth (called organs of speech). Yet speech is psychologically real. It is a sharply defined, measurable, conditioned function of the body, one of the most significant of all psychological realities, one taken for granted by speaking and hearing persons. The most important events in life involve human interactions, and the primary attributes needed for effective interaction are speech and hearing. Speech is not a "thing," but it is a reality of great importance and power. Unlike the hypothetical constructs of mind, intelligence, and the unconscious, however, speech can be directly sensed and measured. It is not hypothetical.

***Mind.*** As psychology evolved from philosophy, its theorists had to contend, as they still do, with concepts that had developed over centuries, one of which is the construct labeled mind. The word *mind* has been used for millennia, usually employed in a way that implies a separate existence from the body, like a parallel concept, soul. For much of the past the mind was thought to occupy space in the heart, along with the emotions. That placement of the mind and emotions in the heart persists figuratively today, exemplified by expressions such as "Learn that by heart" and "I feel in my heart that . . ." The option taken here is not to use *mind** as a noun after this point, because that would lend support to the idea of the mind as a thing, and more usable concepts are available, such as mental processes, thought patterns, cognitive processes, patterns of ideation, and so on. That said, this minor contradiction will be found: use of the word *mental,* which will sometimes be employed as a synonym for *cognitive,* as in mental processes.

Eysenck and Eysenck (1985) identify personality as comprising temperaments and cognition. They see intellect as cognition, but for reasons they justify, they choose to treat intelligence separately from cognition. No matter whether it is assumed that the cognitive domain functions only as an entirety or in subsets of that entirety, cognitive processes are the products of the firing of neurons in the brain.

While it is correct to say that cognitions are not physical objects, they also are not "merely" brain functions, just as speech is not merely lung/larynx/mouth functioning. The inherent nature of cognitions and what their nature is after elaboration by experience make them proactive in a person's dealing with reality. Their dynamism demonstrates that the brain is not a "curator of information gleaned from sense data," a dead-storage warehouse, but is "an active sculptor of experience" (Mahoney, 1988, p. 369).

***Intellect, or intelligence.***    It is odd that the word *intelligence* has been used for years by psychologists and the general public and that decisions have been made about people based on its measurement, yet there is no definition of it that satisfies all who employ the term. Its durability is understood. *Some* concept had to be created to account for those people who demonstrate superiority in the speed with which they acquire verbal and numerical data, the superior quantity of such data, and the superior quality and speed of their reasoning using those data. Such people speak at a younger age, have more extensive vocabularies than their peers, read and understand sooner and more quickly, read materials advanced for their age, remember more facts, and understand complexities in associations more readily. These traits may all reflect the underlying dynamic of speed of brain function, shown in quick reaction time: they get an earlier start and go further than most. Then, too, what accounts for those who show traits opposite to those above? The creation of a construct called intelligence was the answer, a purely hypothetical idea that permitted measurement. This was achieved by creating ways to measure the assumed components of intelligence and spreading the obtained scores on a scale. The scores of gifted people are found near one end of the scale, and the scores of the least able are located around the other end. Most people's scores are distributed along the middle of the scale. In 80 years the concept has spawned an imposing array of measuring instruments, commonly called intelligence tests but also termed scholastic aptitude tests, measures of mental abilities, or other labels preferable to "intelligence."

*In his seminal work on science, Asimov (1981) includes a 49-page chapter titled "The Mind," but the word is used nowhere else in the chapter, let alone defined. Because the chapter's topics are related, apparently readers are to assume that the word *mind* in the chapter's title demonstrates that commonality.

Intelligence is a hypothetical construct, usually filling a gap in theory and thereby giving coherence to the theory. For those who find the concept useful, its employment is justified as providing a short way to express a complex set of ideas, as long as the users remain aware of its potential inaccuracies. Measurement of intelligence particularizes those potential inaccuracies. A major one is the assumption that a numeral given as a person's intelligence quotient (IQ) represents an accurate count of units of some agreed-upon entity called intelligence. "Our child's IQ is 107, but my sister's child's is only 101," typifies this misunderstanding, as if one child has six more of something than the other. Scoring error, in fact, means that the actual scores could be reversed.

A counselor will often need to know about a client's ability in a number of cognitive activities, particularly when applied to education. Data about *specific* abilities acquired by *specific* measures will be most useful, illustrated by the verbal and quantitative scores on one intelligence test, the Scholastic Aptitude Test (SAT). On the other hand, the applicability of an all-inclusive score posing as valid over a wide range has not been demonstrated. In analogy, let us assume that a fictional athletic quotient (AQ) is available. Let it also be assumed that it was obtained by measuring a person's abilities in weight lifting, endurance running, speed swimming, ball throwing, and so on. If a coach responsible for selecting athletes for a specific sport, such as swimming, was provided with an AQ for an applicant, the coach would not be helped by such global data. An above-average AQ, obtained by combining the results of a variety of athletic achievements, could be expected to obscure a low ability in one area of competence.

The general public has no reason to know that a number of the subtests of an intelligence test are also achievement tests. A common subtest is of vocabulary, the one subtest, incidentally, that correlates highest with the total score of those tests. It is apparent that vocabulary is learned; thus, an inventory of the knowledge of word meaning might not measure what a person *could* learn unless other facts were known. If a person of hypothetically high potential ability on this subtest lived in an environment of minimal word use, with limited printed words accessible, a measure of vocabulary would be seriously faulty as an indicator of the person's intellectual capacity. Thus Byrne's Law: a high score is a valid score (if you did not know more or could not do well in what the test measures, you could not attain a high score), but a low score is only a low score. If valid knowledge about one characteristic of a person is sought and all that is known of that characteristic is one low score, that score does not constitute valid information about that person. Data from other sources must be acquired, and these may agree with or contradict that single score.

Early scientific theorists (Galton, 1883; Spearman, 1904) posited the existence of a 'g' (general) factor and special competencies. Others have firmly held the view that we cannot speak of intelligence but only of intelligences, a view that goes back at least to the seven primary mental abilities of Thurstone (1938), with Guilford (1959) offering evidence that there are 120 varieties of intellect. Study continues, and new descriptions appear, such as that of Sternberg (1985), who proposes three facets of intelligence termed analytical, creative, and practical.

Anecdotal evidence from clinical practice tells us that there are discrete cognitive abilities. That fact makes it understandable that an individual can demonstrate a superior literary talent while being relatively innumerate. Another individual is able to see relationships with speed, breadth, and accuracy in a relatively precise physical realm (for example, chemistry) but is baffled by the dynamics of interpersonal relationships. It is a misperception to hold that a person who stands out in one mental process necessarily stands out in all of them, although that is sometimes the case. Functional differences between brain hemispheres theoretically predict the possibility of disparities among abilities.

Measurement of any mental process approximates the functioning of the brain but also taps into the psychological quality of a person's environment, his or her sensory acuity (such as the effect of impairment in sight or hearing), and the person's general health. Until psychologists are able to agree upon and defend cognitive subsets, such as intelligence(s), counselors will be diligent in avoiding the damage done by unjustified interpretations of the nature of intelligence, and they should understand the limits of measurement of this hazily defined psychological construct.

**Consciousness.**   It is axiomatic that humans differ from other life forms in the matter of consciousness. Although there may be no experimental evidence to demonstrate that consciousness is limited to humans, the quality of human consciousness can be assumed to be immeasurably higher than that of any other order of life. At times a counselor deals with client phenomena of which the client is unaware, but to a much larger degree the counselor engages the client's past and present life as it was, and is, consciously experienced. An understanding of the brain operations that create consciousness will result from the continuing study of the phenomenon. At this point study is primarily in the descriptive stages of altered states of consciousness, such as sleep and hypnosis, and deliberately altered states such as drug-induced ones.

**The unconscious.**   The meaning of the unconscious is clouded by associating the word *unconscious* with *the,* which furthers the idea that it is an object occupying a distinct place in the brain. Freud, who popularized the term, did not use it as if implying an attic where painful experiences of childhood could be stored and forgotten. For him the term simply meant any thought that was *unknowingly* inhibited from reaching awareness (was repressed) because it was abhorrent, threatening, or in conflict with other cognitions and thus would cause painful anxiety if allowed to enter into awareness. A related mechanism in psychoanalytic tenets, called suppression, is the deliberate avoidance of anxiety-producing thoughts and desires, a *conscious* effort to forget an unpleasant experience. Many people can understand the concept of suppression because it is so commonly reported.

There is no important need to use these two concepts, with their subtle, negative connotations; they seem as readily explained simply by the term *forgetting.* To simplify the explanation is not to deny that early events in a person's life may have some current significance. In some cases, memories must be deliberately aroused in order to "clean up" a currently distressing condition. The difference between the scientific knowledge available in Freud's time and present knowledge of the brain and its functions and the extensive findings from memory research permit this more parsimonious accounting of forgotten early experiences.

Freud's contributions to understanding behavior include the identification of acceptable psychological defenses in addition to repression and suppression. At some time, most people will be affected by anxiety-producing events, while for others every day will be marked by psychologically threatening conditions, causing them to employ one or more of these mechanisms to defend themselves.

When Shakespeare has Queen Gertrude say, in her evaluation of the actor playing the part of the queen in Hamlet's play, "The lady protests too much, methinks," he is acknowledging through her words that there are such behaviors as defense mechanisms. Shakespeare put into the language through her a phrase still used to convey suspicion of anyone who speaks against a certain behavior too loudly or at too much length without being conscious of doing so. It could be, the phrase cautions us, that the speaker may unconsciously be struggling to keep recollection of his or her past distasteful actions from rising to awareness. On the other hand, a conscious protest, intended to "throw others off the scent," would not be an example of repression or suppression, but of deceit. With complexities like these, it is no wonder that the lives of some people appear as a bewildering tangle beyond the help of clinical psychologists, let alone psychological counselors.

These brief examinations of explanatory concepts may provide nothing immediately practicable for counselors' day-to-day functioning, but they contribute to making counselors-to-be sensitive to unresolved conceptual issues and, it is hoped, increasingly insistent that concepts used in counseling adhere to scientific reasoning and recent evidence.

## The Psychological Variable

### *The Baggage at Birth*

Development can be negatively affected by the birth process, a condition that no counselor is going to modify. For our considerations from here on, descriptions are based on the assumption of a no-problems birth of a biologically normal child.

Parents comtemplating their newborn, particularly if it is a first child, project ideals onto the infant's future that reflect parental wishes and even unmet ambitions of their own. The newborn will surely be an Olympic athlete, the most popular child in school, a community leader, a Phi Beta Kappa scholar, a prominent lawyer, and so on. As the parents gaze with wonder and love upon their infant, it probably will not occur to them that a significant portion of its future is already in place. For example, genes may result in clumsiness instead of athletic prowess and may put limits on cognitive functions, which in turn means that scholastic endeavors will not produce a Phi Beta Kappa key but remedial classes. It is fortunate that the infant cannot foretell that in ten years or so those same parents may complain about the child's laziness, lack of interest, lack of concern for the standing of the parents, and so on, as the reasons why the child has a low level of achievement in school. Additionally, the parents may accuse the child of character deficiencies (the child's fault, of course), including ingratitude for "all we've done for you!" They may consult with a counselor with the intention of enlisting aid in overcoming their child's unacceptable ways. They may present considerable resistance to accepting the fact that the child can do no better in academic matters and that pressures to do so are having a harmful effect. Sensitive, empathic counseling can bring them to that acceptance. However, the counselor may not be able to arouse in the parents a loving acceptance of the child as he or she is, an acceptance that would replace the stance of cool resignation marking their view of the child.

This child, like everyone else, is born with a roughly outlined personality, with proclivites and abilities that will become apparent in a variety of situations and with tendencies and aptitudes that will be modified by environments within those genetic limits. (Counseling may later be one of those environments.)

## Personality: Temperaments and Cognitions

Were 1000 adults selected at random and observed for weeks in a variety of situations, trained observers would note that even though 1000 finely detailed, different patterns of thinking, feeling, and doing were observed and reported, numerous individuals would resemble large numbers of other individuals in certain ways. Greek and Roman scientists noted that fact, identifying four types of what today we call personalities: melancholic, choleric, sanguine, and phlegmatic, each attributed to the predominance of one of four bodily secretions, called humors.

Counselors are able to understand clients using ideas subsumed under the title personality, another hypothetical construct. There is disagreement over the construct intelligence and its measurement, as we saw, but far greater disagreement about personality's definition and measurement. Propositions about personality offered by two authorities, Eysenck and Eysenck (1985), have been selected as reference points, because the Eysencks have researched the topic for years and have made an extensive analysis of others' proposals. This does not suggest that their interpretation of data ought not to be examined with the skeptical and critical eye of science.

The Eysencks find personality to comprise two elements, *temperament* and *cognition,* the former composed of a cluster of *traits,* and the latter of *abilities.* Heredity is an important determiner of both temperament and cognition.

**Temperaments and their traits.**   The Eysencks identify three temperaments, each a continuum, or range. One of these is among the oldest classifications of personality types, extroversion/introversion. The Eysencks chose *extroversion,* one of the poles of the variable, as the label to represent its entire range. Another of the temperaments they identify is also a historic classification, neuroticism, a temperament that locates at one end of a continuum persons who show instability and anxiety and at the other pole those who show an absence of chronic anxiety along with the presence of stability. As the label for this temperament they chose *neuroticism.* The third temperament centers on impulse control, normal at one end and deficient at the other, a variable they term *psychoticism.* These three temperaments are part of everyone's physical constitution and permanently affect behavior.

The Eysencks observe that "these three superfactors do not exhaust the field of personality description in terms of temperament," although up to now no other superfactors (sums of traits) "have emerged that cover such a wide area, are equally replicable, and have some kind of causal explanation in terms of the laws and concepts of academic psychology" (1985, p. 185).

Each temperament subsumes a number of correlated factors called *primary traits,* packages of thought, affect, and behavior that are customarily demonstrated no matter the situation. Even fetuses' behaviors can be attributed to differences in traits, shown by the differences among them in response to environmental changes. In addition to traits, a person can show transient behavior patterns called *states.* Thus, a person's behavior at any moment may show both the traits that make up one of the three temperaments and also those temporary clusters of thought, feeling, and behaving called states. One state may indeed, for the brief time during which states occur, be contrary to a trait that person would normally exhibit. In one situation, for example, a person who normally shows those traits that sum to the E (extroversion) temperament may think, feel, and act in an introverted manner. In counseling this poses the challenge to discover whether a behavior pattern shown or described by a client is customary (a trait), or transient (a state). In the matter of anxiety, for example, there has long been recognition of the need to ascertain whether reported or manifest anxiety is a trait or a state; that determination has considerable counseling significance.

Evidence leads the Eysencks to reach a conclusion germane to this section: "It is found that for practically all traits and dimensions of personality there is a considerable degree of genetic determination of individual differences" (1985, p. 95). One piece of evidence among many is the difference in blood group between extroverts and neurotics. Along similar lines, Kagan (1989) observes that research allowed a prediction that inhibited children would have "lower thresholds of reactivity in the limbic system especially the amygdala and hypothalamus," resulting in greater activity in heart rates, larger pupil diameters, greater motor tension, and higher levels of morning cortisol. "The data support this prediction" (pp. 671–672).

***Cognition and abilities.***    This other component of personality is more stable and more accessible to dependable measurement. It will be examined at frequent places in this book, eliminating the need for elaboration at this time.

# The Environmental Variable

## *The Effect of Environment on Genetic Inheritance*

The infant will increase in physical and psychological complexity to an awesome degree as it increasingly interacts with its environments. The first of these environments is the one called family, with the most significant member being the mother. In the womb the fetus was in a symbiotic (same *bios,* or life) relationship with the mother, and now the infant, bonded with the mother, is in a relationship of psychological mutuality for which the word *symbiosis* is used as metaphor because a parallel word in psychology, *sympsychic,* has not emerged. That relationship is one of transaction in which person and environment are united, in the symbiotic concept, immediately and coextensively affecting each other. Another term, ecosystem, has similar connotations, including the interdependence of elements. If that term is modified to include the interplay of a person in his or her environment, we arrive at the term *psychosocial ecosystems* for the varied contexts within which a person experiences life. The simpler phrasing is just *social systems*.

Psychological symbiotic relationships become diffuse and attenuated as the child ages. The increasing activation of children's cognitive systems produces changes in bondings and other symbiotic relationships as the child's private world enlarges.

It is axiomatic that the quality of family experiences is a variable in development, but perhaps only to the degree that they provide an environment that nurtures and refines the distinctive gene-driven tendencies. In this regard, we do well to recall the observations of Gatz (1990), Rowe (1990), and Baker and Clark (1990) given earlier concerning the limits of family influence on personality development, and why siblings who apparently experience identical environments in a family can have contrasting patterns of cognitions, feelings, and actions.

### *Specific Learning Modalities*

The word *learning* is used to mean any modification of genetic inheritance that occurs as a consequence of experiences in psychosocial ecosystems, modifications that are cognitive, affective, and behavioral, often in inextricable combination. Cognitions refer to conscious thoughts and other mental processes, and how they are acquired through modeling and associative types of learning has been briefly described earlier. (There will be a more extensive treatment below.) Behavior changes, also a form of learning, result primarily from the consequences of behaviors. The variety and degree of emotions are genetically determined, but what arouses them and the ways in which they are expressed are learned partly by associations with cognitions and behaviors. Several learning modalities relating to behaviors and emotions are briefly described in this chapter, but because they are the basis for change procedures employed in counseling, they will be examined in detail in later chapters. A brief description at this point is required to complete a chain of related developmental topics that began with the biological determiners of mental processes, affect, and action set out at the beginning of the chapter. This chain ends in the next chapter, where there is coverage of the numerous characteristics, factors, and variables that constitute the unique person whom the counselor is seeking to assist.

**Modeling.**   Modeling, although akin to imitation, is mostly goal-oriented and is often an intentional effort to act like the modeled person in broad ways. Imitation is the actual or pretended copying of a specific behavior, such as smoking or the pretended gunfights typical of children. Modeling in early childhood can also be an unconscious process. A child who experiences no fear in the presence of a stimulus pattern may acquire a fearful response to that pattern if a parent responds fearfully to it in the child's presence. The child unconsciously models the emotion and the parent's fearful behaviors. Modeling in later childhood can also occur at a relatively unaware level. Speech patterns and accents may be modified as a result of unconscious motivation to conform with those common to peers. Many behaviors, emotions, and ideas in these formative years are acquired by modeling but are limited by the drives and boundaries biologically set at conception.

***Classical (Pavlovian) conditioning.***   Two forms of associative, or con-ditioned, learning are commonly recognized. The earliest (thus classical) form was described by Pavlov (1927) and is now also identified by the term Skinner (1953) gave it, *respondent conditioning.*

Both animals and humans have bodily functions that serve purposes in maintaining the species. Salivation is an important aspect of eating and digesting that occurs when food is put in the mouth. Pavlov found that experimental dogs fed regularly under similar conditions started to salivate at sounds and sights that were produced just before the dogs were given their food, stimuli that would not normally produce salivation. He expanded his research to pursue this phenom-enon by sounding a tuning fork (which would not naturally cause salivation) along with the dog's sight of food, which already caused salivation. In time, just the sounding of the tuning fork caused salivation. Just your reading about salivation may cause it to occur.

The technical term for a behavior that occurs before associative learning happens is unconditioned response (UCR). This term describes a behavior that occurs naturally in certain contexts (for example, salivation while eating), while the stimulus that cues off this behavior is a "natural" one, one that naturally results in a UCR. It is an unconditioned stimulus (UCS). For example, food in the mouth is a UCS that causes salivation, a UCR, but the sound of a tuning fork is not naturally a stimulus for salivation. Its property as stimulus is learned through association and is then labeled a *conditioned stimulus* (CS). The learned response it elicits is called a *conditioned response* (CR).

Salivation is a relatively simple behavior. However, more complex patterns of response, such as those associated with emotions, can also be conditioned in this manner. Eight-year-old Manuel loves cats; his playmate Sonya was badly scratched by one and is terrified of them. Respondent conditioning probably accounts for Sonya's fear. Less obviously, racial or ethnic characteristics, neutral stimuli (UCS) by nature, can acquire the CR characteristics of hate or fear through modeling or other events. In like manner many events, contexts, or situations acquire a lifelong affective coloration that, when sufficiently negative and powerful, may cause a person to seek counseling.

***Instrumental, or operant, conditioning.***   As we saw earlier, the conse-quences of interactions can be either pronouncedly positive or negative, producing either "carrot" or "stick" results (but often both at the same time). There is a surface similarity between the idea of rewards and punishment (the carrot or the stick) and the *operant conditioning* type of associative learning in which the strength of positive or negative response to a behavior affects the probability of that behavior's recurring. The carrot/stick idea is a crude concept, whereas operant conditioning reflects highly detailed and experimentally supported precepts. They not only explain how some behaviors are learned but also provide the procedures for altering them. The research findings related to operant conditioning were gener-ated    experimentally—that    is,    by    controlled    empiricism    conducted    by positivistic scientists. The issue is not whether operant conditioning is valid but whether the procedures used to acquire this knowledge are the only ones that can be defended as science. As with the other modalities of learning, the complexities of operant conditioning receive detailed inspection in later chapters.

Many stimuli naturally cause an organism to respond; stimulus precedes (causes) behavior in those instances. In operant conditioning, the stimulus *follows* the behavior. To illustrate, let it be imagined that a naive person, such as a young child, randomly acts in some way, which immediately results in a favorable response. It is lawful to state that the probability is increased that the act will be repeated. In the technical terms of operant conditioning, the behavior is reinforced.

Vocabulary is acquired through that process. In imitation, a young child says a new word for the first time, resulting in a pleased response from the parents (technically, a social reinforcer), which in turn pleases the child. In addition to social reinforcers, if the outcome of using the word, let's say an approximation of "cookie," leads to the receipt of one, there is an additional reinforcement, likely the stronger one. The stimulus to act is present in the consequences of the act. On the other hand, if the child's action results in an aversive (negative, punishing) stimulus, the probability increases that the act will not be repeated.

The same laws apply no matter the age, except with older people there is an established, complex behavior repertoire that may make acquiring new behaviors or eliminating persistent ones more difficult. Some old behaviors, however, can be extinguished or modified with assistance from a counselor.

## *Learning and Development*

It is important that counselors know the processes by which the rough ore of a person's genetic inheritance and endocrine output is refined and polished by learning. Learning is roughly sequential, or moves in steps as partly determined by the stages programmed into each person. Infants and children are normally active and so are going to learn. Piaget (1952), as we saw, provided evidence that the increase in intelligent behaviors shown by children is an outcome of changes in physical maturity, a developmental epistemology.

***Environments.***    The first environment experienced by a child is the family. Although ideally (in light of evidence) the family includes two parents, single-parent families are increasing. What makes the family so potent in the child's development are the outcomes and lessons learned from interactions within it, such as the bonds created and nurtured and the values set. The family environment typically possesses an intimacy not matched by other environments. In a psychologically healthful family this valuable intimacy is at the same time necessarily asexual. There are different family structures in different cultures, a matter of importance for counselors of children and youths in the United States because school counselors need to know the effects of cultural differences on development.

Data from a variety of academic and practical sources inform us of the general characteristics of ethnic cultures by region of the country and of class differences in and among them. These are useful sociological data of stereotypes but may entrap the unwary counselor into taking for granted that a particular client's family fits the stereotype. Counselors will know the stereotypes and the variability within them, but of most importance, they will know how each family is a unique social system in the same manner as each individual in it is unique.

The variety of environments increases rapidly as a child ages to include neighborhood playmates, extended family, schools, community clubs and teams, and, from pubescence on, informal nonschool peer groups. Each environment results in new or expanded learning about self and cultures. As families differ in a number of variables, so do the wider environments. Sociological data may explain one kind of environment, identifying its stereotypical characteristics. Here too the wary counselor seeks out the specifics of any one environment. The distinguishing characteristics of one religious denomination may be readily identified, for example, but a congregation of that denomination on "one side of the tracks" can differ importantly from a congregation on the other side. One ethnic neighborhood may be expected to differ from another in some important ways even if in other ways they share similar characteristics.

After that period of widening experience, the number of environments narrows for typical people during mate selection and marriage. This major new environment may precede or follow career entry, the latter a typical pattern for members of the middle class and above. Marriage, plus the parenting that follows, establishes yet another new environment for each person, perhaps the last one to provide learning peaks, although these can happen over many years of the marriage. After children mature, parents will restructure their development, with advanced age bringing new challenges that require new learning on the part of a person whose brain and other organs may not be up to those demands. This is particularly true when a radically changed environment has come about—for example, one now bereft of a spouse.

Humankind could not have evolved if each person had to learn a unique response to each situation in his or her daily environments. Conversely, humankind could evolve because common traits permit (require?) generalization from specific learning. As an infant and then a child and adolescent, an individual acquires specific responses to similar situations through associative learning, within the limits set by a trait. These responses become a base learning that can be modified through cognitive interventions and reconditioning, thus permitting adaptation to new experiences through new generalizations, but always within the trait's "territorial" limits.

Study of infant and child development shows the nature of bonding and the imperatives needed to establish bonds, particularly with the mother. Successful bonding in the family facilitates later attachments outside it and leads eventually to affiliations with large groups. These attachments give rise to sentiments of loyalty to "my kind of person," which is, however, a double-edged sword. It usually provides a deeply rooted adult identity and sense of security in patriotism, but at the same time it may lead to intolerance of other ethnic groups. It is commonly held among sociologists that cultural identities acquire such strength that members of a culture prize that identity above all others and are willing to risk death to preserve it, particularly when nationhood and religion are seen as one. The history of any era provides the evidence. In current times there has again been killing in Eastern Europe between citizens of neighboring but culturally different nations, and we are again made aware of the persistence of the Kurdish culture, a nation with no state. A state may be destroyed, but the members of a nation will fight to the death to preserve their culture, as the history of Native Americans demonstrates.

The attributes of adolescence vary among cultures. It has been said that adolescence was invented in the United States, so distinctive have been its attributes here in contrast with other cultures. Nowadays adolescents in some other Western cultures appear to wish more and more to approximate the unique features of U.S. adolescents' public lives. It is a period during which the person critically examines the cultural baggage brought up from childhood, throws some away, retrieves it, and rejects it again, trying to mesh the new with the old (Papalia & Wendkos Olds, 1988).

The common view is that the predominant marker of adolescence is the attainment of independence from the family, meaning from parental requirements and standards. This view holds that such striving inevitably leads to conflict because the parents resist, perhaps leading the adolescent to run away from home or take other drastic action. Developmental experts challenge the view that such harsh conflict is the norm. They point out that while it is true that dramatic rifts between adolescents and parents are noisily notable, family calmness with occasional minor disturbance is the rule. Adolescence is a time when a new self is emerging, a time when the person becomes far more self-conscious and thus aware of restrictions and requirements heretofore accepted with minimal challenge. It is a time for negotiation between parents and child, and that implies compromise. Wise parents, in anticipation of these changes and their accompanying need for new rules, take the initiative in proposing that parents and children plan jointly to make those changes come about smoothly. Such action by parents has the additional benefit of providing examples of maturity to be usefully modeled by the child.

Adolescents do not seek complete independence from their parents. They wish to remain dependent but to transfer some of their dependencies to selected other adolescents or adults while retaining, at least for a while, others rooted in the family, such as financial dependency. If anything, psychological dependency increases in adolescence, culminating in the major surrendering of some of the self that ideally occurs for the majority who marry. Ainsworth (1989) has studied attachments beyond infancy. In her view, "autonomy does not imply cessation of attachments to parent figures" (p. 710). These attachments (affectional bonds) are marked by relatively long-enduring ties, so that even when older and separated, children will have at least an intermittent desire to reestablish some proximity with their family.

Schooling, the physical independence provided by cars, two working parents, and a common subculture with its own music and clothes combine to make a large proportion of naive adolescents experience puberty primarily in the company of their peers. Those experiences provide immature feedback on major issues, such as relationships with parents and appropriate sexual mores. Winnicott (1986) observes that during a critical time of life when the complexities of sexuality must be worked out, adolescents have as models and as sources of associative learning peers who are also struggling. Adolescence is a difficult time, Winnicott remarks, when youths need to work out:

their own immaturity, their own puberty changes, their own ideas about what life is about and their own ideas and aspirations; add to this their . . . disillusionment about the world of grownups—which for them seems to be essentially a world of compromise, of false values, and of infinite distraction from the main theme. [Upon leaving adolescence] boys and girls are beginning to feel real, to have a sense of self and being. This is health. From being comes doing, but there can be no *do* before *be* [p. 25].

Biologically, the end of adolescence is the end of the "teen" years. Cultures in the past—and a few today—did not acknowledge any developmental period between childhood and adulthood; their young were children one day and adults the next, following a ritual that so stated. In the complex cultures of the United States, adolescence is recognized not only as a period of physical change but also, of greater importance, as an extended period of psychological maturation. Levinson (1978) concludes that "[a] young man needs about fifteen years to emerge from adolescence, find his place in adult society and commit himself to a more stable life" (p. 71). He acknowledges that development is not progressively linear but is a backing and filling, the starting, abandonment, and starting anew of adapting traits to the realities of life. There is no smooth motion from adolescent patterns of thinking, feeling, and behaving into adult ones just because time has passed. Some young adults, for example, may move for four years into the labile and impermanent environment of college. This requires learning to cope with an environment that is of limited duration, is dissimilar from the adult world, and postpones major adult commitments. This is not all undesirable, of course. That postponement permits further psychological maturing (rooted in physical maturing) to come about before a commitment is required in the areas of marriage and career. The journey out of adolescence for the men he studied, Levinson says, was not completed until about their mid-30s.

These brief samples of development, which emphasize that critical time of "second birth" called adolescence, are intended to demonstrate that knowledge of development, a topic central to a counselor's function, does not depend solely on a counselor's own developmental history, which, in fact, may contain abnormal experiences and so may be a harmful reference. A counselor needs to know the generous scientific literature that describes and explains life-span development, from which come the life-view criteria the counselor applies.

# Concluding Reflections

The goal of Part I was to describe the functions of psychological counselors and how they acquire their professional knowledge. The focus in Part II is an introduction of the variables that make each client resemble all people in some ways, be like some groups of people in other ways, and be himself or herself uniquely in yet other ways. We began with an exploratory look at biological and environmental variables that affect the lives of all humans. Succeeding chapters of this part will focus on individuals, examining how their unique cognitions, affect, and behaviors are formed.

It is desirable to have warm, fuzzy feelings about clients, but even if such feelings are appropriate, goodwill is an insufficient deck from which to deal counseling cards. In traditional counseling, caring feelings, plus a portion of the adviser's own experience, are all that can be offered. A person placed before the public as a professional counselor by an institution or agency, however, owes society the best that the present degree of scientific information can offer. This knowledge starts with life-span development and the application to individuals of research about it.

Adherence to certain counseling sects or cults that do not attend to life-span development would be turning one's back on this commitment to acquire the best scientific knowledge. Schools, originating in one person's limited perspective of how and why people think, feel, and do as they do, consequently have a limited view of how to help clients manage their lives better. It is appropriate for counseling to be school-less as well as humanistic in its goals, and also to be scientific in the knowledge of how to achieve those goals. These aims call for prospective counselors to be well studied in development and the variables that impinge on it.

■                    **Points to Remember**                    ■

1. People comprise separate organs. These organs interact so that the person functions as a system—all parts reacting simultaneously through feedback to each other part. The psychological aspects of the system—cognitions, feelings, and behaviors—are one with the physical aspects. Whatever "mind" and "intelligence" may mean, they are not something separate from the physical structure.

2. Environments are also systems of varying degrees of structure. The family is a more structured system than casual groups. How people function as systems is affected by the particular environment at any time. The environment's effect on the person-as-system is through the psychological functions of the individual; that is, the environment affects a person's mental processes, emotions, and behavior, which in turn affect the individual's functioning as a system.

3. Environments cannot affect an individual in a completely random way. How an individual will respond to environmental circumstances is directed by the person's genes. Conversely, the genes determine global thought and behavior patterns that are presented in an environment. These global patterns are given their specific expression by what is learned through interactions in those environments.

4. Living in a family does not affect children uniformly; that is, common family experiences do not produce common results. Each individual's unique genetic inheritance interacting with his or her unique experiences produces that individual's personality.

5. The body is a biochemical drug factory, with some secretions distinctive to each person. One variable in an individual's behavior is the secretions by that individual's endocrine system.

6. It has been helpful to create explanations for clusters of ways of behaving. These imaginary explanations are called hypothetical constructs, three prominent

examples being mind, intelligence, and the unconscious. They are useful as explanatory summaries as long as their lack of separate existence is kept before us.

7. Personality is another useful hypothetical construct. The Eysencks posit two major elements of personality, each with its subsets. They are temperaments, with their traits, and cognition, with its abilities. There are three temperaments, each being a range of behaviors: extroversion, neuroticism, and psychoticism.

8. Learning, the modification of an individual's genetic environment through experience, is described as modeling, and associative learning, the latter comprising classical (respondent) conditioning and operant (instrumental) conditioning.

# ■                **Counselor Formation Activities**                ■

1. Identify the systems into which you are locked. If family is one, is it your family of birth or a family comprising your companion or spouse, and maybe children? If you are a member of the latter kind of family, is your natal family no longer a system? If it still is, what is your role in it?

2.a. Think about your natal family. Which of your ways of thinking, emoting, or behaving are different from those of your siblings but similar to those of either of your parents? Is it tenable to consider those ways of thinking, emoting, or behaving as genetically determined? Have you any evidence that such traits run in either your mother's or father's family?

   b. If you have siblings, which of their traits are similar to yours? If they have any traits pronouncedly dissimilar from yours, are those traits also found in one of your parents?

3.a. Where do you classify yourself on a hypothetical seven-point scale of introversion/extroversion (1 = highly introverted; 7 = highly extroverted)? On what basis do you make that classification?

   b. Name up to ten persistent ways you behave that merit being called traits. After you have constructed the list, rank them by a 1, 2, or 3. Assign 1s to those traits that are often present or are most distinguishing; 3s to the least significant, less-often-shown traits; and 2s to the others.

   c. Ask others who know you well to rate you separately on the introversion/extroversion scale and to name some traits they think are distinctive of you. Compare their observations with yours, and discuss differences between them.

4. Pick any one of your traits you designated as 1s. Try to assign some arbitrary proportion of the origin of that trait to genes, modeling, respondent conditioning, or operant conditioning.

5. Trace your history of bonds and affiliations from childhood to the present. Think of persons with whom you are bonded currently. For how long has that state existed, and what of your needs is satisfied by each bond? With whom were you strongly bonded five years ago but are not now bonded? How can you account for the breaking of that bond?

# ■ **Complementary Reading** ■

Students who have recently completed certain majors, such as human development or psychology, will need no further study of the brain/mind topic. If your introductory psychology course was sometime in the past, refreshment and knowledge of current developments is called for. Typical recent introductory texts are useful to this end, such as the one cited elsewhere in this text, Papilia and Wendkos Olds (1988).

It will be useful to study the chapter about physiology and behavior in:

GARFIELD, S. L., & BERGIN, A. E. (Eds.). (1986). *Handbook of Psychotherapy and Behavior Change,* 3rd ed. New York: Wiley.

not just for a cogent article on the topic, but so you can become familiar with other chapters in this useful reference.

To know more about influences on development than is provided here or in introductory psychology texts, I suggest that you examine those topics in which you are interested:

BURGER, K. (1944). *Developing Person through the Life Span,* 3rd ed. New York: Worth.

New research on family influence on children's personality deserves more scrutiny than that given in this chapter. Start with Rowe (1990) to understand further the evidence supporting the view that family child-rearing practices do not have the effect attributed to them.

| 5 |

# Psychosocial Systems and Characteristics of Clients

## Overview

In some ways each client is unlike any other. At the same time each client is like some others, and in yet other ways each client is similar to *all* others. The premise of this chapter is that to understand any one client, one must understand the characteristics common to all humans. Counselors need to be attentive to those common elements, or they may approach each client as if no psychological templates were available for establishing a correct image of that individual.

This chapter and the previous one provide brief descriptions of the psychosocial development of all people. Chapter 4 focused on some major biological and experiential conditions that result in the ways humans are psychologically structured and learn and through which they can be understood, and thus helped. Five psychological structures are the topics of this chapter, with findings of selected scholars summarized for each topic.

The first topic is the systems perspective as an imperative for understanding human functioning. The second, flowing from the first, is a corollary of the systems concept, the functioning of people in an organized manner, partly uniquely and partly in conformance with cultures, with emphasis on the hypothetical construct of self as a way to account for that function. People's selves are made up of both unaware elements and those of which they are cognizant. The conscious element is usually referred to as self-concept, a subset of personality.

I reemphasize in this chapter that life experiences are under the control of cognitions to a significant degree. Other components of cognitions are the chapter's third topic, with an emphasis on maxims, the rules of life to which each person adheres.

People in social systems engage in emotionally tinged cognitions and actions based on their perceptions of themselves and on other components of social systems. These social perceptions are phenomenologically real, whether or not they correspond to objective reality; they are the basis for an individual's thoughts and behavior and are the chapter's fourth topic. The fourth topic also includes the role of an analogous construct, the perceptual "filter system," in influencing what is perceived.

Under the last topic, bonds and affiliations, we consider the imperatives for all people of these emotional attachments, which are the outcomes of social interactions and transactions.

# Introduction

Each client has a unique pattern of cognitive, affective, and behavioral variables. Underlying these variables are determinants of the brain, neural system, and endocrine system that result from the client's genetic inheritance. Although one client's concern may be given the same general label as another's, such as marriage difficulties or career problems, each client will have variables that operate to distinguish him or her from every other person who has a similarly labeled reason to seek counseling. Even though counselors serve individuals, and so will seek out the unique psychological characteristics of each, they also need to know the ways in which some individuals are similar to others. In career matters, for example, some individuals share certain variables that differentiate them as a group from individuals in other groups. Some of these differentiating classifications are gender, cognitive competencies, temperament, cultural characteristics, and developmental age.

Most individuals are identical in their basic psychological structures, which makes understanding these commonly shared characteristics imperative for each counselor. The first of these structures is the individual as system.

# People as Systems

In considering people as systems, we turn again to a car's engine for a partial analogy. When an engine is running, its components work together as an organized unit. In a running engine it is not possible for all major parts except one to be functioning correctly. It is an all-or-none matter.

Three components of human systems have no comparable parts in mechanical systems: (1) mental processes, (2) behaviors that consistently occur in transactions in which humans are embedded, and (3) the element called affect, comprising mood and emotion. Affect is a variable that is physiological in origin but is consciously sensed, although usually without the person being aware of the underlying physiological processes.

I use again the analogy of a car's engine to establish an essential element of a system: communication, or feedback loop. Depression of the accelerator puts into operation a system that operates as an entirety: the flow of gasoline into the cylinders increases; spark plugs fire more rapidly; valves move more quickly; more electricity is generated; air, oil, and coolant flows increase; and, in many new cars, a computer receives data concerning the function of the total system in order to maintain an operational balance no matter what changes occur in subsystems. The system totality is maintained by subsystem communication through feedback.

In human functioning a continuous and instantaneous information exchange among the system's physical and psychological elements is a major characteristic. To adequately understand a person-in-situation, an observer, such as a counselor, needs to be aware that the subsets of the person-as-system are interlocked, functioning as a unit, and communicating through transduction among several body systems.* Counselors will not try to appraise the functioning of the physical elements of the system and cannot directly study the psychological elements of this unitary functioning. Knowledge about the functions of psychological subsystems is acquired primarily through clients' reports, a situation potentially fraught with error. For one, the typical client cannot be expected to be aware that these subsystems are working together. For another, distortion is engendered by client emotions and by inhibitors that prevent (at least at first) clients from recalling painful experiences. An adage holds that in a dispute there will be person A's story, person B's story, and the truth. As one application of this maxim, the advice to psychological counselors is to meet with both spouses at the same time when counseling about marriage difficulties. Not both or none, however; even if one spouse will not attend, the other may learn strategies to maintain or even improve the marriage.

## *Systems and Health*

A person's health is often indicative of how well the physical and psychological components are working as a system. A "competence model of health as an alternative to the illness model" is proposed by Seeman (1989, p. 1099), a system-based model that calls attention to organismic integration of the physical, mental, and social subsets of the system. He goes on to explain that the term *organismic* suggests:

> a pervasive process that encompasses all of the person's behavioral subsystems: the biochemical, physiological, perceptual, cognitive, and interpersonal dimensions. . . . The term integration refers to the character of the transactions that take place among those behavioral subsystems. In the integrated person there is a clear communication among these subsystems such that they generate mutually congruent sets of information throughout the system. . . . As a consequence . . . the person maximizes the probability of effective coping and response [p. 1101].

Based on his practice as a surgeon as well as on medical research, Siegel (1986) describes what he has learned about the interworking of physical, mental, and social subsets. He explains that "every tissue and organ in the body is controlled by a complex interaction among chemicals circulating in the bloodstream, the hormones secreted by our endocrine glands" (p. 67). He cites psychosocial dwarfism, a:

---

*Body systems cannot communicate directly, because they differ in components and structure. They communicate by translating the code of one system into the code of another, a process called transduction.

disturbingly common syndrome in which an unhealthy emotional atmosphere
at home stunts a child's physical growth. When a child is caught in a crossfire of
hostility and feels rejected by his or her parents . . . the brain's emotional center,
or limbic system, acts upon the nearby hypothalamus to shut off the pituitary
gland's production of growth hormone [p. 67].

In contrast to Siegel's calm, scholarly prose, Wolf (1966) slams us with a
journalist's graphic phrasing as he recounts an afternoon observing human behavior in Manhattan with the anthropologist Edward T. Hall. He reports Hall's
observations about the life led by commuters who work in cubicles:

> with low ceilings and, often, no access to a window, while construction crews all
> over Manhattan drive everybody up the Masonite wall with air-pressure gener-
> ators with noises up to the boil-a-brain decibel levels, then rushing to get home,
> piling into subways and trains, fighting for time and space. . . . The whole
> now-normal thing keeps shooting jolts of adrenaline into the body, breaking
> down the body's defenses and winding up with the whole work-a-daddy human
> animal stroked out at the breakfast table with his head apoplexed like a
> cauliflower out of his $6.95 semispread Pima-cotton shirt and nosed over in a
> plate of No-Kloresto egg substitute, signing off with the black thrombosis,
> cancer, kidney, liver, or stomach failure, and the adrenals ooze to a halt, the size
> of eggplants in July.

This tangent into organismic functioning that focuses on health not only
illustrates the significance of systems but also reminds us that health matters may
correlate with a person's psychological concern and that there is some psychological control over health (Cousins, 1979, 1983; Rossi, 1986). A brief psychological
disturbance will probably produce only mild negative health correlates. A continued disruption in the system's corrective feedback loops, however—a consistent
malfunction somewhere in the system that results in sensed psychological disruption—will probably result in malfunctions throughout the system because it
operates as a unit. The client may report physical distress that he or she does not
associate with the developmental imbalances for which counseling is sought. The
counselor needs to be sensitive to this possibility.

## Schools of Counseling and Systems

One counseling school, family therapy,* is emphatically systems-oriented. A
family is "an open system, created by interlocking triangles, maintained or changed
by feedback" (Foley, 1984, p. 447). In similar vein, Wilson (1984), in describing
behavior therapy, writes that, following Bandura, "behavior is based on three
separate but interacting regulatory systems. They are *(a)* external stimulus events,
*(b)* external reinforcement, and *(c)* most importantly, cognitive mediational processes" (p. 240). Multimodal therapy (Lazarus, 1984) also subscribes to Bandura's
three-part system, but, Lazarus observes, his school also draws from Bertalanffy's
*general systems theory* and *group and communications theory*. Multimodal therapy

---

*Comments about tenets of counseling schools in this chapter are offered by the school's
founders or recognized adherents of the school in *Current Psychotherapies* (Corsini, 1984), unless
otherwise noted.

is included here as a school, partly because it is given that kind of treatment in the Corsini text (1984). Lazarus's propositions, in fact, approach the nonschool stance taken by this text.

## The Uniquely Organized Individual

The systems concept offers a general explanation of how humans function in daily life. Counselors typically assist one person at a time, however, so they need to conceptualize how these general principles apply to single individuals.

Each human lives in an organized way, but each person's organization as a system is unique. Normal people make sense of themselves to themselves; they do not appear to themselves or others as fractionated into disparate beings, sometimes a Jekyll, sometimes a Hyde. Others can also see a consistent core of personality in that individual, although in a peripheral way each person appears to present somewhat differing personalities in differing situations. Normal people are aware of their moods and know that they are subject to mild swings. We all experience temporary emotional distress and other episodes that put us "off-center."

A consistent core persists even as a person moves from one social context to another. For example, an architect in a firm may be seen as one "kind" of person on the job, may be seen a bit differently when observed as a homemaker, may show yet other characteristics when on a night out with "the girls," may display still other behavior patterns when observed in temple or church, and so on. At the core, she is an organized, and thus consistent, person over long periods. Only major physiological changes or psychological trauma will alter that core.

It is not just observable behavior that changes with settings but also physiological and emotional responses. For example, a change in one of these subjective states could be expected to result from the fictional architect's recreational night out, which reduces stress and increases the flow of endorphins, followed by the therapeutic benefits of laughter. Throughout those changes, however, there is a core of self that provides the permanent, and thus predictable, organization of the person-as-system.

Engines function as systems but have no being, no aims or intentions other than that given to them by their builders and users. Their organization is simply mechanical. Without the brain, humans would also be just machines, entities without life aims, because those require awareness. Humans function as physical and psychological systems, but enabled by the brain, each has a unique and dynamic organization as part of that system, a structure that affects one's quality of being. Some of that purposefulness is built into the human-as-system through genetic inheritance; otherwise it is learned, evaluated, and sometimes modified through counseling.

### *Self as Organizer of System*

How to explain, how to name this organizing principle? Some say the construct of personality explains, while others think that this construct is too broad to be sufficient. A more adequate explanation is found in the hypothetical construct *self,* a subset of personality. Self is dynamic; portions of it change, usually gradually, thus slowly yielding modified purposes and changes in life's meanings. Adolescence, however, illustrates the possibility of more abrupt and seismic changes in self, such as the major changes in cognitions that result from emotion-arousing experiences.

The construct self permits the counselor (and eventually the client) to make some sense of the information that results from a counselor's formal and informal assessments of the client. Without some organizing principle at work, the relationship of data from one assessment device to the data from another may be difficult or impossible to identify. The concept of self is a major agent for doing so.

Because the root of an individual's personality is found in both inherited and learned elements, self as a subset of the individual must also have genetic and learned origins. The learned part of self, in contrast to the genetically determined element, does not produce a haphazard self for each person, which would result in as aimless an existence as occurs in an animal ecosystem. To the contrary, this part of self is a product of social learning, which is culturally determined, a point emphasized by Cushman (1990). He speaks of self as "the concept of the individual as articulated by the indigenous psychology of a particular cultural group" (p. 599). In this commonly held position, an individual's self is seen not as a fully unique creation but one that is at least partially shared, that "embodies what the culture believes is humankind's place in the cosmos: its limits, talents, expectations, and prohibitions" (p. 599). Selves do not exist outside the culture: "there is no universal transhistorical self, only local selves; no universal theory about the self, only local theories" (p. 599), with "local" including the individual.

Culture, Cushman observes, "infuses individuals, fundamentally shaping and forming them and how they conceive of themselves and the world, how they see others, how they engage in structures of mutual obligation, and how they make choices in the everyday world" (p. 601). His examination of cultural changes in the Western world over the past century leads him to conclude that there has been a historical shift "from the Victorian, sexually restricted self to the post-WWII empty self" (p. 599). The self is empty "because of the loss of family, community, and tradition. It is a self that seeks the experience of being continually filled up by consuming goods, calories, experiences, politicians, romantic partners, and empathic therapists in an attempt to combat the growing alienation and fragmentation of its era" (p. 600). While Cushman's conclusions may be a valid explanation for some selves in the United States, recognition of the large portions of the U.S. population that are indigenous, Hispanic, or African in original culture suggests caution in such a generalization. The "Victorian, sexually restricted self" prior to World War II does not appear to be a trait of some in U.S. subcultures.

The influence of cultures on self is also reported by Kegan (1982). He observes that "Western cultures tend to value independence, self-assertion, aggrandizement, personal achievement [and] increasing independence from the family of origin" (p. 208), whereas Eastern cultures generally instill opposite values. These Western values produce a sense of incompleteness, resulting in the "enormous hunger for community, mystical merging, or intergenerational connection that continually reappears in American culture through communalism, quasi-Eastern religions, cult phenomena, drug experience, the search for one's 'roots,' the idealization of the child, or the romantic appeal of extended families" (p. 208).

Recently, several noted psychologists have praised the highly individualistic, self-controlled self that has emerged in the United States. Other psychologists, notably Samson (1985, 1988), defend their preference for a self more embedded in societies. Samson offers three criteria commonly used to assess the adequacy of self: freedom, responsibility, and achievement. These are goals that those favoring "self-controlled individualism" see attained by such individualism. Samson argues for the opposite position, that those three objectives are more likely to be obtained by selves under some "field control," for whom the boundary of self and nonself is not as sharp as it is for highly individualized persons (1988, p. 16).

***The unaware self.***   Although self is an explanatory concept, not a substance, if for a moment we think of it as occupying space, it is easier to conceptualize it as having a portion of which the client is unaware (likely the lower portion of the visualized self) and a portion of which the client is aware (the upper portion). These imagined portions cannot be quantified, of course, and need not be, because their usefulness lies only in their postulating a match between the way people experience themselves and life.

The unaware self is partly a cultural product, but in our society several cultures may influence any one person, unlike cultural influences in a tribal society. An individual can experience several different social systems during a week and may experience different cultures over time. A single culture informs all selves in tribal societies. At the other extreme, as in our multicultural society, a person's self may be informed by several cultures, each one of which may dominate for a time. The self of an adolescent child of recent Chinese immigrants, for example, will have been structured for years by a relatively compact society. The youth may now attend a school with students from Hispanic-American, African-American, and other ethnic cultures, with his or her self slowly modifying as a function of the need to adapt. If, in addition, there is some traumatic change in the family or racial unrest in the community, the adolescent's self, which is not yet stable, may become less defined as being Chinese because it needs a fluidity to maintain an operational level of ongoing development and purposefulness. A counselor will be pressed to identify a core self that organizes this youth's purposes and behaviors. The counselor may "see" (through the client's report) only the periphery of the hypothetical self, where there may be several somewhat discrete selves. Conflict between any two of those partial selves can be one source of the psychological imbalance that motivates people to seek counseling, particularly when a core self is indistinct.

This unaware portion of self is partly determined by genes, but it is given its operational substance by emotionally tinged, culturally compact experiences. It is an organizing dynamic. If clients are uneducated about their past and about other societies (perhaps not caring about other cultures), they may behave as if assuming that the way their kind of people are is the way one has a right to expect all people to be.

One school, Jungian psychotherapy, holds that there is a collective self from which an individual's self needs to emerge. Jung's use of these words differs from the connotations given above, an expected difference given the psychoanalytic basis of his thinking. This difference in word use is noted in the phrasing employed by Kaufmann (1984) in explaining Jungian therapy. He observes that the self "is an expression of man's inherent psychic predisposition to experience wholeness, centeredness, and meaning in life. The Self is our god within ourselves . . . the internal embodiment of ancient and timeless wisdom" (p. 120). The analytic foundation is reflected in Kaufmann's assertion that at "birth, ego and Self appear as one," with ego dominating for a period, after which "the striving for realization of the Self begins" (p. 120). This seems to be an unnecessarily complex treatment of the topic.

***Aware self, or self-concept.***   We take for granted the existence of an aware self; it occupies most of our conscious moments—our awareness of self-in-situation. The situation may be imagined, as when the person daydreams, conjuring up self-enhancing scripts that make Walter Mittys of all of us, regardless of gender. By adolescence a self-concept comprises intense perceptions that may change slowly, although some never change. These perceptions may be composed of general or specific self-descriptions, but the counselor is more likely to have to deal with the specific views that clients have of themselves in specific situations.

A general perception of self means an encompassing view of oneself, such as "I am stupid," "I am a good Muslim," "I can make people do whatever I want them to," or "I know I'm not a good parent." A specific self-view can report a concept of self as it relates to more specific situations: "I am good in mathematics," "I'm lousy in tennis," or "I dislike . . ."

Bruce excels in aquatic activities. He says, "I'm a very good swimmer." Question: does he swim well because he can make that statement, or is the statement just an objective observation without effect on his swimming ability? This fragment of Bruce's aware self is the ash, the residue of his experience. It can affect his behavior, however, by providing confidence, just as his swimming achievements might be harmed through loss of confidence were he to acquire (improbably) the opposite self-view: "I'm not a good swimmer." Client-centered therapy (now person-centered therapy), in Rogers's (1942, 1951) earlier formulations, hypothesized that a client's self-concept was the active determiner of behavior. The position offered here is that a counselor needs to assess those self-reference statements central to a client's concerns in order to determine which are but a report of fact, like Bruce's confident statement above, and which indeed do significantly affect how the client acts.

An example of a self-statement serving as a determiner of a client's behavior is found in the instance of Edward. He was consistently labeled by his parents and other family members as stupid and therefore thought of himself as stupid. His lack of effort in large classes resulted in poor achievement, confirming for him his self-concept. In fact, objective assessment of his scholastic abilities showed that he had considerable academic potential. Bruce's statement reported fact but may have had only a small effect on his swimming. Edward's erroneous self-statement did not report fact. It did serve as a self-defeating dynamic, a major contributor to his self-debasing behaviors.

Humans act at times in important ways without being aware that an unaware self is causing them to behave in that manner. This does not mean that unaware portions of the self cannot be raised to be part of one's awareness. The converse is fact: humans can become aware of what they do and, in many cases, why. This awareness is one of counseling's purposes, but not the sole purpose as proposed by the Gestalt school of counseling. Awareness and unawareness of self are relative, located at varying points on a hypothetical continuum.

In compact cultures such as tribal societies, in which all members think and act with relative uniformity, people learn behavior in which they can engage without self-monitoring, without cognizance. If there is no awareness, there can be no wondering why the behavior occurred. This applies also to compact cultures within nations that may have several discrete cultures, as in a compactly English culture in India or in large Chinatowns, among many possible examples. Aware selves exist along with unaware portions of self in those cultures, of course, although there is no means available to assess their proportions, nor is there any reason to do so. Counselors will include the concept of self in their matrix of explanatory concepts and be aware that a client's self consists of more than is accessible for either the client or counselor to observe.

***Assessing personality and self.*** Regardless of the explanatory construct employed to account for the tendency of all people to function in a consistently organized manner, there is a need to describe the specifics of that functioning. This becomes possible as information emerges during interviews, sometimes deliberately stimulated by the questions or topics a counselor raises. Published assessment instruments help in this process.

The use of standardized instruments rests on a number of principles, one of which is that they are used only when it becomes apparent that they will benefit the client. In some counseling centers, however, all clients are tested with a battery of instruments prior to counseling. This is done on the premise that the need for the test results may be of use later. In contrast, when assessment needs are discussed with clients who then agree to the use of particular instruments, the likelihood increases that the client will provide accurate responses. Additionally, consultation with clients maintains the principle that clients are participants in all decisions about steps taken to attain their objectives. Counseling is enabling. It shows clients how to take and maintain control of their lives, and it keeps before them the idea that the counselor does not do something *to* them but works *with* them.

One of the difficult technical decisions a counselor faces for each variable to be assessed is the selection of one from among many published instruments. New counselors find that experienced colleagues recommend different instruments or that the choice is made for all counselors by an employing agency. Counselors may become committed to one instrument because it was the one used in their practicum, perhaps the preference of a supervisor committed to a particular school of counseling. Ideally each counselor, through study of measurement principles and scrutiny of the array of instruments available (Hood & Johnson, 1991), selects the best instrument for each client variable to be inventoried or measured.

The choice was made in this text to accept the Eysencks' conception of personality from among the many available. A counselor with that commitment will employ the *Eysenck Personality Questionnaire.* Those who subscribe to Erik Erikson's concept of personality will use the *Measures of Psychosocial Development,* while those oriented to a Jungian view of personality will have clients complete the *Myers-Briggs Type Indicator,* as examples.

When it appears that a client has unclear or conflicting self-views, or if any other condition indicates the value of a systematic inventory of self-concept, the *Adjective Check List* is an appropriate instrument. The counselor may use several theoretical positions to structure the information. Even without imposing any structure, a discussion of the responses can still be valuable. Two other options are the *Tennessee Self-Concept Scale,* which yields eight self-concept scales with clinical interpretations possible, and the *Self-Esteem Inventories.*

# Characteristics of Cognitions

There are several approaches to understanding a client's mental processes and content. Abilities in literacy and numeracy—that is, the knowing of facts and concepts—have long been readily measured cognitions. No matter the categories into which cognitions can be objectively placed, it is the subjective statements that people make about themselves that are significant, because those statements are a major variable in what people feel and therefore do or refrain from doing.

## *Goals*

One subset of these subjective statements is aspirations and goals; their identification is an essential part of career counseling. Goals, a part of self-concept, act like lodestones that draw individuals toward their future and help organize their energies and activities. It is understandable that if the achievement of goals and the realization of aspirations are thwarted, particularly by arbitrary events or institutionalized blocks, clients will experience negative feelings. Goals that are deliberately altered by clients, on the other hand, can be signs of positive change, from hopelessness to eagerness, from unrealism to realism, and from self-centeredness to other-centeredness.

## *Life-View Maxims*

Life views, as mentioned earlier, include assumptions and precepts about major facets of living that partly determine an individual's actions, often exercising their influence in an unaware way. In this section we look again at the effect on behavior of those controlling cognitions of a client's life view, called maxims here.

These unaware elements are internalized from one's culture, at first from parents or parent surrogates, and then are modified, strengthened, or added to in adolescence and later years. If one person subscribes to Red Sander's aphorism that "winning isn't everything, it's the *only* thing," and another is convinced that "it matters not whether you win or lose, it's how you play the game," their athletic behaviors will differ. A person committed unreservedly to certain theological precepts may turn the other cheek if attacked; another may have been acculturated to the tenet of "stand up and fight back, even to the death.".

A counselor will be aware of the potency of these cognitions, of how the absence of conflicting maxims in a client brings psychological composure and conflict-free behavior. The opposite holds: a client's conflicting maxims will probably result in psychological imbalance and conflicting behaviors. The latter may occur when a person holds to a tenet that is contrary to a belief subscribed to by his or her family or by others in social systems of which the person is a member.

The counselor will attend to these controlling cognitions but at the same time will be cautious about imposing his or her values on the client. If the counselor's and the client's values differ on important issues, that difference may be pivotal in the outcome of counseling. Professional ethics require revelation of conflicts so they can be dealt with.

Earlier recognition was given to the impetus that Albert Ellis has given to the incorporation of cognitions and cognitive processes as tenable components of a science of human behavior. In rational-emotive therapy he avers that clients' problems emanate from "should" and "must" cognitions, which he describes as irrational, insane, and absolutist positions.* "All anxiety comes from *musts,*" he says (1984, p. 218). Later, when the client chides the counselor for creating anxiety, the counselor responds that the client is the one creating the anxiety and that other clients have been readily helped because:

> I get *right away* to what's bothering them in five minutes, I've just explained to you the secret of all emotional disturbance. If you really followed what I said, you'd never be disturbed about practically anything for the rest of your life! . . . Everytime you're disturbed, you're changing *it would be better* to a *must.* That's all disturbance is! Very very simple [p. 218].

A position that contrasts with Ellis's is explored by Kohlberg (1976) in an analysis of development in morality. He identifies six stages in that growth, the final one being marked by a person's subscription to universal moral principles. This means that the person's behavior would be strongly controlled by "musts."

Some counselors maintain that adherence to "musts" is the root of all disturbance, but that is not the commonly accepted view. Anxiety is not that simple, and "musts" have not all been proved to be psychologically injurious. Absence of "musts" in a person's controlling maxims may, in fact, betoken an inadequate self.

It is assumed that counselors will acknowledge that maxims, nested in a life view, are one source of controls on behavior, but only one. The counselor will treat maxims in a flexible manner, not ritually. In some instances this may call, on the one hand, for helping a client acquire coping strategies to handle a rule-of-life adage (a controlling cognition or maxim, a "must" or "should" statement) and on the other, the requirements of a situation. This does not necessarily mean removal of the controlling cognition.

### *Affective Nature of Cognitions*

The word *cognitions* covers all aware mental content and can be evaluative, as we have seen. Those evaluations will have some affective tone, perhaps so weak that it is barely noticeable to the cognizing individual or to observers. Other cognitions are wrapped in so powerful an affective web that they are central to the psychological makeup of the individual; they are major determiners of behavior.

---

*Mahoney and Arnkoff (1978, p. 691) cite nine persons who earlier showed this effect of "shoulds." In the 1940s, for example, Rogers explained how "shoulds" determined client negative behaviors.

Religious and political convictions are of this order. Examination of one's own actions or a quick review of friends' behaviors will provide instances of this phenomenon. The power of affect-laden cognitions is recognized in the rule that at social events and even some family gatherings any topic may be discussed except politics and religion because of the emotional charge that customarily accompanies these cognitions.

During a counseling interview a client may state a cognition in an emotionally neutral way, a cognition that in the dynamics of the normal conditions of life could be expected to be strongly emotionally colored. The counselor has to wonder about this. The converse is also possible: a client expresses a cognition with notable positive affect. This may be a pretense, polished by years during which the client was compelled to appear as if such positive affect were true when in fact the client's feelings are at most neutral. A counselor will engage clients from time to time who in first interviews protest much love for a spouse, in-law, or child, because they cannot yet admit to themselves the dislike that they actually feel. The counselor needs to be continuously sensitive to the element of affect and thus to wonder at times if the stated but not demonstrated feeling is accurate.

Other aspects of the topic of affect that are important to counselors will be considered in Chapter 6, including distinctions between the two components of affect, mood and emotion.

How, finally, do we describe what organizes and makes sense of a person's thoughts and actions? It is of less importance to know whether the explanation lies in the constructs of self, personality, life view, or some other variable than to understand that normal people operate as systems in some organized, purposeful way.

Of the schools in the Corsini (1984) volume, several in addition to rational-emotive therapy acknowledge the importance of cognitions. Adlerian psychotherapy, Mosak (1984) asserts, makes a number of basic assumptions, one of which is that to understand an individual "requires the understanding of one's *cognitive organization*" (p. 57), which includes "the *ethical* convictions—the personal 'right-wrong' code" (p. 69). In Wilson's (1984) presentation of behavioral therapy the role of cognitions is recognized, as in the statement that "corrective learning experiences involve broad changes in cognitive, affective, and behavioral spheres of functioning" (p. 253).

In transactional analysis one cognition is emphasized: early in life and continuing thereafter an individual comes to believe that "he is either OK as a person or not OK" (Dusay and Dusay, 1984, p. 395). Lazarus's (1984) multimodal therapy is built on a more comprehensive view of the origins of actions than those of other schools. This therapy may indeed be viewed by some as above classification as a school. Lazarus's position comprises seven elements, which he labels BASIC I.D. The "C" of this acronym is the therapeutic modality of cognitions, which is expressed in action as "*cognitive restructuring* (e.g. changes in dichotomous reasoning, self-downing, overgeneralization, categorical imperatives, non sequiturs, and excessive desires for approval" (p. 515). I agree with these six needs for cognitive change, but the stance of this text in cognitive matters goes beyond them, holding to a need to encompass other emphases such as self-views and goals.

# Perceptions of Self in Social Contexts

You may recall from your introductory psychology course the definition of perception as the brain's reception and interpretation of data about the environment acquired primarily through the sense of sight. The viewer may be aware of what is seen (as interpreted by the brain) or may respond to stimuli at a subliminal level. In any case, the viewer responds to the *interpretation* of perceived material as reality and acts on it as such regardless of whether that interpretation coincides with objective reality.

In this section perception has a wider reference. Perception refers to interpretations that individuals make about themselves in social situations as they sense the nuances among people, things, and actions in that situation. These are likely to be aware perceptions in most cases, received through several senses, probably with sight dominating. The interpretations that people make in this situation are based on self-views and on other cognitions acquired through direct or vicarious experiences.

What a person perceives in the social situation is subjective. It is also real. The subjective perception may agree completely with the objective reality, or it may vary from it anywhere from slightly to completely. That the subjective and objective realities are not in agreement may eventually be of counseling significance, but when a counselor hears a client's report of a social perception, the counselor acknowledges it for the phenomenological reality that it is—the reality on which the client's actions and thoughts were based. This subjective reality may later be compared with the objective reality, if that can be discovered. One of the counselor's immediate objectives may be to determine the objective reality and bring about agreement between the subjective and objective. They can be thought of as two still pictures, each projected on a screen from separate projectors and overlapping a bit, but in the main not matching. Ideally, the counselor seeks to manipulate conditions so that the separate images move closer and closer, eventually appearing as one. The client at first may be too threatened to acknowledge the objective reality, but with patient and adroit procedures that demonstrate competence and sensitivity, the counselor can reduce the inhibitors that prevent acceptance of that reality. In consequence, a hypothetical client, relative to interpersonal concerns brought to counseling, may eventually say the equivalent of "I see now that all along I was the one at fault, not they. I thought they were rejecting me because of my (gender, ethnic membership, and the like) but it was because I was being so obnoxious. I couldn't see that until now."

## *Perceptions "Filtered"*

Although the reports of two persons seeing the same event may be completely similar, they may instead be somewhat dissimilar or disagree completely. This difference in perception may be metaphorically spoken of as a function of differing perceptual filter systems in individuals.* If the filter system of

---

*Mood changes, for example, may cause one person to have different perceptions of identical events at different times.

one person permits consistent gross misinterpretation of data from the environment, the individual may be afflicted with that psychological disorder known as
paranoia. Even normal people, including children, may experience brief paranoid
misinterpretations of data, particularly in stressful situations: the friendly smile that
is misinterpreted as "laughing at" or a sneer.

The full reality of a social situation may not be perceived, only what the
observer would like to be real. This is the phenomenological reality, selectively
edited by brain functions that admit and interpret only data that conform with one's
personality, and particularly with one's self-concept. This means not only admitting
only certain data but also giving them a skewed slant, while filtering out other data.
Variability of perception in nonsocial events can come from so simple a matter as a
shift in visual field, such as when a car's driver becomes a passenger and now sees
frequent dangers in the new driver's performance when, in fact, the new driver is
performing exactly as the original driver did. Although the perception in this
example is of minimal importance compared with the more complex interpretations necessary in a social situation, it illustrates how a physical shift can
change a perception. A psychological perception shift has similar results.

### Learning about People in Social Contexts

In an earlier discussion about systems, it was observed that the separate parts
of a car's engine can be known but that it is not easy to sense how they function as a
system. Similarly, the body's organs, far more complex than engine parts, can be
described as separate entities, but it is far more difficult to sense their operation as
a unit than it is those of an engine's.

People function as psychobiological systems in each social setting they experience, those settings also being systems and somewhat volatile because they are
open. In contrast to the degree of difficulty that mechanics and physicians have in
understanding systems, counselors have more difficulty in comprehending complex, open-system, psychological beings. The counselor will build that sense of the
total person out of pieces of data about such ambiguous, artificial, but logically
defensible entities as personality, unaware self, and self-concept, along with information about the client's controlling maxims, values, and cognitive capacities
and the emotional coloration that may tinge each of these hypothetical variables—
an awesome demand on counselor competency.

Do counselors have to construct the psychologically total individual for each
client they serve? Some answers will be found by briefly examining three hypothetical clients.

To introduce these clients we first recall that a psychological counselor helps
normal individuals seeking to work through developmental requirements, to prepare for their future, or to overcome relatively short-term disruptions in their
development that they cannot deal with using their own resources. This role is well
illustrated by meeting a youth's or young adult's career-decision needs. In some
instances the counselor can fully serve such clients when only skimming along on
their psychological surface. Moment-by-moment assessment determines whether
the client's purposes call for an in-depth inquiry into psychological variables to

permit the counselor's mental construction of the total person, or, on the other hand, for a relatively surface inquiry, one that nonetheless presents an adequate sense of the operating individual.

***Marie: client no. 1.***   The first of the three hypothetical clients is Marie, 19 years old. She tells the counselor that she has just about concluded that she will go all-out to be a veterinarian but wishes to check out that decision. She discussed the possibilities with a different counselor in the previous year and then followed up with intensive investigation of veterinary medicine and of two alternative choices. Although she has to act now and is confident that her choice is correct, she is seeking one more evaluation of her conclusion.

The counselor reviews the material that Marie has collected—data acquired from recent career-oriented standardized assessments and information about the three occupations to which she has narrowed her options. He listens as she recounts the reasoning process she has followed. The counselor is ever attentive to affective tone as explicitly expressed or as implied in voice tone or body signals, but in the end he notes nothing that suggests anything but straightforward motivation and sound logic leading to Marie's occupational decision. Other than information about herself that she offers as she discusses her concern, the counselor sees no need to inquire about her self-concept or other components of her psychological makeup in order to help her. His conclusion is reflected in his statement to Marie, in the slang of the day, "Go for it!"

***Shelia: client no. 2.***   Shelia, also 19, comes to a counselor for help in making an occupational choice. Her history differs somewhat from Marie's. In the first interview the counselor deems Shelia's life to be marked by pervasive developmental disruptions and immaturity, of which she is aware. The counselor in time leads her to see that a sound career decision cannot be made without some resolution of these other matters, and she wonders if Shelia would care to consider them. Shelia is eager to do so; she has been aware of a general dissatisfaction with life and a sense of coping deficiencies, but they were so vague, the counselor determines, that they had insufficient motivational strength to lead her to consult with a counselor about them. The need to make a career decision was specific and provided the motivational drive, and therefore she welcomes the opportunity to examine these other facets of her life.

There ensues an examination of portions of Shelia's developmental history, her views of self-in-situations, controlling maxims, emotional history, instances of unsuccessful and successful coping, with strategies employed for the latter, her career-related history, and other imperatives that let the counselor help her understand herself as a psychological system insofar as that relates to an occupational decision. All that, with the additional data from use of career-related instruments, leads Shelia to aim for an eventual specialty in data processing, but to do so along with military service.

***Ramon: client no. 3.***   Ramon, age 37, begins consulting with a counselor for notably different reasons. By his early 30s, his behavior had become increasingly erratic, with alcohol used compulsively and to excess, although for a long time he denied it. Eventually his wife left him. He managed to hold on to his small manufacturing company for a while but then lost that. After a period of severe depression during which his alcohol use was unabated, with savings gone and parents less able (and more reluctant) to help financially, he acceded to a friend's insistence and sought help from a drug-abuse clinic. In time a small benign growth on his brain was discovered and removed. This was followed by increasingly positive changes in personality, changes abetted by Ramon's overcoming his alcohol problem with the help of a clinical psychologist at the clinic.

Clinic personnel and Ramon saw that sufficient change had occurred to enable him to put his life back together, taking up normal modes of living after years of abnormality. Consequently, he was referred to a rehabilitation center. There he is receiving assistance from a psychological counselor (who might be a counseling psychologist if he or she has completed doctoral-level training and is licensed), a person who is experienced in recovery cases of this sort. The counselor helps Ramon repair a disrupted psychological system by enabling him to restore broken development lines and to restructure his disorganized general sense of self, which is also negatively colored. His self-concepts in general and perceptions of self in social situations are examined so that changes could be induced if they were persistently negative (which is not the case because of the changes in his life). On the positive side the counselor sees a person now in a constructive mood, eager to move on despite doubts about his ability to do so. Training and experience inform the counselor that as difficult as it may seem at the outset to help a person reconstitute normal development, given Ramon's motivation and potentials, progress to that end will accelerate.

In Shelia and Ramon's instances, the counselor was required to lead the clients in an examination of constituents of the personality. There was a requirement to sense out the way in which these constituents functioned as an entity, whereas in Maria's case the counselor sensed scant need to inquire into the client's functioning as a system.

In sum, people behave in situations partly on the basis of their perceptions, both genetically influenced and learned, and of their moods (see Chapter 6). Each of the three clients above tried to manage their lives for self-enhancement purposes. Personality structure and developmental history permitted only one client to move forward in life effectively, judged by mental-health criteria.

To seek self-enhancement does not mean that only immediate, hedonic goals are sought; people may choose to bring disagreeable circumstances on themselves if, in the long run, those circumstances will lead to major self-enhancing experiences. On the other hand, if disagreeable consequences appear likely to follow an action that has no foreseeable benefits in the long run, individuals will protect themselves by physical or psychological escape. In any situation a person's behavior is determined in general by personality and specifically by unaware self and self-concept, maxims, values, goals, cognitive capacities, perceptions, moods and emotions, and whether the consequence of the actions taken will be desirable or undesirable.

# Bonds and Affiliations: Development Imperatives

To help us address the topic of bonds and affiliations, essentials for mentally healthful growth, a few more comments about development will be useful. Development can be continuous, although not at a uniform rate. It slows as age advances, and sometimes there may even be temporary regression to an earlier developmental period. In typical adults of middle age and above, only a little change is possible compared with earlier years, and that at the periphery of self. I say "periphery" because the core of personality has been continuously firming up so that after a time it changes only a little if at all. One's personality, genetically roughed in and then modified by experience, comes to be a permanent psychological nucleus that provides the stability essential for mental health.

Childhood and adolescence are the periods when the struggle to build developmental strengths onto the genetic inheritance is lost, at one extreme of a hypothetical range, or maximally won at the other extreme. Most children and youths occupy places along the middle of the range and can benefit from the development-enhancing programs that counselors organize in schools. These "for all students" activities can be compared to clothes bought off the rack that are designed to fit all people of a designated size. Supplementing these activities, a counselor will meet with some students individually to adjust the activity to the individual, just as a tailor will make minor alterations to the fit-all clothes.

Even if some counselors serve only youths, they also need to know developmental matters that characterize adulthood, because the foundations for a satisfying adulthood are laid in childhood and youth. This need is demonstrated in bonds and affiliations, which while important for adults, are equally important for children and youths.

The words *bond* and *affiliation* are used synonymously by some. Others use *affiliation* as an overarching term under which there is the special category called a bond. Here the word *bond* is used to convey a more intense personal intimacy than the word *affiliation*. An affiliation usually means an individual's loose attachment to members of a group, with some of whose members the individual is probably also bonded.

In this section we again consider the social nature of the mentally healthful life by looking at the developmental function of people's past and present bonds that emotionally weld one individual to another. Children may have long-lasting bonds with parents but at the same time be affiliated with their second-grade peers and teacher in a less intense and only temporary way. In adolescence some long-lasting affiliations will be established but only a few bonds, with school and nonschool peers. Evidence of the power of high school affiliations can be seen in the reunions that large numbers of people attend throughout their lives. Adulthood brings newer affiliations with fellow employees and with members of secular and religious groups, while some bonds made in prior years are retained, bonds with spouse and children and perhaps a few others are added.

An individual's few bonds and larger number of affiliations are developmentally important because they provide psychological security by maintaining personal identity, or self-completeness. Bonds and affiliations have affective coloration by definition. Scenes of zealous groups in various parts of the world inform us of the intense emotion that marks bonds and affiliations, particularly when they call for the submergence of self to claims of nationhood coupled with religion—an example of self imbedded in society (Samson, 1988). In the United States there are ethnic groups just as tightly woven, with codes that require complete submergence of the individual to the group and make death the price of disloyalty.

There is reasonably certain evidence that the ideal bonding for a child is with both parents and that children who mature in a situation with the parents bonded to each other are generally less susceptible to developmental difficulties than those who have experienced the rupturing of the parental bond. Bonding also occurs with other family members, although antipathy between certain siblings may result from competition for parental love when the parents have not assured the maintenance of an emotional bond with each child. Anecdotal evidence informs us that imbalances in mental health can sometimes be attributed to day-to-day living in a family within which emotional bonds among individuals are feeble or nonexistent, with even antipathy marking interpersonal relationships.

Intense bonding in same-gender small groups is common at puberty and during early adolescence, with the most intense bonding occurring with a person identified as one's best friend. The small group in which an individual is embedded may in turn be embedded in a larger social system to which adolescents, in particular, develop a strong affiliation, most pronouncedly to their secondary schools and groups in them. Although the bonds in the small, same-gender group can persist for life, by midadolescence the majority of girls and boys are starting to pair off with members of the opposite sex, while a minority retains a same-gender orientation.

Some specialists have called attention to a need for men to maintain strong bonds with other men, to establish new ones, or to reestablish lost ones. Bly (1990) proposes that men in highly technical societies have deficient or distorted masculinity as a result of social changes that started almost a millennium ago, a state accelerated by the industrial revolution. One cause of this diminution, he asserts, is the loss of father as mentor. To counter these deficiencies Bly proposes that men engage in extended (weekend or longer) bond-establishing, self-exploring, rugged experiences with other men, a notably different experience from being with a group of men watching with frenzied intensity a professional football game on television, often to the puzzlement or annoyance of female partners.

Keen (1990), in a more controversial analysis of the male psyche, contends that men spend a large amount of time reacting to the presence of women in their life and too little in sorting out the mysteries of their own identity. This attention to concerns about the male psyche is comparatively recent, and the evidence is scant in contrast to the much-needed and now-extensive study of the female psyche, which has a history of several decades of intense scrutiny.

### *Sexual Component of Some Bonds*

Following the sexual ambivalences, insecurities, and ambiguities besetting many (if not most) adolescents, a permanent bond with one other-gender individual is a common outcome, with sexual activity a major or even the sole motive. If it is, sociological data foretell an approximate duration of five years for the bond.

In ideal maturity, a permanent bond requires relinquishing parts of one's self and taking on parts of the other's self, in consequence of which pleasure is found not in sex alone but in looking out for the partner's welfare and in sharing parenthood and some major delights, antipathies, values, goals, and other commonalities that favor a permanent union after the attractions of sex have declined to a lower intensity.

Among humans, sexuality is more than a procreational drive; it is enjoyed by both genders. Men, with hormonal urgencies that differ from women's, are more driven, a potential for casual mating. A characteristic of Western civilization has been the legal and ecclesiastical pressure to ensure that there will be but one lifetime mate. Even though this pressure has changed considerably in some Western societies, social pressure for permanent bonding is still maintained by a bonding contract formally and publicly entered into, often in a religious ceremony. There are other benefits that accrue to formal, public bonding: elimination of traditional, competitive mate-seeking by men, and psychological security and personal validation for both parties, even if financial support of the woman by the man may no longer be central.

Acknowledgment of these crass-sounding but factual attributes of marriage does not diminish the desirability and existence of emotional bonds between mates, including the shared feelings of love for their children. The issue under consideration is not romantic love or the permanence of marriage in societies that place no value on love. The issue is the identification of the variety of bonds that provide a satisfying life, including awareness that sexual and parenting urges in both genders can lead to an adolescent's bonding with another adolescent. Although this is seen by both youths as a permanent bond (to some parents' dismay), these commitments are usually soon seen for what they are: temporary, sexually driven bonds, even if not physically acted on, that indeed may lead later to permanent union but typically do not.

### *The Bond of Nationhood*

Bonds are existentially validating. When they are few or weak, the existential disorder labeled anomie can result, in which a person senses rootlessness, purposelessness, and aimlessness. When this idea was touched upon earlier, two conceptualists were cited, one noting post–World War II self-seeking, in which emptiness has been filled by things, calories, experiences, politicians, romantic partners, and empathic therapists (Cushman, 1990). Another identifies a hunger for community and mystical merging, which people try to satiate with communalism, quasi-Eastern religions, cult phenomena, drug experiences, and the search for one's roots (Kegan, 1982).

Sociologists, philosophers, and psychologists have long noted that even in culturally stable societies, one aspect of modern occupational life contributes to anomie: the separation of daily labor from the finished product of that labor. Although that remoteness is not characteristic of most crafts and of farming, the changed occupational structure in the past century has reduced the number of craftspeople and farmers. Thus, there is a decreased proportion of income earners whose sense of importance is nourished by a finished product. This is particularly reported for assembly-line workers.

Nations, whether or not they are also states, are the largest groups that provide emotional attachments, prevent anomie, and fill selves. Use of hard drugs is found in almost all societies, but current data point to Americans as the proportionately largest users of nonalcoholic drugs. An acceptable hypothesis holds that a culturally uniform nation, particularly when its nationhood carries with it a subscription to a sharply defined religion, is negatively correlated with hard-drug use.

This tangent into nationhood was taken to complete the range in which bonding and affiliation occur, from bonds with a few individuals to bonds (or affiliations of almost bond strength) with all in a nation, bonds so strong that individuals are ready, willing, and in some cases even eager to die to preserve their culture.

## *Career as Affiliation*

For some professional counselors, the word *career* refers to the several modes of persistent activity employed by a person to achieve maximum fulfillment. An individual's money-producing occupation is so major a part of his or her career that the two words are often equated, a usage that occurs in this text at times. The use of *career* by some to mean only that kind of occupation is understandable, given the importance of wages or salary in an individual's life. Of course, instead of limiting the use of the word *occupation* to income-producing activities, it can be used broadly to refer to any organized activity to which an individual is committed and that provides a sense of identity—psychic income—whether or not it also provides a monetary income. To use the term *occupation* in this broad sense lets us see the tasks, skills, and responsibilities of the homemaker as an occupation, as well as the activities of those engaged in unpaid public-welfare activities, the Andrew Carnegies of the world. In this sense the term *occupational career* is applied to whatever answer is given when people are asked, or ask themselves, "Who [what] am I?"

A major criterion of a mentally healthy life is the quality of bonds. For children, this quality depends mostly on the bonding initiative of adults. The individual who experiences good and lasting family bonds as a child can model them in adolescence to initiate bonds with others and be able to control their quality. By adulthood the individual is potentially in full charge of maintaining old bonds and initiating new ones, a condition maximally expressed by surrendering part of one's identity to one other person and taking up some of the other person's identity.

A career commitment is an affiliation of oneself with like people. Careers are cultures, attracting those who are similar on a number of variables. This is clearly so when the career is a lifetime commitment that requires lengthy preparation. Crafts and professions are examples.

## Concluding Reflections

A counselor cannot adequately serve clients without knowing the sweep of lifelong development, some aspects of which have been examined here. The need to see that people operate as systems has been established, and we have also seen that any individual, as a system, functions in an organized manner. For some, personality is the organizing element, but the construct of self, a component of cognitions that are part of the concept of personality, may have more explanatory power. This potency lies in those cognitions called self-statements and maxims, the rules of life that over a person's lifetime increasingly provide controls over behaviors.

Humans are social creatures in both their public and private lives, finding themselves in a variety of social systems during the course of days or weeks. Their thoughts and behaviors in any one social system are not to be understood solely by the objective realities of that social system, if at all, but by the subjective ones. These phenomenological realities are the "true" ones for any individual.

Social units are systems too, and therefore counselors also need an understanding of how they function as such. Social systems, starting with one's family, are the source of bonds essential for mentally healthful development. Part of understanding some clients will entail finding out about the quality of their bonds.

The construct of existentialism is deemed useful as a summarizing term for specifics that can be examined under the title of mental health, although the term *existentialism* conveys a unifying dynamic that would be lost were mental-health criteria alone examined. Humanism, likewise a summarizing concept, catches the thrust of existentialism along with phenomenological processes. Counselors, then, may be enriched by contemplating the origins and current thrusts of those two concepts. The adequately committed and prepared counselor is an existentialist and humanist, both of which categories, if not fully compatible with the epistemology of science, are not in opposition. It follows from that judgment that there is no need for separate counseling schools labeled existentialist or humanistic.

■                    **Points to Remember**                    ■

1. One person's psychological operation is in some ways similar to that of all other people. In other ways it is like that of some people but not others. In yet other ways, significant for counseling, each person is unlike any other person.
2. One way in which all are alike is that each person functions as a system; that is, the physiological parts and their psychological expressions in all people transact so as to work as a total unit.
3. The psychological element, through cognitions, organizes this total operation. Self is a hypothetical construct that is commonly accepted to account for this organization.
4. An individual's self comprises two components, the aware and unaware selves. The aware self, a function of cognition, is composed of concepts of oneself (self-concept), is part of one's life view, and is one variable that determines behaviors.
5. As the organized person functions in social situations, the perceptions of the potential mass of data from those situations are unconsciously "filtered," a

process that provides the individual with selected data. These data are subjective but nonetheless are psychologically real.

6. In conjunction with self-as-system, the bonds and affiliations that develop in the individual's life become major variables in the person's cognitions and behaviors. These may be as specific as a bond with one person, or much broader, including a sense of bonds with all others who make up a nation-state.

■                    **Counselor Formation Activities**                    ■

1. Into which systems are you locked? They may include family, occupation, social groups, and a coterie of friends, among others.
   a. What behaviors are expected of you in one system that would not be tolerated in another?
   b. What contribution to your satisfaction in life does membership in each system contribute?
   c. In what system were you strongly entrenched in the past but no longer are? What caused the change?
2. Think of some recent contentious event that lasted for a half-hour or more—perhaps a discussion with peers in which there was much disagreement (as in politics or religion) or a dispute with a superior. Recall the event in detail: what you thought, said, and did. Try to describe what aspects of your self were operating, particularly self-views—the consistent ways in which you think about yourself.
3. If you are employed:
   a. Are your co-workers like you or different? If different, in what ways?
   b. Does your occupation validate your view of self, enabling you to become more yourself?
   c. Does it conflict with your self-views, requiring you to find validation and enhancement elsewhere?
4. Think of people whom you see often, such every day or every week.
   a. With which ones are you bonded? Has each bond a unique characteristic or origin, such as being familial, sexual, spiritual, occupational, friendly, or dependent? Or are there several features of a bond with any one person?
   b. With which of the persons you see would you say you have an affiliation rather than a bond—a lesser psychological union? Are the relationships you have with people in organized social groups bonds or affiliations?
5. With which living person were you bonded at one time but are no longer. What caused the bond to atrophy? What was the bond's chief characteristic at its strongest: being familial, spiritual, political, sexual, friendly, or something else?
6. Think of your national and ethnic affiliations.
   a. Which is paramount, race, religion, or country?
   b. If you are an American citizen, do you see that affiliation as paramount, equal, or lesser to your feelings for your ancestral country.

■                   **Complementary Reading**                   ■

Two brief chapters, this one and Chapter 4, in effect address the sweep of human development, a topic so immense that it generates an overwhelming amount of literature, making the suggestion of complementary readings temerarious.

In addition to the adequate coverage for beginning students found in introductory psychology texts or the more thorough coverage in life-span texts, such as the one by Burger cited at the end of Chapter 4, there are the specialized texts and journals that focus on each developmental stage.

One illustration of literature that attends to a single developmental stage—in this case, adolescence—offers a counterpoint to other reports and case experiences that inform counselors of the *risks* faced by adolescents in their development. This counterpoint is found in a number of research articles reporting on the *opportunities* of adolescence in:

"Adolescence" [Special issue]. (1993). *American Psychologist, 48*(2).

The article "Development during Adolescense" will be particularly informative.

J. Seeman's (1989) article about a competence model of health, as opposed to an illness model, deserves a complete reading. Challenging thoughts, about not only health but also a wide range of topics of major interest for counselors is provided by:

THORESON, C. E. (1980). "Reflections on Chronic Health, Self-Control, and Human Ethology." In *The Present and Future of Counseling Psychology.* Pacific Grove, CA: Brooks/Cole.

In this highly recommended chapter, Thoreson also shows why counseling is humanistic and existentialist.

$$\boxed{6}$$

**CHAPTER**

# Affect in Clients' Lives

## Overview

Let an equilateral triangle represent any human, as in Figure 6-1. The eye naturally focuses on the figure as a whole. Its sides represent facets of an individual's total psychological being, one facet representing behaviors, another, cognitions, and the third, affects. The error in this instructional device is the representation of these facets as if they had discrete existence.

To understand the individual, we assume each side to be permeable—we can move inward through any one side in an effort to get the sense of the total figure. Counseling typically requires entering through not only one side but also one or both of the others, separately or simultaneously. How far that reach is to be depends on variables that will become known only during counseling.

Because of a counselor's need to know about humans in general, we will metaphorically reach into the geometric figure through each side in separate chapters. In this chapter we enter through the side labeled affect, in Chapter 7 we examine behaviors, and then in Chapter 8 we look at cognitions.

After earning scant attention for many years, research on affect has surged in the past two decades. There is an inevitable lack of unanimity at this early stage, given the relative recency of scientific thinking about affect and the paucity of evidence. The position advanced here, for example, is that a meta-analysis of current research justifies the identification of mood and emotion as two aspects of affect, although not all agree. Counselors will probably not often be called upon to work with mood, but they do need to be aware that it serves as ground against which emotions, cognitions, and behaviors are set off as figure, and that mood influences the quality and intensity of emotion.

Because the topic of emotion is more familiar to counseling students than mood, the chapter begins there. After then exploring the theme of mood, we return to complete the topics related to emotions.

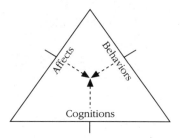

**Figure 6-1**
Construct of an individual's psychological structure

## Introduction

It is rare for a counselor to be asked to help solve a solely rational dilemma. It may happen in a high school, for example, when a teenager seeks help in making a decision about an occupation to enter, an uncomplicated, rational decision like Maria's in Chapter 5. Or a parent or student may also consult a high school counselor about options among colleges. In the vast majority of counseling instances, however, some affect is involved, perhaps in only a minor way, but it needs to be considered. Often affect is central to the client's concern.

The importance of affect is expressed by Tompkins (1984) this way: "The affect system is . . . the primary motivational system because it combines urgency and generality [and] . . . it lends its power to memory, to perception, to thought, and to action" (p. 164). That being so, it remains a puzzle that affect (emotion and mood) could have received only peripheral attention in psychological research even in the days of equating science with positivism. In the counseling field Rogers (1942, 1951) did attend to emotion, but from the limits imposed by an exclusively phenomenological standpoint. Ellis, as noted earlier, also raised affect as a topic central to clinical practice beginning in the late 1950s but based on conclusions from only his own experience—that is, from uncontrolled empiricism. Only recently has a sufficient body of science-generated knowledge about affect been available. The coverage of the topic here acknowledges that two occupations provide psychological help: counseling, which attends to the normal development of normal people, and clinical practice, which attends to those with severe or abnormal distress. Clinical practitioners need knowledge about affect beyond the scope of this chapter.

## Emotions

Emotions have evolved over time because they contribute to survival. Variables affecting survival of the human species today differ from those at the time when emotions were first genetically encoded tens or hundreds of thousands of years ago. Although certain emotions from primitive times will continue to be transmitted, others may diminish or disappear, a process that may have been continually occurring. Based on the same evolutionary criteria, new emotions may evolve over the next thousands of years. In any case, emotions are a normal part of living—both positive ones (those perceived to enhance) and negative ones (those perceived to be threatening)—potentially contributing to mental health and thus to survival. Although negative emotions, such as anger, are frequently considered undesirable, they often serve valuable purposes, being undesirable only in excessive intensity or length. The inability to place a line that separates excessive from normal reflects the unavoidable imprecision that marks studies of emotions.

In the time when psychology was committed to logical positivism, it was understandable that this topic was considered inappropriate for research, because feelings are subjective, definitions and terminology are imprecise, and the intensity of the emotional experience cannot be measured according to the precision required by logical positivism. Some study of emotion must rely on subjective reporting, although more precise study can also be made by measuring physiological responses through an electroencephalogram (EEG), galvanic skin response (GSR), blood pressure, and heartbeat. Definition is imprecise, as shown by panels of trained observers who sometimes are unable to agree about emotions that are being experienced by others. Despite such lack of agreement, it is the consensus that emotions sometimes dominate behaviors and mental processes, just as either of those two at other times affect emotions.

We begin our inquiry by addressing the matter of definition, and to this end we eavesdrop on Romeo. We find him approaching the balcony under Juliet's window and, with deft toss of pebble, calling her forth. "Romeo, oh Romeo, how art thou Romeo?" she breathlessly asks. "Dearest Juliet, I am undergoing a physical departure from homeostasis, and I am subjectively experiencing strong feelings of ecstasy. This homeostatic departure manifests itself in neuromuscular, respiratory, cardiovascular, hormonal, and other bodily changes preparatory to overt acts, which may or may not be performed. I am thus impelled to inquire, art thy parents to home?"*

In this uncharacteristic, pedantic manner, Romeo has informed his love that he is experiencing a positive emotional state, a powerful motivator of gross and refined behaviors that are likely to be impulsive because emotions are more potent than rational, planful actions and therefore override them. Plutchick (1984) puts it this way:

> An emotion is an inferred complex sequence of reactions to a stimulus, and includes cognitive evaluations, subjective changes, autonomic and neural arousals, impulses to action, and behavior designed to have an effect upon the stimulus that initiated the complex sequence [p. 217].

From Darwin on, students of emotion have considered perception to be an essential ingredient of an emotion, occurring before and during it. In Lazarus's (1991b) theory, emotions include two elements, one a "clear, personally significant

---

*With only slight modification to comport with the drama of the moment, Romeo's statement is identical to the definition in *Webster's Third New International Dictionary*.

relational content" and the other a potential for action. To arouse emotion, a situation must elicit "an appraisal of personal harm, threat, challenge, or benefit" (p. 822), which in existential terms means a perception of the significance of the event for the person's being. It logically follows from this relational content and appraisal of prospective harm or benefit that emotions "are always about person-environment relationships" (p. 819). In any such relationship, an individual appraises the presence of a clear, personally significant relational content, which can then be further appraised as to the harm or benefit that will result from that relationship, an appraisal that produces an emotion.

In Lazarus's (1991b) view, these appraisals are cognitive—although not necessarily in the sense of being "coextensive with consciousness, deliberateness, and rationality" (p. 361)—but are probably automatic and involuntary. He favors Buck's (1985) distinction between *analytic cognition,* in which meaning is built up bit by bit at an aware level, and *syncretic cognition,* in which meaning is instantaneously achieved without reflection or awareness. It is this unaware type of cognition that lets an individual implicitly appraise situations for their potential harm, threat, challenge, or benefit. If any of these is identified, an emotion occurs.

Lazarus (1991a) names some emotions that result from harms, losses, and threats. These "are also referred to as negative emotions because the cognitive-motivational-relational process involved in their generation is based on thwarting" (p. 827). Other emotions are labeled positive for the opposite reasons: they enhance the individual. Lazarus further proposes that emotions are similar across and within cultures, illustrated by 14 universal emotional families, such as being slighted or demeaned, facing existential threats, and experiencing irrevocable loss. In our culture these result in the emotions labeled anger, anxiety, and sorrow.

Theorists do not agree whether cognitions are necessary in emotions and, if so, when and how they function—as causal prerequisites or only as correlates *after* an emotion has been caused by a noncognitive stimulus. Only a few subscribe to the notion that emotions are aroused by cognitions of which the person is aware. Most maintain that an unconscious cognitive process occurs prior to the elicitation of the emotion.

## *Three Categories of Emotions*

Analysis of theories of emotion therapy, coupled with their own experience, have lead Greenberg and Safran (1987) to identify three classes of emotion: primary emotions, the sort that have been our consideration to this point; secondary reactive emotions; and instrumental emotions.

The *primary emotions* are those that result from immediate experience when a person senses either threats or positive outcomes. *Secondary reactive emotions* are those not normally expected in response to stimuli, such as, in Greenberg and Safran's illustration, people feeling and expressing anger when their primary emotion in response to a stimulus is fear. Most usefully for counselors is their identification of the category of *instrumental, or learned, emotions,* "those that people have learned to use to influence or manipulate others" (p. 172).

Primary emotions are autonomic—the natural, understandable, affective responses people have to situations. Although primary emotions cannot be eliminated, living experiences or counselor-induced experiences can result in extinguishing emotional responses to certain stimulus packages. The anger-producing effect of experiencing a certain specific stimulus can be eliminated through counseling, but the primary emotion of anger remains available for other appropriate situations.

Secondary and instrumental emotions are learned and therefore can be more readily "unlearned."

## Identifying and Naming Emotions

There is no agreement about the categories of specific emotions and the names given to them. One can find in both popular and professional literature incidental mention of emotions without knowing how the writer defines them. It is as if readers are expected to know what is meant by the label used. A common misuse of one term for an emotion that is common in popular usage is to speak of a person being "anxious" to do something. The appropriate word would be eager or avid, but of course a person can experience the emotion of anxiety while at the same time eagerly waiting to engage in an activity (adience/abience responses), such as a first-time bungee jumper.

Thompson (1988) identifies four emotions that have been extensively studied: anger, anxiety, depression, and fear. Some empirical study has been made of disgust, excitement, embarrassment, guilt, happiness, humor, sadness, shame, and surprise, whereas less study has been made of contempt, jealousy, loneliness, love, and pride. Other writers add grief and elation (joy, happiness, glee) to this list.

Plutchick (1984) suggests that there is a better way to conceptualize emotions than the customary list of apparently equivalent terms. He proposes, instead, eight basic *adaptive reactions,* each with its own three-part hierarchy of related emotions that show differing degrees of intensity. For example, annoyance is less intense than anger, which in turn is less intense than rage, but each is within the same adaptive reaction. Pensiveness, sadness, and grief are in a hierarchy, as are the triad of apprehension, fear, and terror. Plutchick sees the figure he uses for illustration as comparable to a color wheel: eight "colors" (adaptive reactions) with three shades (related emotional states) in each color. These emotions can be expressed in the primary way defined by Greenberg and Safran (1987) or as secondary reactive and instrumental emotions.

## Anxiety from Existential Threat

A negative emotion usually originates in the perception of a specific threat, especially a physical threat that is perceptible to other people. A person can also experience a psychological threat: a threat to the essential being that is not readily noticed by others. This kind of threat can result in disruptive anxiety, a condition the master counselor learns to identify and address.

It is a mental-health principle that a person needs a clearly defined sense of self. That is a valid rule, but it may not be adequately stated; it could mean that a self can be defined by other people and institutions. It is imperative, by mental-health criteria, to go beyond that reactive way for self to be defined. The need is better met if a person is conscious of his or her being, chooses what that being will be, and asserts and preserves it. This is the essence of an existential position.

Choosing is the heart of this position. Its maximum expression occurs when people acknowledge that the opposite of being is nonbeing and that they have made a choice between them. Most people do not confront that option, just as they may make few or no life-significant choices based on the wish to define themselves. Their lives have been reactive, letting self be defined by others, by circumstances, by institutions. It is likely that a self that is at least half-formed in this way is the state of being for most people.

A self that was formed predominantly by others and institutions nonetheless acquires some sense of being, even if it is not the product of aware choices. Any person, therefore, can experience anxiety that is aroused by a threat to being but may have a difficult time expressing to a counselor just what the nature of that threat is. At different places in this text are descriptions of clients who are experiencing existential challenges but are unable to conceive of them that way because they have not lived existentially. They lack a being defined by major choices made over time.

I devoted considerable attention earlier to knowing, the topic of epistemology. Existentialism is nonepistemological—it does not deal with concepts. It does attend to aware or unaware cognitions, but not knowledge. It acknowledges the perceptive and aware responses that people make to conditions they face, one of those being the state of nonbeing, of death. Vandenberg (1991) observes:

> Death is a core phenomenon for the existential perspective and provides an example of how an exclusive focus on epistemology fails to consider important existential issues. The uncertainty surrounding death not only prompts anxiety, but also leads to various strategies that are a response to the basic unknowns of existence. These existential uncertainties are not necessarily eliminated or diminished through the use of logical-mathematical thought. Indeed, these uncertainties may give rise to other ways of considering the world, ways that may be nonlogical in nature [p. 1279].

Whereas "traditional epistemological approaches to development treat death as a concept" similar to other concepts such as space, time, and causality, "the existential perspective . . . argues that the meaning of death encompasses more than its logical properties" (p. 1279). Study of individuals with terminal illnesses reveals that:

> The enormity of the burden of terminal illness lies in the weight and immediacy of the existential themes it evokes: fear of death, regret and guilt about past life, mourning the loss of the future and of one's self and loved ones. . . . Although these issues are likely to surface in their most stark form during times of travail, they nevertheless exert a formative influence on the human psyche throughout life [p. 1279].

Although classic existentialism views nonexistence (death) as the fundamental source of anxiety, counselors will engage clients whose anxieties are attributable to more immediate but still vague threats. These anxieties, Lazarus (1991b) observes, are also:

> existential, that is, centered on meanings and a sense of identity that the individual has constructed. . . . Although an uncertain threat . . . may be

concretized as an upcoming examination or social confrontation, the basic threat is to existential meanings that are vague and symbolic. . . . Perhaps this is why anxiety has so often been treated as *the* basis of psychopathology. In anxiety, the threat is not insult [which would result in other emotions, such as anger] but the potential loss of meaning and uncertainty which makes us feel . . . powerless [p. 829].

An existential viewpoint carries with it the obligation for each person to be accountable for himself or herself. This responsibility starts with knowing oneself, proceeds to enhancing one's uniqueness, and in turn results in an increase in the sense of purposefulness, of becoming, and thus of one's ontological substance.

Existential insecurities, Vandenberg observes, drive individuals to "religious beliefs that often involve nonlogical forms of thought," beliefs that "reflect the felt limits of science and technology for answering questions about meaning, value, and being" (1991, p. 1284). He further reports the relationship that attachments to other people have in establishing and maintaining some degree of existential certainty:

It is through shared meanings and beliefs that children remain close to trusted caregivers. The power of beliefs [defined as *fervent hopes*] is derived from their existential implications. . . . They are efforts to establish some sense of stability, and they serve as a buttress against existential uncertainty [p. 1284].

Vandenberg concludes that viewing human development through an existential filter:

raises significant issues, such as the importance of beliefs and will; gives new and deeper meaning to familiar topics like attachment; provides grounding for the ethical nature of our relationships with others; and points to the limitations of an exclusive, epistemological focus on scientific reasoning. Our lives are dominated by central existentialist concerns, and the recognition of the importance of these issues greatly expands and enriches our understanding of development [p. 1284].

It may sound as if a counselor can be overwhelmed by client emotion, particularly when it arises from an imprecise existential source. There is, indeed, an ever-present need to know one's limits as a counselor and to help a client find an appropriate professional when one's own competencies are overchallenged. A counselor may be spiritual but religiously agnostic and thus may be overchallenged by a client whose existential anxieties are of a kind best addressed by a person with a religious commitment. Counselors will more commonly serve clients who are afflicted with emotional distress other than the existential. But they may nevertheless feel inadequate in some of those instances and thus be obligated to refer those clients.

Alleviation of a client's distressed emotional state may require personality restructuring or other drastic steps outside the scope of most subdoctoral psychological counselors and some counseling psychologists. The boundary between normal and abnormal emotional dysfunction, as is the case with many psychological variables, is imprecise, requiring counselors to make ethical judgments about the kind of assistance required.

# Role of Emotions in Mental Health

When judged by either mental-health or social criteria, the ability to experience some emotions, such as happiness and sorrow, is desirable. Such negative emotions as anger, jealousy, and fear are generally characterized as undesirable by social criteria and, at times, by mental-health criteria. Mental-health criteria would hold, however, that negative emotions may be healthy. It would be therapeutic for a habitually submissive person to experience anger toward someone who is consistently degrading (assertiveness training generally is a better alternative), or for a sociopath to experience sorrow, guilt, and embarrassment. Ultimately, the desirability of an emotion is relative to its context.

Cultural and gender variables are part of our emotional context. In some cultures males are expected to show no negative emotion toward fear or pain, to adhere to a stiff upper lip code. In some cultures crying is seen as a female trait; males are expected not to cry and are so trained from their earliest years by parents and male peers. One beneficial outcome of counseling is that it may counter that training. Counselors-to-be learn about their own emotions and the values they place on them, particularly how they respond to the negative emotional states of others. This awareness is essential. It allows the counselor to be empathic, to stand in a client's emotional shoes and see the world through the client's eyes. The empathic counselor accurately senses what an emotional experience means to the client, but does not experience the same emotion. Emotions are active when they result from transactions with real persons in real contexts where overt acts are required.

The importance of emotion is put this way by Thompson (1988):

> Emotions are integral components of human experience. Most people report that their everyday subjective experiences consist of a kaleidoscope of positive and negative feelings. . . . Intuitively we realize that emotions are literally the subjective spices of life. Without [them] life would be a barren experience [p. 3].

He also observes that "from a psychiatric viewpoint, emotions are considered 'healthy' *unless* they represent very extreme and/or inappropriate reactions" (p. 1).

Before continuing the examination of emotion it is appropriate to introduce the other element of affect, mood.

# Mood

Not all theorists, as mentioned, find emotion and mood to be two distinct subsets of affect. Kaplan and Sadock (1985) refer to affect as the immediate experience of emotion and to mood as a pervasive, or sustained, emotion (p. 499). I find that the evidence supports the view that emotion and mood have noticeable and significant differences but that both are part of the category labeled affect.

In response to Romeo's inquiry about Juliet's parents being at home, Juliet might have responded, also in dictionary-speak: "Aye, Romeo, they are within, experiencing a mood; that is, they are wrapped in a distinctive atmosphere, a negative state of mind of pervasive and compelling quality." Romeo would have been pleased had Juliet reported them as being in a positive state, because mood comprises both states, but then the drama would have suffered. Although counselors will be called on to attend mostly to client emotion, mood's effect on emotion is one reason to address that topic.

Moods fall in a range marked by the extremes of depressive and manic syndromes, which by the fact of being at the extremes of a hypothetical scale are thus identified as abnormal states, and therefore outside the typical counselor's expected competence. Between those extremes is a range marked at one end as "down," or depressed (feeling "blue"), and at the other as "up," or happy—the range of moods, approximating 12-hour periods, that are termed normal. Figure 6-2 conveys that concept visually, but it should be recognized as a teaching device portraying a rough picture of mood range, not as a definitive scope of the subtleties and permutations of that topic. The scale of 1 to 10 is arbitrary yet typical of devices that permit more precise assessment than "none, some, or most."

Morris (1989) regards mood as a construct that is distinct from emotion. He sees emotion as a state of *sharply focused* and *relatively sudden physiological change* caused by or directed to specific persons or events. Mood, in contrast, is a *low level of diffuse physiological change that persists for an extended period* (in contrast to the shorter life of an emotion) *and colors responses to events and persons:*

> Moods may be defined as affective states that are capable of influencing a broad array of potential responses, many of which may seem quite unrelated to the mood-precipitating event. As compared with emotions, moods are typically less intensive affective states and are thought to be involved in the self-regulatory processes [p. 3].

Personality gives gross direction to patterns of cognition, feeling, and behavior, actuated by the individual's genetic endowment. Moods define these gross patterns by giving an affective tone, or color, to experiences. The quality and duration of an emotion is affected by the quality (nature and intensity) of the mood.

To explain the function of mood in daily life, Morris offers a comparison to the concept of figure and ground from studies of perception. A perceiving person focuses on one small portion of all that is potentially visible; the bit focused upon is figure, and all else in the range of sight, but not focused upon, is ground. A painted portrait places the subject in figure; in the background are indistinct features placed by the portraitist to convey a mood by which the subject is given further meaning.

Mood, says Morris, is "the formless backdrop against which we experience events." (p. 8) and a "context which frames and colors what it 'surrounds,' namely

| Abnormal | | | | Normal | | | | Abnormal | |
|---|---|---|---|---|---|---|---|---|---|
| 1 | 2 | 3 | 4 | 5 | 6 | 7 | 8 | 9 | 10 |
| Depressive syndrome | | "Down" or depressed | | | | "Up" or happy | | Manic syndrome | |

**Figure 6-2**

A range of moods

our ongoing focal experience [the figure to which we are attending]" (p. 21). A person in a nonclinically depressed, or "down," mood (ground) will respond to a focused-upon person or event (figure) in a way influenced by that mood. For example, if Patsy is in a depressed mood, she will probably respond to a friend's negative comment differently than she would if she were in an "up" mood, one in which there was a sense of confidence and control over events. The event is differently "framed and colored" by the differing moods. Memories, perceptions, judgments, and behaviors of an individual in an "up" mood, Morris says, reflect that mood, and conversely so for a person in a "down" mood: "People who are in a bad mood often demonstrate bias in memory such that negative items are more likely to be retrieved" (p. 161).

Whether or not people are aware of their current mood, Morris finds, the evidence "suggests that [moods] can nonetheless subtly insinuate themselves into our lives, influencing what we remember of the past, perceive in the present, and expect from the future" (pp. 8, 9).

Clients can come for counseling in a readily recognized state of heightened physiological response, one that identifies the presence of an emotion. Lack of emotion does not mean that no affect is present. The client will still be in some mood, one that may not be readily identified by either client or counselor. That mood, however, will color how the client experiences interview events and will affect what is recalled and how the client sees his or her future. It may be appropriate to assess the developmental health of the client by exploring the frequency and duration of typical mood states and how mood may bear upon the concern the client has brought for counseling.

The counselor, indeed, needs to monitor his or her own mood before an interview, to be at least aware of it because of its potentially harmful effect. A counselor at an 8-level "up" mood may be less empathic with a client experiencing a 3-level "down" mood. Or the counselor may be experiencing a minor "down" state—which occurs as part of the normal 4-hour cycling of moods within the more pronounced 12-hour cycle—while interviewing a client who is in an "up" mood. A counselor may not be able to postpone an interview if self-monitoring shows the presence of undesirable affect, but by being aware of those states, he or she will be better able to insulate the client from their potentially harmful effects. Moreover, the desirable traits of genuineness and authenticity may lead the counselor to tell the client candidly of the emotion or mood he or she is experiencing.

## *Sources of Mood*

To what degree the source of mood is exogenous (external) or endogenous is a question of continuing study. The meta-analysis conducted by Morris (1989) led him to conclude that mildly pleasant and unpleasant events, and imagined emotional events, are antecedents of short-lasting moods. The actual events are exogenous, while the imagined ones are endogenous. Schnurr (1989), however, conducted a meta-analysis of research on the extremes of manic and depressive behaviors that led her to observe that although she would like to be able to conclude that moods were indeed solely of an endogenous (biological) origin, the evidence requires her to state only that biological "abnormalities seem to *permit* maladaptive responses to environmental events" and thus that the hypothesis is still tenable that "everyday moods [not abnormal ones] that seem to 'come out of the blue,' whether extreme or mild, arise from unidentified environmental sources" (p. 69; emphasis added).

The assumption that moods result from internal sources is ancient. We recall the observation of the ancient Greeks that there are four personalities that result from the secretion of one of four "humors." Although these views are not now accepted, current knowledge about personality shows that there are genetically based physiological causes for personality differences and, by extension, for moods. Moods are a minor explanatory construct that provides a useful refinement to the major construct, personality.

Eckman (1984) suspects that moods originate in changes in the organism's biochemical state or may result from repeated elicitation of a particular emotion over a short period. Whybrow (1984) is more specific about the physiological correlates of mood, postulating that the thyroid axis is a major modulator of mood, acting in synergism with the catecholaminergic messenger system. You may also recall the proposition stated in Chapter 4 that the quality of mood is modulated by the secretion of seratonin in the brain's midline raphe nuclei and norepinephrine in the reticular formation. Data of this order serve generally to inform counselors of the lawfulness of human conduct, decreasing the probability of their viewing clients' abnormal mood states as mysteries or, worse, as willful actions to be addressed by whatever procedures the counselor has an impulse to use. The knowledge of the physiological sources of mood, on the other hand, does not provide counselors with intervention strategies designed to deal with the endocrine origins of moods but only with their cognitive and behavioral consequences.

One example of an exogenous source of mood has been increasingly reported in the past few years: the depression experienced by millions in higher latitudes during the period from late autumn to early spring when there are long periods of diminished sunlight. A psychiatric classification has been established to account for the depression, labeled seasonal affective (mood) disorder. This imbalance responds favorably to treatment by extensive exposure to artificial sunlight.

In Figure 6-2 the two extremes were identified as abnormal mood states. These are labeled in the *Diagnostic and Statistical Manual of Mental Disorders* (3rd ed. revised) (DSM-III-R), published by the American Psychiatric Association (1987), as full or partial depressive syndrome and full or partial manic syndrome. People frequently cycle between these two states, a condition labeled bipolar disorder.

Subdoctoral counselors do not deactivate abnormal moods; this is done only by specially prepared doctoral-level practitioners. Based on this résumé of studies showing normal moods to have environmental determiners, however, it is within the counseling warrant to deal with the undesirable results of such moods. As noted earlier, the use of prescription drugs to combat abnormal moods is limited to licensed medical practitioners.

## *Degrees of Moods*

Some people may see moods as occasional deviations from an individual's normal level of psychological functioning in the same way that an emotional act is an exception to normal behavior. This incorrect view that moods are a brief, transient state may result from the fact that usually only extreme moods catch one's attention, such as a person's behavior when afflicted with "the blues." In fact, individuals have little occasion to be aware of the mood states in the midrange of the 1–10 scale in Figure 6-2. They become aware of mood when it moves from ground to figure, as when a mood that had been in the 5–6 range is now of a strength that places it at a more extreme point, such as a 3 or 8. Individuals are not likely to sense a need for counseling if they are consistently in the 5 and higher range (in an "up" direction), but they may be motivated to confer with a counselor when aware of a persistent negative mood.

### *Homeostasis*

Each individual acquires a feel for what is a comfortable level of psychological balance and functioning, a state of equilibrium of the psycho-physiological system spoken of as homeostasis. This balance is maintained by the use of symbols to effectively self-regulate the several biological "clocks" on which all humans run. The capacity for such equilibrium has evolved as a defense against constant and random fluctuations in mood that would occur if those biological clocks were not coordinated. Constant behavior changes in response to frequent mood swings would make it impossible to have an organized personality, and that would prevent the development of any kind of society.

Disruption in an individual's comfortable mood state, particularly the intrusion of an emotion, produces some degree of stress and distress, which results in actions to restore homeostasis. At the same time, the mood of a distressed person can be lightened by a positive emotion, perhaps deliberately induced by someone seeking to ease the other person's depression.

## Origin and Characteristics of Emotions

Whereas mood is marked by a relatively long period of consistent disposition of which a person may not be aware, an emotion is a relatively abrupt event producing feelings that fall within a range for that emotion for that person, and of which the person is usually cognizant. Individuals vary in the behaviors that express a particular emotion. One person's maximum emotion of anger may be observed as behaviors of a lesser degree of severity than those shown by another also experiencing maximum anger. Everyone experiences grief (except the psychopath), but for any person the severity of the experience varies according to differences in events causing the grief and in the person's mood, physiological variables, and learned responses.

Emotions, the subjectively experienced and objectively expressed results of abrupt and extensive physiological changes, are of different kinds, as we saw earlier, each resulting from different patterns of the physiological change. These patterns, in turn, result from the person's assessment of the potential of a transaction for beneficial or harmful outcomes.

Some negative emotions can be experienced with damaging frequency, as we learn from reports of children living for years in fear of harm by an abusive parent.

A few children are innately able to defend themselves psychologically against such environments and develop normally.

A counselor determines whether a client is in an abnormal negative emotional state partly by assessing the reality of the seriousness of the perceived harm, loss, or threat that produces the emotion; partly by determining the duration of symptoms; and partly by assessing the effect on the person, such as the inability to relate to others and to carry out functions that typify normality for that person. The identification of abnormal positive emotional states also requires judgment informed by experience. Linn (1985) finds that there are four levels of pleasurable response to positive emotions, similar in a way to the hierarchy of three degrees for eight affective respones that Plutchick (1984) identifies. The first two of Linn's levels, euphoria and elation, are normal responses to normal situations, but they are abnormal when the judgment can be made that they are not appropriate to an observed or reported setting. The next two levels, exaltation and ecstasy, may be elicited by truly exceptional positive events in a person's life, but otherwise they may represent some degree of abnormality. A person in a manic mood may present exaltation and ecstasy behaviors for no discernible reason.

Biological and cultural intervening variables lie between a noticeable external stimulus and a person's emission of emotional behavior. Counselors will deal with emotions that normal people experience, and thus they need to understand the role of these three sources of variables, although counselors' intervention strategies will be with psychological variables.

## *Biological Variables*

Emotions have been attributed to survival responses favored by evolutionary developments. Certain emotions, Izard proposes, appeared in advanced genera and species as motivators for approach by serving defensive and reproductive purposes, just as other emotions developed as motivators for avoidance (Izard, Kagan, & Zajonc, 1984). In Greenberg and Safran's (1987) terms, "emotion exists because it contributes to survival. If it did not, it would have been eliminated from our repertoire." Natural selection "would logically favor certain emotional experiences over others" (p. 115).

Both brain hemispheres contribute to emotional experiences, although the "perceptual processing of emotional stimuli is primarily under the control of the right hemisphere" (Greenberg & Safran, 1987, p. 122). Approach motives apparently lie in the left hemisphere because it is more involved with positive experiences, while the involvement of the right hemisphere with negative experiences gives rise to avoidance motives. Thompson (1988) believes that the frontal lobes are paramount, with the cortex playing a complex role relative to emotional response and awareness. Not all emotions resulting in approach behaviors are thereby of necessity positive emotions; anger is an approach motive when defending territory or driving off a rival suitor.

Thompson notes that a crude and tentative map of the emotional circuits of the central nervous system (CNS) is now available:

> These circuits are connected in a hierarchical fashion so that each level of the brain contributes to a more organized level of emotional behaviors and emotional states. The hindbrain elicits somatic [muscular and skeletal] and visceral

[internal-organ] activity during emotional reactions and forwards sensory reactions to higher brain centers. The midbrain contributes to emotional reactions by stimulating cortical arousal (via the RAS [reticular activating system]) and providing the pleasure-pain aspect (hedonic tone) of emotions (via the MFB [medial forebrain bundle]) and the PS [periventricular system]. The limbic system contains a number of separate excitatory and inhibitory centers for specific emotional experiences . . . and behaviors. The frontal lobes of the cortex integrate ongoing sensory information from both the external environment and body with images, plans, and memories and then decide whether to excite or inhibit specific emotional behaviors. Moreover, the cortices appear to be the locus of conscious emotional experiences, whereas the limbic system (and perhaps the right hemisphere) are the locus of unconscious emotional experiences [p. 41].

There is variability in emotional arousal at the biochemical level, which "may represent genetic variability . . . a variety of transient biological factors (diet, drug use, health, menstrual cycle, sleep-wake cycle, etc.), . . . environmental history, [or] individual differences in cognitive coping strategies" (p. 331). Additionally, there are clear patterns of autonomic activity—blood pressure, heart rate, and stomach activity—for anger, fear, happiness, and sadness but perhaps also guilt, humor, and embarrassment (p. 332). Examination of external responses shows distinct facial-muscle patterns across cultures in the emotions of anger, disgust, fear, happiness, sadness, and surprise (Davis, 1985). Izard proposes that such facial expressions are an integral part of the emotional process, not merely a muscular leftover (Izard et al., 1984).

### *Cultural Variables—Conditioning*
Although the neural and biochemical processes of all individuals may be similar for any one emotion, with bodily processes not differing among cultures, the overt manifestations of identical emotions do vary among individuals as a result of cultural influences. Differences in overt emotional responses can be stipulated by class and by occupational differences within a culture, Thompson observes. Herders are to show bravery, aggressiveness, tolerance of pain, and face-saving. Farmers demonstrate such community-oriented traits as amiability and industriousness. Some occupations call for displays of bogus emotions, as in acting, and in dealing with the public. Flight attendants must present one kind of positive affective face to the public. Bill collectors must be able to show simulated impatience and anger or perhaps false empathy with the debtor—whatever produces results.

An emotional response can be conditioned to a stimulus regardless of the context in which the stimulus occurs, a case of response generalization. An example of response generalization is found in the person who dislikes all members of certain ethnic or racial groups. The generalizing of a negative emotion toward a class of people can be conditioned by one's parents in the earliest years and then reinforced by relatives and neighbors or perhaps even by the culture at large. In this process, modeling is a major shaper of emotions, or "monkey see, monkey do." In Chapter 4 we briefly considered the conditioning of behavior and emotions by the associational process known as classical, or respondent, conditioning, which can either be deliberately carried out or result from a chance association of an unconditioned response with an unconditioned stimulus. Generalization of the emotion to all members of a class can result from such conditioning.

Watson and Rayner (1920) reported that 11-month-old Albert had been conditioned to fear a rat and had later generalized that fear to a rabbit, a fur coat, and a dog. This case was long accepted as the classical illustration. Although that research is now questioned, anecdotal reports appear from time to time about young children who have been terrorized by a particular dog after having shown some affection for dogs in general. If the dog behaved in a threatening way, the child's great fear of that specific dog was appropriate. Fear, acquired during the evolutionary development of humans, serves to activate avoidant (self-preservation) behaviors. What follows in those reported instances is not rationally defensible: a now-generalized fear of all dogs. This illustration has specified young children because the ability to discriminate cognitively between a specific instance and a class is age-related. An adult is able to process the experience symbolically, to reason that only Rex is to be feared while dogs as a class may still be viewed affectionately.

An excessive, irrational, generalized fear is called a phobia, a condition some clients will ask counselors to eliminate. Removal of some phobias is within the scope of counselors who have had an introductory level of education and training in their removal; other phobias are resistant to change, and the client may need referral to a specialist.

It is difficult to discern the affective web that wraps so much adult behavior, particularly in those who learn to screen their emotions from others behind an overlay of reasoning or by learned suppression of the outward signs of emotion. This kind of deceptive practice can produce later problems that bring clients to seek counseling assistance not only because of an inability to express outward signs of inwardly experienced negative emotions but also because of an inability to express positive feelings toward others. Some families condition their progeny from earliest childhood not to express such positive feelings, and perhaps any feelings. Occasionally, one learns of a father who beats his preadolescent son and who stipulates that the beating will be lengthened if he gives any outward sign of pain. Suppression of outward signs of negative emotions is called stoicism, prized in some cultures but not by mental-health specialists.

Let us assume that two children are conditioned by their parents and others to experience loathing of any member of a certain ethnic group or race. This emotional response remains throughout the life of one child, an unsurprising outcome. For the other child this loathing response disappears without any deliberate deconditioning or single cause, an outcome that may be puzzling. It may be impossible to find the reason why this change in a conditioned emotional response would occur in any one person, but theoretically one accounting is that it results from the changing loyalties and dependencies typical of adolescence. Up to adolescence the child is dependent on the family for economic support and psychological formation in value matters; the child is in a (diminishing) symbiotic relationship with the family. Adolescence brings a shifting of psychological dependence from the family to peers, and perhaps to nonfamily adults, such as an esteemed teacher, coach, or youth-group leader. Some parents who hold certain values know that this shift can occur. When circumstances permit, therefore, they act to prevent the potential value shifts at adolescence by ascertaining that their children associate only with "people like us" during the formative years. They do this by living in enclaves of similar people and then by sending the children to schools, camps, and colleges that maintain those values. This preservation of beliefs and mores, when duplicated by many people, results in nationhood, an "us" who must be leery of a variety of "them" against whose contamination the nation must arm itself and be ready to fight to the death. History records over 4000 years of this circumstance; daily newspapers record its bloody persistence today.

Despite efforts by the parents of the second child to maintain the rejecting response into which they have conditioned their child, during adolescence he or she may have had positive experiences with members of this rejected group. Additionally (it can be theorized), the adolescent has been led to examine values through academic (objective) study and by some esteemed others of his or her own ethnic group or race, those who not only have not been similarly conditioned against a group but also hold opposite values. The deconditioning occurred as a product of the natural process of living.

The family provides other influences on emotional development that are more subtle than ethnic or racial prejudice. For example, Thompson (1988) reports studies that "found that the mother's personality rather than child-rearing practices *per se,* appears to be the primary causal variable" in a child's emotional development (p. 292). Mothers who were "emotionally cold to their children and had high levels of sexual anxieties tended to punish their children severely for *any* behavioral infraction and thus might form (or deform) their children's personality in their own image" (p. 292). Even birth order may affect emotional development. Parents are more demanding of their firstborn, so it is no surprise that firstborns are more anxious and experience fear of failure. Those born later are more likely to engage in dangerous activity, with higher levels of aggression.

At a basic biological level, all humans experience the same emotions. At a higher level, those physiological changes, sensed as emotions, differ noticeably among individuals because of mixes of the overlapping variables of heredity, family training, accidental or deliberate conditioning, and exposure to cultural and sub-cultural values.

## Concluding Reflections

This chapter is not designed to provide you with intervention strategies for easing or changing negative affect; such strategies come later. It carries the message that clients' affective states are central to helping them with the concerns they bring. Affect cannot be thought of as an epiphenomenon that will be "taken care of" by attending only to mental processes or behaviors, the opinion implied by lack of consideration of the topic by all but two counseling schools. The evidence says otherwise.

In keeping with a scientific orientation, the chapter explores the physiological nature of affect, particularly emotion, not because such information is required by counselors in their working with affect but to more broadly educate counselors-to-be, to reduce any misunderstandings about affect, and thus to increase counselors' sense of professionalism. Following, in summary, are some considerations for counselors when dealing with a client.

## Counselor Affect

Counselors need to monitor their current mood and emotional state before each interview and to cancel the interview if they deem their level to be extreme or are aware of an emotional state that could negatively affect counseling. A counselor's anger-producing confrontation with a colleague prior to a counseling session, for example, may result in displacement on the client.

Just as prospective counselors need to become aware of the life views they bring to the counselor-preparation program and to engage in exercises to modify those portions that would be incompatible with counseling, so could the preparation program lead to examination of the mood states typical of the prospective counselor. A more important awareness is of the persistent (and therefore unresolved) negative emotions or emotional deficiencies—those that are potential "psychological land mines"—that would suddenly be activated by a client's inadvertent facial expression or statements. These lurking snares may be of little significance in professions such as medicine or in other arts, but they are of critical significance in psychological counseling.

## Client Mood State

It is to be expected that numerous clients will appear to be dejected when appearing for a first interview. They will have come because something is not right in their lives; they are beset with developmental difficulties they have not been able to resolve on their own. The counselor, however, will in time seek information from the client to judge whether the client's "down" state is indeed specific to the difficulty faced, whether it has been persistent, and how the client's mood is typically affected by adversity. The counselor will be aware that the client's negative mood will color the person's perceptions of the precipitating events that brought him or her to counseling and thus may seek to induce a mood change to bring about a more realistic appraisal by the client of the precipitating events.

## Emotional Content of Interviews

With the exception of the relatively rare event of a client's concern being solely cognitive, counselors will expect any concern that a client presents to have emotional content. This content is always a matter of significance, requiring skill in analyzing the origin and potency of the emotion and the effect of the client's mood on the emotion. The emotion may be motivated by an event that bears immediately and directly on the client, such as an appraisal of a direct threat. Or the emotion may reflect a threat to a loved one, and thus be a vicarious threat. Yet again, emotions may be present not because they are motivated by some definable present event but as expressions of unresolved emotions from the past. The first two of these cases involve developmental concerns within the scope of psychological counseling. The latter may require personality restructuring, which falls within the domain of the clinical psychologist or those counseling psychologists prepared by training and experience for this advanced form of therapy.

This brief recapitulation of the emotional facet of counseling, to repeat, is not designed to provide counselors with intervention strategies. Emotions do not exist separately from actions and mental processes, and therefore intervention strategies will typically incorporate those latter as well. The union of emotion and cognitions is stated this way by Greenberg and Safran (1987): "Emotions and cognitions are inferred entities. We can distinguish between them for conceptual purposes, but in reality they are fused together and are inseparable" (p. 122). Only when we deal with cognitions later in this text can procedures for modification of emotions be considered.

In a similar fashion, behavior and cognitions are often fused, which leads us next to examine behavior in a discrete conceptual fashion, after which attention will be accorded to the fused entity comprising cognitions, affect, and behavior.

# ■ Points to Remember ■

1. Two human conditions of counseling significance are emotion and mood; together they are termed affect.
2. Emotions are primarily abrupt, sharply focused responses to external stimuli. Moods are diffuse and long-lasting states of a biochemical nature, set off by either internal or external sources.
3. The gaps in knowledge and disagreements among scholars about emotion can be attributed to the recency of the study of it. It was long considered to be outside the scope of psychological study.
4. Emotions evolved into the human repertoire because they were useful in preserving and advancing humans over a long evolutionary period. In the complex societies of today, some emotions needlessly work against individuals. Counselors will be called upon to help clients determine which of their emotions are useful and which are harmful.
5. There are two classes of emotions, positive and negative. The positive emotions result from a perception (but not an aware cognition) that an external stimulus will have enhancing effects. Negative emotions are those that result from a perception that an external stimulus will have threatening or thwarting effects.
6. An emotion is a genetically based potential that can be cued by external stimuli. How intensely and in what other manners it will be expressed are determined by physiological and cultural variables that intervene between stimuli and the emotional response.
7. On the physiological side, both brain hemispheres contribute to emotional arousal and manner of expression. Numerous cultural variables impinge, including the individual's unique, respondently conditioned cognitions and behaviors.
8. In their general manifestations, emotions are alike across cultures. Cultures affect specific ways in which emotions are expressed.
9. There is considerable disagreement in the labeling of emotions, but some uniformity is slowly appearing.

10. Plutchick's analysis of emotions produces eight adaptive reactions, each with three levels.
11. Existential anxieties are distressing, a cause for people to seek counseling assistance, although most do not conceptualize their concerns as existential.
12. An individual's mood can be expressed as an imprecise spot on a continuum that runs from mania at one end to depression on the other. Normal people are in the midrange. Those at either extreme of the range are clinically manic or depressed and not within the range of most master's-level psychological counselors' assistance.
13. Mood has counseling significance because it serves as ground for and colors experiences. A client's evaluation of an experience has to be understood as being affected by his or her mood. Therefore, to assess the meaning of an event for a client requires understanding the person's mood at the time.

■ **Counselor Formation Activities** ■

1. a. Think about the past hour. If you judge that your mood has been consistent in that time, where would it fall on the scale in Figure 6-2? Think about the rest of the day. Was your mood different at other times? Where on the scale? If it changed, can you judge why?
   b. Work backward a few days and try to recall moods you experienced during those days, placing them on the scale. If they changed, can you see why they changed?
   c. Try to describe your average mood over a long period, such as a year. Where on the scale would you place your typical mood state, if you can identify a typical one. Think back over most of your life. Can you identify a typical mood state over that full period, or most of it? Where would it fall on the scale?
   d. Thinking of recent days, was there an experience to which you reacted in a way that might have been different had you been in a different mood?
2. Think about today again. What emotions have you experienced, giving them names you customarily do? Was each emotion of short duration (a fleeting pleasure), longer (perhaps a half-hour), or quite lengthy (perhaps several hours, such as anger directed at someone or disappointment)? What cued each emotion? In what way was the emotion affected by your mood at the time? Were you angry with someone because you were somewhat depressed, or did you experience only slight anger because you were in a positive mood? Reverse the question to ask if you can identify a positive emotion that you did not experience as positively as you might have because of your being in a negative mood at the time.
3. Moods can affect cognitions, too. Can you identify any time when your thinking was affected by your mood; that is, were you experiencing negative cognitions because of a negative mood when normally your thoughts would not have been so negative? Conversely, did you experience positive cognitions along with a positive mood when you expect you would otherwise have had negative thoughts?

■                       **Complementary Reading**                       ■

Unlike the study of behavior, which has a long history, or of cognitions, which
has a history of shorter length, psychological science is in a relatively beginning
stage in its study of affect (emotion and mood). To deal with affect that clients bring
to counseling, counselors will need a solid base of knowledge about affect. From
among the chapter's references, I call particular attention to Greenberg and Safran
(1987), particularly Chapter 5, "Emotion, Cognition, and Behavior: An Integration";
Lazarus (1991b); Plutchick (1984); and Thompson (1988). Also recommended is:

FRIJDA, N. H. (1988). "The Laws of Emotion." *American Psychologist, 43*(5), 349–358.

Sources pertaining to dealing with affect in counseling will be found at the end of
Chapter 13.

7

**CHAPTER**

# Clients' Operant Behaviors

## Overview

For decades psychological science focused primarily on observable behavior; cognitions and emotions were deemed to be unacceptable research topics. Counselors, however, saw that behavior patterns, often a client's presenting concern, were usually interwoven with the ways clients thought and felt. Clients, however, may not see that cognitions and affect are inextricable parts of a behavior pattern.

Just as the affective aspect of behavior and cognition can be separated out for academic examination, as we did in Chapter 6, we can focus on the behavioral component of cognition and affect. These separate inquiries ultimately provide richer understanding of the synergistically operating client whom the counselor seeks to assist.

This chapter's goal is to examine the second kind of associative learning, or conditioning, of behavior, called instrumental, or operant—one process to help clients manipulate their lives to produce desirable outcomes.

Some writers speak of operant-based counseling procedures and techniques as if they were distinct counseling schools, such as applied behavior analysis. In the view espoused here, those approaches are specialties or particular emphases of a larger body of principles and techniques that counselors learn. Those approaches do not constitute separate systems, or schools.

Another distinctly labeled approach that employs behavioral techniques is social-learning theory. Its emphasis on external stimulus and reinforcement includes cognitive mediation of external events (Bandura, 1977), and therefore reflects this text's systems emphasis.

The most scientifically empirical knowledge about behavior per se has come out of laboratory experiments on operant conditioning, followed by experiments in applied settings. This chapter addresses in a selected and summary fashion a portion of the body of operant principles and their application as generated by both laboratory and nonlaboratory study. The primary topic is the two kinds of consequences of behavior: reinforcers, which increase the probability that a behavior pattern will be repeated, and those which reduce that probability. These latter are called punishers, aversives, or aversive stimulae. A later chapter will show the behavioral techniques employed to help clients, whose behaviors, affect, and mental processes operate as an integrated whole in a systems relationship with their environments.

## Introduction

The effect of the carrot or the stick on the donkey is well known. Do this, and you will be rewarded with a carrot (the carrot is the stimulus and follows the hoped-for behavior), a positive outcome; do that, and the consequence will be a beating, a painful outcome. Crude as the aphorism is, it states the essence of behavioral principles: the probability is increased that behaviors will be repeated if they are associated with desirable consequences, and the probability of their being repeated decreases if they are associated with undesirable outcomes.

Evolutionary changes reflect that law. The goal of primitive existence is simple: to stay alive long enough to reproduce one's kind (the purpose of an egg is to produce more eggs). Staying alive requires energy; energy requires food. Some individual primitive organisms chanced upon food and ways to ingest it and thus they lived and passed this behavior on through genes. Other individuals of the species did not adapt, and died without reproducing. As vast amounts of time passed, better ways of being nourished and of reproducing were discovered, and further changes occurred, based on the law that behaviors that produce favorable consequences will strengthen, whereas those that do not will extinguish. The extinction of some species and the survival of the fittest of any continuing species was (and is) a continuing process.

Humans as well as donkeys comply with that law, but for humans the law is immeasurably more complex because, unlike the acts of animals, human actions are intertwined with cognitions and with a more complicated array of emotions. Of these, it is cognitions that are the defining human characteristic. Although some advanced animal species show emotions, and it is a defensible conjecture that some may have primitive cognitive ability, the greater variety of human emotions and their incredibly more advanced cognitions provide humans with their enormous adaptive capacity. Emotions and cognitions give humans a purpose, a moral sense, and allow them to enjoy a rich quality and diversity of interpersonal relationships. That mix also provides the *potential* for humans to create caring civilizations and to prevent harmful emotions from dominating a society. It is apparent, however, at the present state of evolution, that the realizaton of those potentials is occasional at best.

There has been a century of psychological research in this area. Freud was earnestly seeking to establish a science of behavior, although his data collection was limited to relatively uncontrolled investigations. The Russian physiologist Ivan Pavlov (1927) conducted studies that can more tenably be described as scientific.

While experimenting on salivation in dogs, as we saw, he accidentally discovered the associative-learning process that came to have psychological significance— conditioning. Although B. F. Skinner's term, respondent conditioning, is now commonly used, it is also called classical, or Pavlovian, conditioning.

At about the same time in this country Edward L. Thorndike was studying learning effects on animals, and John B. Watson, building on Pavlov's findings, began studying the relationship between Pavlovian conditioning and human behavior, as did Joseph Wolpe in South Africa. Meanwhile in England Hans J. Eysenck and M. B. Shapiro undertook experimental studies, based on learning theory, of the treatment of psychiatric patients.

Animal experiments, like those Thorndike carried out, were also the characteristic of Skinner's laboratory studies. He became recognized as the psychologist who for 50 years most strongly held to the need for research on behavior to be conceptualized and studied in an uncompromisingly objective, empirical (positivist) manner. He recognized that associative learning was of two differing modes, classical, which he termed respondent, and that form of conditioning Thorndike called instrumental, which Skinner labeled operant. The research by Skinner and his colleagues and students is acknowledged to be the origin of the substantial knowledge about operant conditioning of animals that also constitutes the solid core of behavioral principles now applied to humans.

# Studying Behaviors' Consequences

Advanced animal species provide clear evidence of the operation of the law of operant conditioning—particularly, species trained to provide public entertainment, such as aquatic animals. Television has informed us about the astonishing feats performed by dolphins in entertainment centers, and it equally informs us about operant conditioning because we see trainers providing food after each trick.

A more readily observable outcome of operant conditioning is enjoyed by the many dog owners who take their pets to training or obedience schools. There they learn about the need to promptly provide positive consequences for a desired behavior in order to increase the probability of the recurrence of the behavior.

## *Increasing Response Likelihood*

The two kinds of responses that increase the likelihood that a behavior pattern will be repeated, positive and negative reinforcers, and the two that reduce that likelihood, punishment and extinction, are portrayed in Figure 7-1. The two vertical columns show the outcomes, or consequences (identified by the letter C), that result from a behavior. One column shows behavior-strengthening consequences, and the other column those Cs that weaken or eliminate behaviors. Arrows are placed at the top of each column to show strengthening (pointing up) or weakening (pointing down) of behaviors.

The two horizontal rows show two kinds of consequences. The top row shows consequences that are "added to," or follow, a behavior (thus the + sign placed in front of the Cs). Provision of positive reinforcers is shown in the left cell

| Out-comes / Pro-cess | Start, increase, or maintain behavior. ⬆ | Reduce or eliminate behavior; prevent new behavior. ⬇ |
|---|---|---|
| Add or provide (+): | C+<br><br>A positive or rewarding outcome; reinforces behavior. | C–<br><br>Punishment: social or physical pain; loss of a pleasure; reduces behavior. |
| Remove or subtract (–): | C–<br><br>Avoidance or escape from hurtful consequences; reinforces behavior. | C+<br><br>Reinforcers no longer provided (extinction); no consequences for new behaviors. |

**Figure 7-1**

Consequences of behavior. Based on an A-B-C model of cognitive-behavioral counseling developed by Wallace Kahn. See "Cognitive-Behavioral Group Counseling: An Introduction," 1988, *The School Counselor, 35,* 343–351. Reprinted by permission.

of the top row (+C+—that is, a desirable consequence following the behavior). The right cell of that row shows a punishing consequence following a behavior (+C–).

The bottom of the two rows shows subtractions, or removals—thus the minus sign in front of the Cs. The bottom-left cell shows the taking away, or prevention, of a harmful consequence, a C–; therefore, the consequence can be described as –C–. The right-hand cell of the bottom row shows extinction, which means removal of a positive reinforcer, C+, which has customarily followed a behavior. The full symbol, then, showing that removal, is –C+. This symbol is also used here to show that no consequence, positive or negative, followed a behavior. When a person's behavior is punished by another person, the latter person is attending to the first one. The attention received by a person who glories in it can make a consequence more desirable than the punishment is painful. In that case, as will be seen in an illustration later, it is best to provide no consequence but just to let it die for lack of attention.

***Positive reinforcers.***    Two kinds of consequences increase the probability that a behavior will be continued, and two enhance the probability that a behavior will be discontinued, preferably by replacement with a desirable behavior. One of the consequences that increases the probability that a behavior will be strengthened is called *positive reinforcement* (+C+ in Figure 7-1). Among animals, potential reinforcers are few, the most powerful being food. Mammals engage in the same two primary behavior patterns as did their primitive ancestors, food-seeking and reproduction. Both of these require another evolved behavior that is maintained because of its favorable consequences: establishing and defending an eating territory and, for some, a mating territory.

Wild animals spend their days looking for food. Some, such as squirrels and beavers, even store food against lean times, a learned behavior passed on to progeny through their genes. The food-seeking behaviors of most large mammalian species is typically interrupted once a year for a rutting season, after which food search again becomes paramount until bearing time. If humans control the food supply of animals, they can control many if not most of a species' behaviors, a fact apparent in the behavior of trained dolphins and dogs. Food, then, is a primary positive reinforcer for animals and humans, a desirable consequence that follows and thus maintains food-getting and eating behaviors. It is termed *primary* because it is a requirement for life, as are water and adequate shelter. Equally primary among animals are reproductive behaviors, annually or more frequently in lower orders, with a permanent or accidental mating partner. For many species in which males keep harems, sexual activity on the part of the male continues as long as female pheromones invite sexual activity. Humans, on the other hand, engage in sexual behaviors in addition to those intended for reproduction.

***Negative reinforcement.***    The other kind of behavior strengthener, or reinforcer, often confused with punishment, is termed *negative reinforcement* (–C+ in Figure 7-1). That it cannot be synonymous with punishment is apparent in the opposite meaning of the two terms *reinforcement* and *punishment*. Punishment is a consequence that serves to extinguish a behavior. It may be an accidental consequence, such as a naive animal experiencing the outcomes of a porcupine's or skunk's defenses. The animal is no longer naive; the punishment received reduces the probability that the animal will attack porcupines or skunks. Some behaviors of children just starting to walk and to manipulate their environments are eliminated by single punishing experiences that are consequent to their random actions, such as touching hot appliances.

The significant word in the phrase *negative reinforcement* is "reinforcement." It always means that the consequence of a behavior will strengthen the behavior. When a behavior is followed by a desirable consequence, the behavior is positively reinforced—the probability is increased that the behavior will be repeated. Negative reinforcement is the term to use when a behavior is followed by the *removal or avoidance of an unpleasant consequence* that was occurring or could be expected to come about. Some drug-taking behaviors are negatively reinforced (strengthened) because they result in the *removal* of psychological or physical pain that may mark much of a person's daily life. Some children who experience physical punishment learn to lie, a behavior negatively reinforced because it prevents physical hurt.

Avoidance behaviors (diets) related to certain foods and drinks or their quantities are begun and maintained because people's awareness of the consequences has risen from ground to figure: excess weight, digestive distress, or prospective poor health. These avoidance behaviors are negatively reinforced because of the expectancy that they will prevent unpleasant consequences.

Positive reinforcement of a behavior, in brief, results if desirable consequences follow that behavior. Negative reinforcement of a behavior results if
engaging in that activity results in avoidance of unpleasant consequences. In both
instances the behavior is reinforced (strengthened) by its consequences.

## Decreasing Response Likelihood

Similarly, there are two procedures for reducing or extinguishing a behavior.
The one, briefly mentioned above, is punishment, an unpleasant consequence of a
behavior (+C–). The other is extinction.

**Punishment.**    Punishment has two forms, one called here *positive* punishment
(the technical term is aversive stimulation), which results in a directly hurtful
consequence. This consequence may be social, such as scorn or ridicule, which is
psychologically punishing, or physical hurt. The other kind of hurtful consequence,
labeled *negative* punishment, refers to the loss of a pleasant experience. (In
negative *reinforcement* there is a "loss" of an *unpleasant* experience.) One human
may physically hurt another (positive punishment), as young children sometimes
do to each other or as parents may do to their young children because that was the
way their parents treated them as children. Negative punishment is preferable to
striking a child, both because it accomplishes whatever positive punishment brings
about and because it prevents long-run psychological damage that may follow
physical punishment. There is a better way to change a child's behavior, which we
will look at shortly.

Two examples of a parent's employment of negative (depriving) punishment
are in the phrases "You may not watch your favorite television show this evening"
and "Because you hurt your brother, you may not go out to play after supper."
Withdrawal of social contact is another example of negative punishment, the
"freeze treatment" not being uncommon between two individuals who seek to
punish each other by not speaking.

Any supermarket provides opportunity to see positive punishing consequences administered to children. That source, along with observing parent/
child interactions in neighborhoods and reading survey reports, informs us that
parental administration of physical harm or hurtful social behaviors (slapping,
shaking, screaming, name calling, shaming) is not a rarity. These parental behaviors
probably represent modeling of behaviors used on them by their parents or show
ignorance of how desirable behaviors can be established and maintained by
positive reinforcement.

Positive punishment of children is sometimes sanctioned when parents get
together and inevitably discuss child-management techniques during which
"spanking" behaviors are socially reinforced. Sometimes physical punishment is
institutionally supported. Advertising for sturdy canes for whipping children
appeared in the education journals of other countries as recently as ten years ago. A
number of years ago the headmaster of a private Maryland school was sued for
physically abusing a student. The court hearings revealed that all teachers at that
church-based school were required to whip children for any infraction of the
school's severe rules. In court the headmaster was quoted as saying that the only
way to eliminate undesirable behavior was to follow God's orders to beat children.

Four negative outcomes of positive punishment (physically or psychologically hurting another) are provided by Nemeroff and Karoly (1991), who
observe that this kind of punishment first:.5

> seems only temporarily to suppress [the undesired behavior], rather than
> permanently removing it. This implies that when punishment is discontinued or
> is avoidable, the punished behavior may reappear. . . . [W]hat punishment often
> teaches is simply how to avoid punishment. Second, punishing stimuli can
> create fear so that the person administering it and the situation in which it is
> administered can themselves become classically conditioned aversive stimuli.
> Third . . . it may in fact serve to demonstrate or model the use of violence as a
> way of coping with problems. Thus, while the behavior may be suppressed in
> the presence of the punisher, it may actually *increase* elsewhere. Finally,
> punishment procedures are . . . uninformative in that they only indicate . . . what
> *not* to do (and sometimes the substitute behavior that emerges is as problema-
> tic as the behavior being treated) [pp. 131–132].

**Extinction.**   The other procedure for reducing or extinguishing a behavior is a
bit more complex because there is a classical, or typical, mode and also a subsidiary
mode. The usual, or classical, mode, that for which the word *extinction* has long
been applied, is the withdrawing or withholding of a positive reinforcer (–C+) that
had been maintaining a behavior. If an animal has been given food each time after
performing a certain behavior, with no other reinforcing consequence happening
at the same time, and then is no longer given food after engaging in the behavior,
the theoretical likelihood is that the behavior will extinguish. Of course, the
behavior may have become associated with some other unintended and un-
recognized reinforcer and thus be maintained even after the food reinforcer is
stopped.

A subsidiary of this extinction is employed when there is *no extrinsic consequence* (response from outside the individual) that follows the behavior. This is an
infrequently needed option for deliberate use, but because this form of extinction,
absence of any environmental response, occurs all the time in the real world, it
needs to be understood. The phrase *no response* will be employed here because its
purpose is not extinction in the classical sense, since no behavior has been
regularly occurring. The intent is to prevent the likelihood that a behavior that has
just occurred will become established. Even if the environment does not provide
any positive consequences to a random or accidental behavior, there may be
intrinsic (within the individual) positive consequences that will strengthen the
probability that the person will repeat that behavior.

Any of us can perform a vast number of possible behavior patterns. The
relative psychological law says that, other things being equal, those patterns that
produce positive outcomes will have an increased probability of recurring. If no
desirable condition is consequent to a behavior in which a person may inadvertently (but not necessarily so) engage, the probability is high that the behavior
will not recur. Why should it? No positive consequence came from doing it.

That principle of "no response" is sometimes knowingly applied by
knowledgeable (and patient) parents of young children who have engaged in
undesirable behaviors: they ignore the behavior. To illustrate, let us imagine a first
home visit by a family's religious leader to a parent and a 3-year-old son. Despite

the parent's (useless) prior admonitions to the boy to "behave" because the visitor is important, he may quite naturally show off. He brings toys into the living room (not normally permitted there) and while pretending to ignore the adults, engages in loud imaginary behaviors addressed to the toys accompanied by throwing them about, all in the hope of being rewarded by attention from the adults.

Some parents may employ punishing behaviors right then or, worse, after the visitor leaves—worse because the punishment is not an immediate consequence of the undesired behavior. If the child is alone playing quietly after the visitor leaves, and the parent, now experiencing the anger that had been restrained while the visitor was present, seeks out and "spanks" the child for his earlier, disruptive actions, the parent is also inadvertently punishing the quiet playing, reducing the probability that such desirable behavior will be continued.

The knowledgeable parent, however, would quietly ask the visitor to "just ignore him and he'll stop." The parent is correct in meaning that the attention-seeking aspect of the child's activities may stop for lack of reinforcement, but the play itself may continue because it is intrinsically reinforced, as shown by the many times a child engages in play when not seeking attention. Attention is often a reinforcing consequence, whether it is doting praise for the child's imaginative play, even if it also annoys (a sure route to brathood), or disapproval of behavior. Some children engage in negative actions to get attention if they have learned that such behavior is the only way to get recognition of their otherwise unacknowledged presence. Existentially, for this period of their lives, they have no being unless indulging in negative actions.

## Variations in Positive Reinforcers for Humans

"Food" is a primary reinforcer. People may eat "food," but individuals do not, and a counselor's concern is with individuals. The word *food* was put in quotation marks to connote an abstract concept. Individuals, however, eat specific foods and avoid others, which leads to another aphorism: one person's meat is another's poison. This axiom introduces an essential characteristic of positive reinforcers: they must be identified for each individual. All people indeed do eat, but if food is to be employed, it had better be known that Loraine not only dislikes chocolate but is severely allergic to it. On the other hand, it is a favorite of Jeff. A behavior of neither Loraine nor Jeff would be positively reinforced by the treat Ibrahim receives in his homeland: sheep eyes. These three children were born with a need for food; the kind of food each prefers is physiologically (genetically) and culturally determined (conditioned). Furthermore, the potency of these reinforcers may change for several reasons. Thus, what reinforces an individual now cannot be assumed to be a reinforcer later.

Those points also apply to another form of positive reinforcers, called secondary, which are learned, or acquired, reinforcers, such as a material thing or a reinforcer still more remote from primary ones, money. Money has no intrinsic value except for the miser or numismatist. It is symbolic: it stands for the purchase of desired services or things. It can even be replaced as a reinforcer by another level of symbolism in which checks are employed instead of money, or just a statement that money has been deposited in an account held by the person.

Such a regular infusion of funds for many people, called a salary or wages (the technical term: fixed-interval reinforcement), maintains their employment behaviors. Stop the wages or salary, and the individual's occupational behavior patterns are extinguished, a case of –C+. The extinction results not from withholding a life necessity, such as food or water, but from withholding a learned symbol, a secondary reinforcer.

## Social Reinforcers

Primary reinforcers relate to biological essentials; secondary reinforcers are learned and are often symbolic. Receipt of attention, affection, and approval are pleasures at all ages. If audiences no longer applauded (–C+), acting and other forms of public performance would probably disappear. Signs of affection, particularly physical ones like hugs, praise for achievements, or any kind of positive statement from significant other persons makes any of us feel pleased and gives us a sense of significant meaning in life. These powerful reinforcers are social ones, of course, because of their interpersonal nature.

Are social reinforcers primary or secondary? Mortality is high among institutionalized orphaned infants whose only attention is sanitation and feeding by a bottle held at their mouths by slings. Those infants who live show retardation along numerous variables. Attention and affection are surely life-significant for those infants, and therefore are primary. Whether a reinforcer is primary or secondary is of some technical interest, but for our consideration it is sufficient to recognize that certain social responses have a powerful influence and that they can be deliberately used. The power inherent in social reinforcers is a reason to advise parents not only to ignore undesirable behavior when possible but also to notice when children are acting desirably and to promptly socially reinforce those behaviors. A not-infrequent complaint of adolescents is that their parents are quick to find fault but never offer praise.

## Behaviors and Behavior Patterns

In a few instances a precisely defined behavior is established and maintained when followed by positive consequences. In a hypothetical electronic game, for example, the pressing of a button within a second after a light appears, if it is accompanied by a tone, enables the player to accumulate points. If the button is pressed when the light comes on but is not accompanied by the tone, points are lost. A first-time player may have a zero average score because the desired behavior has not yet been established and there are equal correct (C+) and incorrect (C–) responses. With a speed that varies among individuals, the player learns to push the button when both light and tone are presented (the behavior is positively reinforced, or +C+) and to avoid pushing the button when the light is on but not accompanied by the tone (the behavior of restraint is negatively reinforced, or –C–).

Most human actions are not that simple, however. Consider a simple act like cigarette smoking; it is not a single behavior like the button-pushing act above; it is a behavior pattern, a chain of a number of behaviors. For example, something cues an urge to smoke. The first behavior of a chain can be to reach into a pocket or purse for a pack, followed by bringing it into the open, tilting or tapping it, grasping the cigarette, extracting it, moving arm and hand to the mouth, getting and then using a lighting device, and, finally, drawing in the smoke.

Illustrations in this chapter are sometimes chains of a number of behaviors or otherwise multiple behaviors occurring simultaneously. These are more accurately called behavior patterns, but for ease of reading the word *behavior* alone will usually be used.

## Mixed Consequences of Behaviors

To understand a client's operantly conditioned behaviors, we must identify the consequences that maintain those behaviors. Even a simple behavior may be followed by two or more consequences that compete, but it is more likely that competing responses will follow complex behaviors. Even if consequences are separated by time, they can nonetheless become associated with a behavior. An adolescent, for example, is new to the community and school and has been feeling lonely, avidly hoping to be accepted by a clique of high-status peers. By chance, she may engage in a behavior that is contrary to family and other adult mores, but it receives powerful social reinforcement from that clique, creates a sense of euphoria in her, and brings about repetition of the behavior.

Given this girl's sense of not belonging, the positive consequences that immediately follow her chance behavior are powerful reinforcers, more potent than the negative consequences that may follow if her parents hear of her actions— future consequences of which she is only barely aware as she relishes the immediate positive consequences of her behavior.

Another adolescent, however, faced with the identical wish for acceptance by that clique, is inhibited from emitting that behavior because the prospect of punishment is more potent. Many adolescents must struggle with the presence of two competing consequences of a behavior, such as a positive peer consequence and a negative adult consequence. It is through these struggles that the adolescent matures, even growing positively from an occasional violation of a long-held moral or ethical principle.

Animal experiments also demonstrate the effect of competing responses to an act. A rat can be trained to get food by pressing a lever. A grid that can be electrically charged is placed in front of the dispenser from which the rat gets its food. The rat is deprived of food, is therefore motivated to eat, and then is released. It goes promptly to the lever and depresses it to receive the pellet, a behavior that has been strongly reinforced. But now when the lever is pressed, an electric current of sufficient strength to be painful is also run through the grid. There are now two competing stimuli: press the lever for food, which would be a positive reinforcement for lever-pressing, or do not go for food, thereby escaping the shock, a negative reinforcement of the withholding behavior.

Individuals of an animal species differ as do humans, so there can be differences among individual rats in their responses to these competing stimuli.

For one, the need for food may be paramount so the rat, therefore, will continue to press the lever, despite the shock. When the rat's hunger is at least partially sated, it will discontinue feeding. Another rat may leave the feeding point at the initial shock, and others may leave after a shorter or longer time.

In human lives the mix of positive and punishing consequences is vastly more complex because of different but simultaneous mental processes occurring, and it is further complicated by affect. These tangles challenge the counselor's knowledge and skill when a client asks for help with a behavior. The counselor will set about acquiring a detailed description of the behavior and the context in which it typically occurs, and will assess the positive and negative reinforcers and the punishers. The behavior will not be understood until the cognitions that are an integral part of the behavior are examined and the significance of concurrent moods and emotions are appraised.

# Results of Behavior Research

## *Schedules of Reinforcement*

There is more to the understanding of reinforcing consequences of behaviors than identifying only that they occur. Consequences have been studied in both laboratory and other settings relative to "how quickly, how regularly, after how many discrete responses, or after how much elapsed time, reinforcement is applied" (Nemeroff & Karoly, 1991, p. 129). This inquiry led to the identification of four schedules by which reinforcement in laboratory studies can be provided: *fixed-interval* (reinforcement will be provided for a behavior the first time it appears after a predetermined amount of time has elapsed), *variable-interval* (the periods between reinforcements are more random but occur around a predetermined average), *fixed-ratio* (reinforcement will be provided after a set number of times the behavior occurs), and *variable-ratio* (the number of occurrences of the behavior before reinforcement is not set, but an average number is predetermined, and the number of reinforcers is fewer or more than that average).

A particular form of fixed-ratio reinforcement that logic would apparently call for as the best schedule is *continuous reinforcement.* A desirable consequence is provided every time the target behavior (the one planned for reinforcement) occurs. Logically best, but experimentally not so. Continuous reinforcement does build the target behavior quickest, but extinction of that behavior is more rapid after withdrawal of the continuous-reinforcement schedule. To build the behavior quickly and to maintain it, continuous reinforcement should be faded into the more effective schedule, *intermittent* (random) *reinforcement.*

## *Shaping Behaviors*

A behavioral technique, *shaping,* illustrates application of some behavioral principles. The assumption is that a certain behavior is desirable but the animal or human does not behave that way. The desired behavior is described, and because it is the one to be realized, it is called the target behavior.

The target behavior for animals may be complex. Skinner, for example, trained pigeons to play table tennis, at least to move the ball over the net. This filmed achievement is a dramatic example of behavior established and maintained by reinforcement, but incidentally it also led Skinner to hope that he was not to be remembered chiefly as the psychologist who had taught pigeons to play table tennis. This target behavior had to be attained by training the pigeons to engage in a simple behavior, which was established through reinforcement. Then a new behavior could be added to that first simple one, and reinforced, and so on until the target behavior was reached through a process called shaping.

How much more complex the behaviors of humans, welded as they are to affect and cognitions. Yet the same principle of shaping applies, illustrated by the target behavior of studying in the case of Paul, a high school junior. He is a person of academic potential but had no disciplined study habits, and consequently had a poor achievement record. He had recently acquired an urge to achieve, a wish long held by his parents, who, after years of nagging, had given up on him. There may have been a number of reasons for the absence of study behaviors, but in any case these behaviors were not going to be acquired simply by his willing them to exist or by parental nagging.

Paul asked his counselor in school how he could elevate his grade-point average. The interview quickly brought out the absence of a disciplined approach to studying, and that fact along with other information that Paul provided showed the counselor the appropriateness of a shaping procedure. With Paul's approval, the counselor explained the plan to his father (his mother could not attend). The plan also called for teacher cooperation. Parent and teacher support were necessary because they controlled the external reinforcement of behaviors for this plan.

During an earlier conference with the counselor, Paul revealed that he was eager to have new stereo speakers, but he knew his parents would not buy them for him because of his poor grades, and he had no job. This wish for speakers became central to a contingency-management contract that the counselor prepared in consultation with Paul and his father and then explained to the appropriate teachers.

Under the provisions of the contract, Paul would carry out certain highly specific requirements over a nine-week span, starting a week before a new grading period began. For the performance of each required behavior, the parents would pay Paul a predetermined sum, to be used only for the purchase of the agreed-upon equipment. The contract was begun by the youth merely sitting at a clean desk in a quiet room at home for a brief period (no phone calls permitted). No other requirement; just sit at the clean desk. For this behavior he received the stipulated sum. The desk-sitting periods were extended. (The quantity of the secondary reinforcer, money, remained the same—the effort needed to earn it was slowly increased.) New behaviors were added one by one, with increased time required for each one; each was followed by positive reinforcement. The contracted progression: having school books on the desk, having one book open to a teacher-assigned spot, reading assigned pages, taking notes on assigned pages (several days or even more than a week passed as each of these steps was reached), and eventually study of all assigned texts and submission of required written work. The plan called for teachers to acknowledge success in each of these latter steps by notes to his parents, reporting when he had met assignments and had fruitfully participated in class activities. Meanwhile, the counselor monitored his progress and provided social reinforcement. Paul saw (and felt) the continuing increase of funds for his eagerly desired purchase.

During the planning conferences with the counselor, the idea of cognitive controls over studying behavior was explained, and specific cognitions to employ were established. As Paul took each step, he was to tell himself before the step what he was to do, how it was to be done, and how nothing would distract him from the step. After taking each step, he would tell himself what he had done, how important that was to good studying habits, and how well he had behaved. Those cognitions produced positive changes in Paul's concept of self, changes that would contribute to the attainment of his counseling objective. These cognitive steps were monitored and socially reinforced by the counselor during the period of this contract. The counselor saw no need to attend to emotion except to provide social reinforcement of Paul's increasing confidence and enthusiasm.

By the end of the contingency-management contract, good study habits had been shaped and chained (behaviors locked in a sequence), and Paul's goal of improvement in academic achievement had been reached. Those behaviors were maintained after parental material reinforcers were no longer supplied, because social reinforcers increasingly took over: not only parent and teacher praise but also acknowledgment from students, particularly the welcomed comments from Kitty, whom Paul had recently found it important to impress. Also potent in maintaining his new study behaviors were intrinsic reinforcements: changes in cognitions that let him think differently, and now positively, about himself, praising himself for specific achievements and seeing that higher-education goals were now far more likely to be attained. Oh yes, and enjoying his new stereo speakers.

This illustration shows the importance of the behavioral maxim "Think small." Many of us are accustomed to thinking about behavior patterns as just one behavior and attempting to reinforce or extinguish "that behavior"—studying or smoking, for example. Change in these behavior patterns requires attention to the discrete behaviors that each comprises, so, Think small.

## *Choice? Take Reinforcement over Alternatives*

When I discussed punishment I offered two alternatives for a parent to reduce or eliminate an undesirable behavior, adding a note that a better way would be examined later. The alternative: rather than using either type of punishment, *replace* ("overprint") the undesirable behavior with a desirable one. For any undesirable behavior, there is one or more preferable alternates. The principle: instead of "attacking" the undesirable behavior, an activity that may have the undesirable side effect of conditioning the child against the "attacker," select an incompatible preferred behavior, induce its appearance if it does not appear spontaneously, and reinforce that behavior. The energy employed is used constructively, not in fighting the unwanted actions. If an older child acts resentfully about a recently born sibling, instead of punishing the older child for the harmful actions he or she may exhibit, design a preferred opposite behavior, or hope for the spontaneous emergence of one, and reinforce it. If the reinforcers are sufficiently strong (and appropriate cognitions are employed), the new behavior will replace the undesirable behavior.

An earlier comment deserves repetition and elaboration: some parents and teachers are quick to notice a child's "bad" behavior, perhaps because that kind of behavior either is a direct personal (psychological) attack on the adult, such as "talking back," or disturbs the smooth functioning of the household or classroom. Some adults' approach to changing that kind of behavior is to punish it, possibly resulting in the unwanted effects explored earlier. Counselors in schools, in addition to helping individuals develop plans or work through developmental problems, also help teachers learn how to manage classes, when asked. They remind teachers to be watchful for times when children are doing "good" things and to reinforce those behaviors. The confident teacher and parent can occasionally overlook a child's "bad" behavior, explaining to the child why that behavior is not to be done while at the same time reminding the child how he or she usually does the correct thing.

By reading, through parenting classes, or in consultation with a psychological counselor, parents become aware that they have been practicing behavior management from a child's earliest days, without using that term, of course. If concern is expressed about a child's undesirable behavior, parents can find out if their behavior-management system has been faulty and how it can be corrected. Just telling parents (academic instruction only) is not enough for them to reach the goals of good parenting; assisted practice enables them to replace undesirable child-rearing procedures with desirable ones. Parenting programs, therefore, help parents learn to manage their own behaviors and to reinforce their desirable child-management practices. They see that their behaviors are under the same laws of reinforcement or extinction as their children's, although, of course, cognitive approaches can be more effective among adults than they can be with young children. A parent who is skilled in child-management techniques (these supplement, not replace, love and tender nurturance) is a comfortable, confident parent.

### *Bribery?*

Some people when learning about behavior-management procedures find at first that certain behavioral principles appear to contradict values they internalized early in life and to which they are strongly committed. In the shaping program used to build Paul's study habits, and therefore improve his academic attainments, he earned money from his parents and saved it throughout the management contract, then used it for an agreed-upon purpose. Some object that payment of money to a child to do what he or she "ought" to do as a matter of character or principle is bribery. (Paul "ought" to study, and if he doesn't, he is showing bad character.) The response is twofold. Bribery customarily means payment for an illegal or unethical action, which does not fit this instance. The other rejoinder is more general and emphatic: *all* behaviors are engaged in to obtain the rewards they provide. The employed parent receives money regularly from an employer, but that is not thought of as bribery, although it does maintain the employee's occupational behaviors. A parent's behaviors for a full day can be recorded, and in each instance a reinforcer can be identified for that behavior. The goal of having a child learn to study, a learning need built on a sound psychological principle (shaping) and no different from those employed to learn to play tennis, is a highly desirable outcome. The use of money as reinforcer is merely a modification of Grandma's Rule: "Eat all your vegetables, and Grandma will give you a piece of her peach pie." The Donkey Rule we recall: "Do all these tasks, and you'll receive a carrot." The Sales Rule is not bribery: "For every one of these you sell, you'll get a commission." Behavior management, whether self-initiated or initiated by others, is similar to employment. "If I do each of these little steps that leads to a big goal, I will pay myself in some fashion" (self-initiated), or "As you do each of these small steps towards a larger goal, you will be paid materially and socially" (behavior managed by someone else, as in Paul's case). The goal in behavior-management programs that begin with contrived reinforcement is to arrive at the time when the behavior pattern will be maintained by reinforcers naturally available in daily life so that the contrived ones are no longer needed. Behaviors that can be identified as "good character" are built this way.

## *Alienation*

Alienation, the existentialist term for the separation of a person from his or her culture, from a life purpose, is one of the first modern explanations for humans' discontent. Indeed, early psychotherapists were called alienists, but that term is now used only in forensic psychiatry. Alienation is not a term that gives clear counseling clues, but it does convey the difficulty. In behavioral terms, it describes the useless feeling and despairing state of people who are cut off from positive consequences, who are prevented from having a sense that their life makes a difference or has meaning. One is a stranger—an alien—in one's own psychological country. Alienation is more likely to be an affliction of those urbanites in occupations whose outcomes are not tangible or knowable. How common is this state? No data have been collected. In the early days of psychiatry, only economically well-off urbanites knew about it, could afford the fees, and would have been likely to sense severe alienation. Those few could patronize an alienist in hopes of being restored to the citizenship of personal meaning.

If not alienated, in what state are the permanently unemployed men living in city cores, devoid as they are of the positive consequences of being effective in occupations and interpersonal relationships and without hope of change? For most of them there are no opportunities for reinforcement of socially useful, personally constructive behaviors.

It is not only the permanently poor who can experience alienation. A well-paid white-collar worker may receive papers from an unknown other person on which he or she performs some routine action and then sends them on to some other unknown. Such an employee is active all day long but does not experience the reinforcement that comes from seeing that each bit of daily effort is contributing to an outcome in which pride can be taken, the sense of accomplishment that is the reinforcing experience of a cabinetmaker, for example.

For many adults a major sense of personal meaning, of having an identity that results from creating worthy consequences, comes from creative participation in their children's formative years. If economic necessity requires both parents to be employed and have long trips to work, opportunities for enriching and reinforcing experiences with their children are diminished. If their employment is as unfulfilling as that of the white-collar worker described above, they are both occupationally and parentally alienated from conditions that would provide reinforcement for their behaviors.

### *From Laboratory to Life*

The empirical evidence on which behavioral principles have been established emerged primarily from laboratory experiments, primarily on animals, for well over a half-century. More recent experimentation with human subjects in both laboratory and real-life conditions has progressed to the point where a substantial body of evidence now supports the employment of operant-based procedures with clients in a variety of settings and with varying concerns about specific behaviors.

As noted earlier, decades ago Eysenck conducted single-subject-design studies at the Institute of Psychiatry of the University of London, and experiments in psychiatric hospitals in the United States have been continuous. Wilson (1984) reports the studies by Paul and Lentz of hospitalized mental patients that "produced a wealth of objective data, including evidence of cost effectiveness, showing that behavioral procedures . . . are the treatment of choice" (p. 264). Nemeroff and Karoly (1991), reviewing the topic of behavioral medicine, demonstrate the extensive spread of applied behavioral techniques to numerous physical and psychological concerns. They summarize with the observation that "the degree to which behavioral medicine has become a major focus of interest for applied behavioral analysts is illustrated by the fact that an entire recent issue of *Behavior Modification* was devoted to the topic" (p. 152).

Wilson (1984) reports on other problems for which the efficacy of behavioral therapy has been demonstrated by controlled, clinical investigations in various countries. These include phobias, depression, sexual disorders, interpersonal and marital problems, cardiovascular disease, and a number of childhood disorders. O'Leary and O'Leary (1976), among others, have demonstrated the application of operant principles in elementary schools.

In the concluding comments of their chapter, Nemeroff and Karoly assert that "a strain of old-fashioned positivism, operationalism, and reductionism is still quite dominant among many behavioral investigators" (1991, p. 155). Other clinicians, who at one time may have subscribed to such positivism as the antidote to including mental processes in research or practice, "now recognize that careful analyses, beyond the level of instrumental [operant] performance, can and should be employed if a complete picture of the adaptive process is desired" (p. 155). Wilson offers a comparable comment:

> Behavior therapy emphasizes corrective learning experiences in which clients variously acquire new coping skills and improved communication competencies, or learn how to break maladaptive habits and overcome self-defeating emotional conflicts. In contemporary behavior therapy these corrective learning experiences *involve broad changes in cognitive, affective, and behavioral spheres of functioning; they are not limited to modifications of narrow response patterns in overt behavior* [p. 253; emphasis added].

# Concluding Reflections

Counselors who function at full competence know the importance of operant principles in all people's daily lives, but at the same time they know that clients' concerns cannot be dealt with from an operant basis that would ignore the affect and mental processes associated with an individual's functioning in a systems relationship with the environment. In this critical issue the "new" psychology, which is humanistic as well as empirical, differs from the material sciences.

"Humanistically oriented psychology is correct," Manicas and Secord (1983) aver, "in insisting that because phenomena of consciousness are real, psychology constitutes a different level of stratification from the material sciences" (p. 406). Causal mechanisms are the heart of science, they note, so it is correct for psychology to study the causal properties of psychological structures and processes, as happens in positivism. In psychology, however, it is erroneous to construe such causal statements as showing invariance between antecedents and specific behaviors.

In Chapter 4 a child psychiatrist, Winnicott (1986), is quoted as saying that for the developing person "there can be no *do* before *be.*" A behaviorist may counter, "We are what we do, and thus there can be no *be* before *do.*" Is either of those statements "the truth"? Each surely bears a portion of truth. It may be more correct to say that "do" and "be" transact, are instantaneous cause and effect of each other, but in any case counselors need to attend equally to being and doing.

The relatively recent attention of academic as well as applied psychologists to mental processes has been noted here numerous times. This change has come to be commonly called the cognitive revolution. At the same time another counterforce, a humanistic revolution, has occurred in psychology. Just as cognitivists do not find adequate a science that does not account for mental processes, humanists cannot find a science to be adequate that does not attend to humans' intentionality, to the existential nature of human life. Positivist science addresses human concerns with the same objective aloofness that scientists employ in material areas of inquiry. This condition is viewed by some psychologists as erroneous because humans' lives center on values, aspirations, and other distinctively human cognitive characteristics. Humanistic psychologists help identify to *what* cognitions psychology should attend. The cognitivists and humanists thus complement each other.

Some psychological theorists and counselors remain committed to positivism, of course. For them, the only defensible study and application of psychology comes from experiments on observable phenomena. On the other hand, some practitioners are so committed to either cognitive or humanist positions that they ascribe no usefulness to what the science of positivistic psychology has so rigorously tested and demonstrated in the past half-century. Commitment to either indefensibly exclusive stance would result in counselors of diminished vision and competence.

There is an irony in the existence of any present discord between humanism and science. Thoreson (1973) has observed that "many contemporary humanists now oppose the scientific world view" that was initiated by Renaissance scholars, a world view that originated "as a reaction against the revealed truth of the Church and the dominance of Aristotelian thinking" (p. 386), the antihumanistic forces that dominated life for over a millennium. Science created humanism; now the humanist must oppose the postivism that has come to mark the science that studies humans as psychological beings.

I offer a final observation to sum up this topic: the laws of operant conditioning, the product of positivism, must be applied to counseling concerns when appropriate because they are indisputable, and counselors must always employ empirically demonstrated procedures. Their application to the development (shaping) of behavior in animals and young children is a boon to those concerned with either population. When the developmental concerns of older children and adults need to be addressed by counselors, consideration of cognitions and affect take on increasing significance. If operant conditioning were put under oath, it could swear with clear conscience to be "the truth and nothing but the truth." It could not swear without perjury to be "the whole truth."

# ■        **Points to Remember**        ■

1.  Every person's waking day is filled with "doing" something. Even "just sitting" is doing something. Science provides a substantial base for knowing why people act as they do.
2.  Emotions serve to defend or enhance one's psychological being. An individual's behavior similarly amplifies desired outcomes and minimizes undesired ones.
3.  In the terms employed by psychologists, behaviors that have desirable results are reinforced (strengthened) by those results. Conversely, undesirable (punishing) consequences weaken the behavior. What science has done is specify the conditions under which actions are strengthened or weakened, enabling counselors and others to use those techniques.
4.  Two kinds of consequences of a behavior reinforce it: the direct positive consequence ($+C+$), called positive reinforcement, and a consequence that permits avoidance of present or prospective pain ($-C-$), called negative reinforcement.
5.  There are two kinds of positive reinforcements ($+C+$): primary, or natural, consequences, which satisfy biological needs or provide pleasures to the senses, and secondary, or learned, reinforcers, such as money and praise.
6.  There are two kinds of punishers ($+C-$): positive punishment, which refers to an undesirable consequence directly sensed by an individual, and negative punishment, which is indirect, usually in the form of a loss of a pleasure.
7.  Punishing consequences ($+C-$) result in a decrease in the likelihood that an action will be repeated. Another way to decrease the likelihood is to withhold positive reinforcers ($-C+$), a process technically labeled extinction.
8.  A subset of extinction calls for the withholding of *any* kind of reinforcement. This does not appear in Figure 7-1, but it would be symbolized as (0.C.0). This process is designed to minimize the likelihood that a behavior that has just appeared in a person's repertoire will be continued. It is called ignoring.

9. Punishment of one person by another may result in the elimination of a behavior, but there are often secondary, undesirable consequences. The preferred action is to reinforce a behavior that competes with and therefore eliminates the undesired behavior.

10. The consequence of an action is most often mixed; that is, desirable and undesirable consequences result from the action. Whether or not the action is strengthened or weakened depends on the potency of the positive or negative consequences, the context in which the action occurred, and the cognitions and emotions associated with it.

11. Alienation, an affliction of urban economies, can be understood as the consequences of daily behavior that are inadequate as reinforcements, both in quantity and quality.

■                 **Counselor Formation Activities**                 ■

1. Think of your life as a child and adolescent. Recall the actions your parents took to train you in the behaviors they considered desirable and their actions after you did something they did not want you to do.

   a. Were their procedures mostly punishment (+C–), generally ignoring the times when you were behaving desirably? When they acknowledged the times you were doing well, doing what they valued, what was the nature of that reinforcing reaction (+C+)? In which ways did your mother and father differ in their reactions to your behaviors? How did that difference affect the continuation or stopping of any behavior? Were the responses to your behaviors made by both parents consistent over time?

   b. Classify any punishments you received as positive or negative. Did your parents' punishing or reinforcing responses affect your behaviors?

   c. If regularly or at times you are now in a position of responsibility for younger persons (as parent, teacher, child-minder, youth leader), do you generally manage their behaviors similarly to the way you were reinforced or punished by adults when you were a child and adolescent? What positive reinforcers do you use to maintain good behavior, and what punishment, negative or positive, do you use to extinguish undesirable behavior? What have you done, or could you do, to *strengthen* desirable behavior through *negative reinforcement* (–C–)? What evidence have you seen that these particular procedures are developmentally sound? Do you ignore undesirable behavior (–C+) on the premise that if not attended to, it will extinguish?

2. Think of a friend of your generation with whom you frequently spend time. You do so because you "like to."

   a. Determine what makes that time together likable; that is, identify the specific reinforcements provided you by being with that friend.

   b. If you had a long-lasting friendship that no longer exists, identify specific examples of +C– and –C+ (refer to Figure 7-1) that contributed to extinguishing that friendship.

3. Think about your current or recent employment. What were the positive (reinforcing) consequences that occurred as you did *specific* tasks in that employment. Were they primary or secondary reinforcers? If you cannot identify reinforcers for specific tasks but you continue(d) in that employment, what general reinforcer caused that continuation?
4. Recall one or two of the numerous behavior patterns in which you have engaged as recreation for a long time (a hobby or sport, for example). Identify the positive consequences that have maintained those behaviors. Recall a behavior that existed for some time but no longer does. Identify the specific consequences of that behavior that caused it to extinguish.


■                      **Complementary Reading**                      ■

Although study of the principles of behavior has generated numerous texts that give a comprehensive treatment of the topic, introductory psychology texts offer adequate coverage. If your introductory study of psychology was done more than seven years ago, you will profit from examination of a newer introductory text.

Ultimately, a counselor's concern is in the application of those principles. Before reading one of the comprehensive texts, and as a brief substitute for material in any recent introductory text, I propose study of a brief exposition of how behavioral principles are applied to bring about client change. This will introduce behavioral principles and illustrate them with application procedures. I suggest either Nemeroff and Karoly (1991) or Wilson (1984).

# 8

**CHAPTER**

# Client Cognitions

## Overview

Clients bring cognitive, affective, and behavioral concerns to counselors. Counseling relative to any concern is cognitive, because it is by ideas expressed in words that counselors make a difference.

A number of educated laypeople, asked to say what the word *cognition* connotes, would respond that it refers to isolated thoughts or ideas of which an individual is cognizant and can express in words. Cognitive content and activities, for them, are solely rational. Theorists and other scholars of mental activities analyze cognitions into a more complex array of content and process. If prospective counselors were later to employ this central tool of counseling with no further understanding of its theoretical and practical complexity than that of the layperson, clients would not be adequately served. This chapter examines theoretical and other issues related to cognitions that are germane to counseling.

We will explore the organization of cognitions into structures and schemata. At times, bringing about changes in clients will require the restructuring of cognitive systems.

Laypeople may see cognitions as rational activities falling within the philosophy of rationalism (though they might not use the term), but theorists conceptualize cognitive content and process differently, using the term *developmentalism,* or *constructivism,* to be defined in the chapter. As this text is committed to the concept expressed by either term, the topic is covered in detail.

After examination of these theoretical issues, I will present an analysis of cognitive process and content, identifying three processes and six modes of content, with functional descriptions of each. Counselors' positive views of clients may lead them to accept client statements as valid. At the same time, counselors will be alert to the possibility that those statements may actually be distortions of reality or show faulty cognitive analysis. The last section of the chapter, then, considers some of the origins and appearances of cognitive distortion.

# Introduction

The term *cognitions* does not refer to a unitary concept of mental processes and contents; rather, it incorporates a number of both broad and specific constructs. It covers an assembly of words that have not yet acquired precise meaning. Indeed, anyone who acknowledges the importance of cognitions in counseling can be envious of the radical behaviorist, who is not faced with the task of extracting meanings from that pile of semantic jack straws. The variety of labels and descriptions found in the professional literature, Dobson and Block (1988) conclude, is overwhelming. They offer this list, described as partial: "cognitions, thoughts, beliefs, attitudes, ideas, assumptions, rules for living, self-statements, cognitive distortions, expectancies, notions, stream of consciousness, ideation, private meanings, illusions, self-efficacy predictions, cognitive prototypes and schemas" (p. 31).

Mental activity is not carried out in fragments casually employed. That activity, comprising cognitive processes and contents, is organized into a related and interdependent whole called cognitive structure.

# Cognitive Structures, or Systems

Each human functions as an organized whole and acts to maintain that organization, a ship holding to course despite storms. Guidano (1988) writes of the self-organizing paradigm, the fundamental invariant of each individual that symbolically manipulates self and environment to maintain his or her own organization. This is done "through an ongoing and generative process of self-renewal in order to assimilate incoming information and to cope with perturbations arising from [the individual's] exchanges with the environment" (p. 308). The cognitive system, in this view, "is characterized by its basic feature, namely the ability to construct models of self and the world capable of arranging and regulating reality itself" (p. 308).

The cognitive system is not present at birth but develops over time, probably with some genetic influence. Guidano (1988) provides a brief examination of this growth, with emphasis on the role of attachments because they nurture the development of one's uniqueness, serving as "a sort of template, [to provide] the child with a framework within which otherwise fragmentary information about self and world can be organized into a structured whole" (p. 312). As the child internalizes the characteristics of attachment figures through modeling and imitation, those figures become intertwined with the representation of the child's self and have long-range effects: "If children extract an image of themselves using their parents as a mirror, this image does not remain mere sensorial data but instead directs and coordinates self-recognition patterns until the children become able to perceive themselves consistently with that image" (p. 313). Attachment, then, because of its integrative power, helps the child organize the continuing and increasing flood of perceptions of self and environment.

The process of identification with others, Guidano comments, also provides cues to children by which their diffuse feelings are shaped into emotional schemata that give a sense of stability and of continuity. These schemata, in turn, give direction to cognitive abilities that affect the child's interactions with the world and thus the content of their self-knowledge. "The available content of cognitive processes can, in turn, change the intensity or quality of emotional experiences . . . influencing . . . further emotional differentiation" (p. 313).

Emotional schemata interacting with the cognitive process become elements in one's personality about which there is an inertial homeostatic urge. Despite that urge, changes can occur. Changes occur more frequently on the surface of personality than at the core of personality, "surface" and "core" being metaphorical and relative terms for which Lyddon (1990) speaks of first- and second-order changes. The surface changes permit easy adaptation to contingencies without the need for a major reconceptualization of the self. The core, or deep, changes, however:

> correspond to changes in patterns of attitude toward oneself as a result of the reconstruction of [deep rules about self]. The changed attitude toward oneself will consequently produce a modification of personal identity, which will in turn entail a restructuring of the attitude to reality through which the world can be seen and dealt with in a different manner [p. 322].

Both surface and deep changes are cognitive changes.

Does a psychological counselor become involved with bringing about second-order changes? A counseling psychologist might, but each counselor must ask, "Am I able to do that?" And the answer must always be determined by whether training and practice have given him or her the competence to do so. All counselors, being knowledgeable about development, know that a person who has not had to grapple with problems is an underdeveloped person. Said conversely, development into a mentally healthful adult requires, in Lyddon's (1990) words, periodic encounters with impediments to development, obstacles that lead to the necessary restructuring that is normal and necessary for psychological growth, particularly during adolescence. This imperative can occur "through some temporary increase in disorder—in other words, the experience of dis-order, dis-equilibrium, or dis-ease is necessary" for necessary changes to come about. Any desirable developmental change "is often preceded by system jolts, turbulent environmental stresses, or internal conflicts. . . . The course of human development [is] an ongoing process of organization, disorganization, and reorganization" (p. 123).

It would be an error in counseling practice not to recognize the normal need for restructuring of portions of personality from time to time during the developmental years, particularly in adolescence and extending into young adulthood. It may be that a client approaches a counselor for relief from the painful symptoms of change. It will be an error if the counselor becomes party only to the symptom relief the client seeks instead of providing support while the needed but psychologically painful cognitive restructuring occurs.

No matter if a cognitive content overlaps with other contents or is completely distinctive, no cognitive element functions as a separate entity. Cognitive elements are woven together into a cognitive structure that is unique for each person even though the elements of that individual's cognitions may be shared with many. The need in counseling generally is to assess cognitive *structure,* the interrelatedness of each client's cognitions, instead of focusing on a single cognitive content independent from other contents. Among Dobson and Block's list above, for example, the counselor might tap and deal with the content of beliefs, automatic thoughts, and values separately without knowing that they are actually elements of an interrelated whole—a structure—that requires a different (higher) level of assessment. Dobson and Block hold that cognitive structures are basic to clients' developmental continuity, that people who will come for counseling are those "struggling to maintain a particularly dysfunctional cognitive organization in the face of continuously challenging environment[s]" (1988, p. 29).

### *Schemata*

As there is a stable core of personality and then potentially unstable personality components that one may think of as lying at the surface of personality, there is not a single cognitive structure but a core structure and a number of substructures. Beck (1964; Beck & Freeman, 1990) labeled these substructures as *schemata,* rules that govern information processing and behavior in such categories as family, religion, culture, and so on. Cantor (1990) also describes schemata as "organized structures of knowledge about particular domains of life and of the self" (p. 736), a useful way to conceptualize the more specific cognitive structures whose processes and contents are more likely to be addressed by a counselor.

Thus, the potential role of clients' cognitions is usually not the simple one of a rational employment of words in an impulsive, off-the-top-of-the-head manner but, rather, a role that will require more extensive appraisal of clients' cognitive structures or schemata so that these can be restructured, if necessary, to meet clients' needs. In addressing some clients' concerns, such as in career planning, the need to appraise and change cognitive structures and schemata may be minimal.

## Rationalism versus Developmentalism/Constructivism

Long before scientists had amassed the vast knowledge of brain structure and function that exists today, philosophers and other educated people knew of the brain's existence. The brain was viewed as a thinking machine, and rationality was the maximum distinction between humans and animals, rationalists believing that "thought is the most powerful domain of human activity" (Mahoney, 1988, p. 364). An equally pervasive view, one still tenable to respected scholars, is of reality as objective, with relatively fixed characteristics that can be perceived. In Western society the pervasiveness of rationalism has more than abstract historical interest for counselors. It requires that they must commit to either rationalism or to a competing view called *developmentalism* by Mahoney, or *constructivism* by Lyddon (1990).

Numerous theorists have contributed to the developmentalist position, and the various topics of this text are based on one of its subtheories. Mahoney (1988) is one of its more cogent protagonists. (Also recall Steenbarger's views, recorded in Chapter 1.) You may recall from Chapter 4 Mahoney's comment that rationalists view the brain as a curator of information about the real world as a person perceives that world, whereas developmentalists are inclined to see the brain as an active sculptor of a person's experiences. Mahoney's developmentalist position stresses the importance of the qualities of flexibility, generativity, complexity, and resilience. In contrast with rationalism, developmentalism holds that even if a client clings to technically inaccurate beliefs, such beliefs may still bring about adaptive behavior patterns, while well-supported beliefs may bring about maladaptive behavior patterns (p. 370). Adaptation and development are the criteria by which cognitive process and content are to be evaluated, because the value of any mental representation lies primarily not in its objective accuracy but in how well it contributes to those two purposes. Thus, one's personal symbols that disagree with reality only *may* be, not must be, appropriate topics for a counselor's efforts for change when they are judged by the criteria of adaptation and development.

Lyddon (1990) sees that a problem-versus-process distinction marks the difference between the views of rationalists and developmentalists, or in his term, constructivists. A rationalist approach deals with a client's immediate concerns, with easing the client's distress, whereas "constructivist approaches are founded on the assumption that humans, as self-organizing, developing systems, actively construe or create their personal and social realities." The counselor, therefore, seeks to "facilitate clients' *self*-construction of new meanings in the context of a safe, caring, and, at times, intense relationship" (p. 124). Constructivists, therefore, tend to conceptualize client concerns as "developmental challenges that are typically accompanied by episodes of emotional disequilibrium" (p. 124). Disequilibrium is helpful to the client in the long run because it brings about needed restructuring; constructivists, therefore, "tend to encourage emotional experience, expression, and exploration" (p. 124). The counseling relationship is appropriate for dealing with emotion, Lyddon (1992) observes, because it is "the primary crucible for change and [constructivists] accordingly seek to establish a secure and caring relationship" (p. 453). Lyddon cites Neimeyer's (1990) view that counseling from a constructivist stand is more a *creative* than *corrective* enterprise in which the counselor "helps the client invent new and perhaps more viable understandings rather than directly challenging the validity of the client's belief system" (p. 453).

Rationalists believe that there is a stable reality that can be authentically known. That requires the fractioning of the cognitive process into two components: the knowable real world and the knower who acquires the knowledge. The constructivist, or developmentalist, takes the position that knowing, feeling, and acting are a unified expression of adaptation and development. "From this perspective," Mahoney observes, " 'knowing' (scientific and otherwise) is seldom technically logical, but always pervasively psychological" (1988, p. 370).

Mahoney sees differences between rationalist and developmental views in their philosophies, theories, and practices; these are presented in Tables 8-1 and 8-2.

**Table 8-1**

Theoretical differences between rationalist and developmental cognitive theories

| Concept/Area | Rationalist View | Developmental View |
|---|---|---|
| 1. Basic functions of human nervous system | It *controls* and directs action and feeling via *valid mental representations*. | It *orders* and organizes experience via *viable mental representations*. |
| 2. Nature of representation | Representations are accurate *copies* that *correspond* to the "real" world. | Representations are predominantly *tacit constructions* of order that constrain but do not specify plans of action. |
| 3. Body/brain relationship | *Cerebral primacy:* the brain leads and the body follows. | *Somatopsychic unity:* body and brain are inseparable and interdependent. |
| 4. Cognition/behavior/affect relationship | *Rational supremacy:* "higher" intellectual processes can and should direct feelings and actions. | *Holism:* thought, feeling, and action are structurally and functionally inseparable. |
| 5. Nature of emotionality | *Emotions as problems:* negative and intense affect are to be controlled or eliminated. | *Emotions are primitive, powerful knowing processes;* disorder and affective intensity are natural elements of development. |

*Note.* From "The Cognitive Sciences and Psychotherapy: Patterns in a Developing Relationship" (p. 372) by M. Mahoney, 1988, in K. Dobson (Ed.), *Handbook of Cognitive-Behavioral Therapies,* New York: Guilford Press. Reprinted by permission.

**Table 8-2**

Practical differences between rationalist and developmental cognitive therapies.

| Issue/Theme | Rationalist View | Developmental View |
|---|---|---|
| 1. Intervention emphases | a. Ahistorical; b. Problem-focused; c. Control-focused; d. Teleological | a. Historical; b. Process-focused; c. Development-focused; d. Teleonomic |
| 2. Conceptualization of problems | Problems are deficits, dysfunctions, or their emotional correlates; they should be redressed, controlled, or eliminated. | Problems are current and recurrent discrepancies between challenges and capacity limits. |
| 3. Conceptualization of affect | Affect, especially intense, and negative, *is* the problem; irrational and unrealistic cognitions are its cause. | Affect expresses a primitive and powerful form of knowing; emotional experience and expression and exploration should be encouraged. |
| 4. Therapeutic relationship | It entails technical instruction and guidance. | It entails a safe, caring, and intense context in and from which the client can explore and develop relationships with self and world. |

*Note.* Abstracted and condensed from "The Cognitive Sciences and Psychotherapy: Patterns in a Developing Relationship" (p. 376) by M. Mahoney, 1988, in K. Dobson (Ed.), *Handbook of Cognitive-Behavioral Therapies,* New York: Guilford Press. Reprinted by permission.

# Cognitive Process and Content

The mental (cognitive) world is awesomely complex. The congeries of terms or labels used by theorists to describe the elements of structure can be organized into two subsets, process and content. This division can be instructionally useful as long as it is remembered that process and content in reality function simultaneously. Some commonly used terms are summarized in these lists:

| *PROCESS* | *CONTENT* |
|---|---|
| Analytic thinking | Concepts |
|   (internal dialogue) | Data (information, knowledge) |
|   Logical reasoning | Convictions about self and |
|   Recalling (memory) |   world (life view) |
|   Problem solving |   Beliefs |
| Attributing |   Values |
| Imagining | Automatic thoughts |
| | Behavior-controlling rules |
| | Aspirations, goals |

Add to the admonition that process and content function inseparably the reminder that the terms used within each category are not fully discrete. Similarity between beliefs and rules can be noted, for example, yet there is sufficient difference between them to merit separate labeling.

Underlying all mental process and content is the fact of awareness, or consciousness: when awake, normal people continuously represent themselves symbolically—that is, by words and images—as they experience their environmental context moment by moment, with the context also symbolically represented. These symbols may be erroneous, of course, and the help of a counselor may be appropriate to correct some of them. One responsibility of counselors, therefore, is to seek out discrepancies between symbols by which clients represent themselves and their worlds and the realities of those clients and their worlds. When significant discrepancies are found, the counselor may see the need to restructure that portion of the clients' cognitions if, as in Mahoney's view (1988), such a challenge will contribute to adaptation and development. Consciousness permits humans to bring their past and anticipated future to bear on immediate events. Without awareness there would be no history to be employed when trying to cope with events being currently experienced.

## *Cognitive Processes*

***Analytic Thinking.***   The process of analytic thinking is built upon perceptions at the moment, on memory of bits of knowledge, on information comprising words or numbers or both, on rules, values, and aspirations, and perhaps on other content. Analytic thinking and its contents, such as vocabulary, are the subject of intelligence tests.

Analytic thinking, which is internal dialogue, is engaged in by all people of all intellectual levels but with obvious differences in the subjects addressed and the quantity and quality of content employed. The quality of the process and outcomes of the analytic thinking of a physicist or a psychologist as each ponders theoretical questions, for example, differs from that when either thinks about how to repair the toaster or about which course of action to take to achieve some simple satisfaction. Other people are limited by genes and environment to engaging only in limited forms of mental processes.

Analytic thinking results in analytic cognition, one of two kinds in Buck's view as reported by Lazarus (1991a). One kind of cognition results from a "buildup of meaning from originally meaningless bits in a stimulus display through linear scanning and digital analysis" (p. 359); that is, from reflective thinking about verbal and numerical information. Buck labels the other cognition syncretic. This is instantaneous awareness of the adaptive significance of an event—that is, the spontaneous interpretation of the event's meaning for that person at that moment in that context without internal dialogue. Instantaneous awareness permits people to act without reflection, or going through deliberate (volitional) cognitive stages (p. 359), as occurs, Lazarus writes, when emotions are elicited. He holds that the instantaneous appraisal a person makes of an event, which results in emotion, includes cognitive components but that these are not deliberate, rational, or at an aware level. They are automatic and involuntary.

***Attributing.***    Through the process of attributing, clients provide themselves with a reason they can accept as the cause of their behaviors. Clients may be accurate in their attributions, of course, but a counselor may also expect that clients' needs for psychological defense are present, requiring them to attribute the cause of their behavior to events or other people instead of themselves. Clients attribute causality to someone else or to some vague generality such as "the system" with a logic that convinces themselves and their psychologically unsophisticated peers or relatives of its accuracy. A counselor can be expected to reserve judgment about the accuracy of attributions, according them status as hypotheses.

***Imagining.***    Cognitive processes include imagining, the mental creation or representation of experienced events, fictional ones (fantasies), or a mix of both. Imagery is a mental process of counseling importance, employed in cognitive restructuring, manipulation of emotions, and modifications of behavior.

## Cognitive Content

***Concepts.***    The content of mental processing includes concepts that are broad abstractions acquired from experience: nationhood, fidelity, justice, and other areas of concern that are of wide significance.

***Data.***    Specific verbal and numerical data are employed in most cogitation, that kind of material often spoken of generically as knowledge.

***Convictions about self and world.***    The concepts of self and world that make up a person's life view are frequently employed in mental processing, particularly self-views. Some of these are beliefs (knowledge accepted on faith), and some are values (beliefs colored by affect). A person can believe without any affect that thunder causes milk to turn sour because "we've always known that; I have faith in the people who say that's true." A belief is tinted with affect when, for example, an individual maintains that "my kind of person" is better than other kinds, "as I've always been told." The individual can state that belief with emotion and will take emotionally driven action based on it if necessary to maintain what the belief posits. The emotional component of affective-tinted beliefs becomes apparent when such views are challenged.

Among beliefs about oneself, Bandura (1989) observes that "none is more central or pervasive than people's beliefs about their capabilities to exercise control over events that affect their lives." This purposefulness reflects the fact that "people are . . . intentional cognizers with a capacity to influence their own motivation and action," instead of being neurophysiological computational machines (p. 1175). Bandura notes that most behavior, being purposive, is regulated by foresight—not to remote aims but to defined goals. A major purpose of thought is to enable people to predict events of personal significance and create means to exercise control over those that affect their daily lives. Imagery has a role, too: "Those who have a high sense of efficacy visualize success scenarios that provide positive guides for performance" (p. 1176).

Self-efficacy beliefs determine motivational strength and thus bear on the amount of effort and perseverance shown in the face of obstacles. On the other hand, perceived self-inefficacy can result in various forms of undesired consequences, including depression, and occurs from having to cope with tasks outside one's perceived self-efficacy range. "After perceived coping efficacy is strengthened . . . coping with the previously intimidating tasks no longer elicits [those undesirable consequences]" (p. 1177). That this is a developmentalist, or constructivist, position is borne out by Bandura's statement:

> Through their capacity to manipulate symbols and to engage in reflective thought, people can generate novel ideas and innovative actions that transcend their past experiences. They bring influence to bear on their motivation and action in efforts to realize valued futures. . . . The self is thus partly fashioned through the continued exercise of self-influence [p. 1182].

In parallel comments, Seeman (1989), in reporting how cognitive processes affect health, observes that two themes regularly emerge from the empirical literature, one related to affirmative self-definition and the other to "a sense of personal mastery and control over significant components of one's life" (p. 1105).

Belief about self-efficacy is but one among many beliefs about self, and obviously an individual will have many beliefs about the world. Bandura's observations accord with the thrust of this text that beliefs about self-efficacy are elemental in every person's effectiveness and thus are of particular importance in counseling.

***Automatic thoughts.***   Beck et al. (1990) employ the term *automatic thoughts* when they write about the specific suboral evaluative thoughts that course through anyone's awareness even as the person may be speaking with another about a different topic. These thoughts are one expression of a person's belief system as it relates to competencies and other expressions of self-worth. They are a factor in affect and behavior and thus are significant for counseling. Unlike openly expressed judgments about self, however, automatic thoughts exert a subtle influence. When exploring clients' cognitive worlds, a counselor will attend to their speech mannerisms for a variety of reasons, one of which is to look for clues of suboral thoughts coursing alongside their oral statements. At times a counselor's professional judgment will lead him or her to ask a client to record automatic thoughts as they occur at selected times between interviews.

A counselor also has automatic thoughts, which must be monitored for mental-health maintenance in general and counseling effectiveness specifically.

**Rules.**    Through experience each person comes to construct mental models, or rules about how "the world" works and how to interact with and manipulate it safely. These are a vital portion of one's life view, called world view by some others. Johnson-Laird comments (in Restak, 1988) that:

> The brain exists in order to construct representations of the world. Very simple organisms have no brains, construct no representations of the world. And the reason we probably have such large brains is in part because we live in a very complicated world, a complicated *social* world. We're social animals. So the brain has to do a great deal of computation in order to solve the very intricate problems that social life poses for us [p. 235].

Although rules by which people govern their behavior have been listed as a distinct content of cognitive structure, their overlap with other content is apparent. At times, however, a counselor will find it useful to facilitate increments in client self-knowledge by focusing on this topic. There may be similar outcomes if a client is asked to focus specifically on values.

**Aspirations, goals, and fantasies.**    Just as awareness permits clients to tap into their histories by memory, it permits them to look to the desired future by joining emotionally tinted self-views with imagery. Although no relative weight can be ascribed to the several contents, it can readily be seen that aspirations, goals, and fantasies about one's future can be powerful centripetal forces in a client's cognitive structure, related, of course, to self-efficacy beliefs.

Some theorists call the sum of cognitive contents and processes mind, about which, Searle (cited by Restak, 1988) writes:

> There is nothing more mysterious or mystic [about mind] than there is about digestion. What the brain does for the mind is what the stomach does for digestion. [Mental life and consciousness are] just an ordinary part of the physical world like anything else. [The mind is not a separate thing] but rather the sequence of thoughts, feeling, experience, and so-called mental phenomena that go on in it. "Mind" is the name of a process, not a thing. . . . We have this tradition that makes [the concept of mind] spooky, but there's nothing spooky about it. It's part of our biological life. The thing is, it's what matters most about our biological life. We can give up [body parts] [b]ut if we give up our consciousness, that's it. We're dead [p. 26].

# Cognitive Distortions

Client distortion of cognition, which can occur in either processes or content or both, is to be expected as long as it serves adaptive and developmental purposes. One can be staggered by the prevalence of superstitious belief in the Western world despite the availability of accurate information. Distorted self-views are reported despite experiences that should have provided accurate images of self, of which inaccurately debasing automatic thoughts are an example. The rules by which one lives may be not one's own but the inappropriate ones of others, and a client's aspirations and goals may be distortions of reality.

Beck, Rush, Shaw, and Emery (1979) identify six types of cognitive distortions: arriving at logically unsupportable conclusions; focusing on specific details while ignoring context; overgeneralizing (arriving at conclusions based on single experiences); over- or underevaluating the significance of events; personalization—that is, the relating of external events to self in the absence of any objective connection ("If I wash the car I just know it will rain"); and classifying experiences in extreme categories: either good or evil, all or none, and so on. These distortions, Beck and his colleagues find, are not autonomic, unconscious, primitive responses to events but are conscious. They serve an adaptive function, permitting the individual to cope with life's complexities. The counselor may avoid direct removal of such distortions, working instead to enable clients to rebuild their lives so that the need for such distortions is eliminated.

# Concluding Reflections: Part 2

Each client differs psychologically from all others in particulars just as each person's face differs from all others. At the same time, all humans resemble all others in some ways. As counselors we begin to understand the psychological functions of a particular client by being sensitive to the biological and cultural forces that shape the cognitions, feelings, and behaviors of all humans.

Part 2 was designed to strengthen concepts that were introduced earlier but whose significance for counseling may not have been sensed. One concept is that humans function as interrelated wholes, as systems. Cognitive processes and content, affect, and behaviors readily lend themselves to observation as distinct facets of a client's life. Although we may think of them as separate entities, these elements function as a unit, just as separate bodily organs function as systems, even as they are available for study as unique entities.

Similarly, each of us is locked into social systems, featuring psychologically vital affiliations and bonds. Daily experience may erode our awareness that our clients are biologically and psychologically imbedded in systems and that some of their concerns result from disruptions in those systems.

Cognitions are a major variable in the system that includes the client's affect and behaviors. A person's psychological functioning may be maladaptive as a result of distorted cognitions just as his or her physiological functioning may be negatively affected by a distorted heart. Counselors-to-be learn how to identify disruptive cognitive processes and content and will acquire the skills necessary to help clients (as explained in Chapter 10).

All individuals are affected by the environmental consequences of their behaviors in conjunction with the simultaneous control exercised by cognitions, mood, and emotions. This axiom does not reveal how a particular client will be so affected. Just as counselors must understand the role of cognitions and affect in clients' concerns, they also need to assess the affect of environmental consequences on behavioral patterns. Ultimately, counselors need to know each client's functioning as a relatively unique system comprised of interlocking elements.

Counseling that attends just to interlocked cognitions and behaviors is still not attending to all that bears on clients' concerns. Complete counseling takes into account individuals' affective states, their moods and emotions, two potent forces that have a bearing on cognitive functioning and behaviors. To think about affect is to again be made aware of the biological element in all human functioning: affective behaviors are overt expressions of biological functions, operating with other elements in a systems manner.

A primary professional characteristic of a master counselor is the ability to acquire accurate assessments of clients' complex lives—their cognitions, affect, and behaviors—and to use language that enables clients to reach their objectives by overcoming obstacles. Through words, humans "create and construe their personal and social realities" (Mahoney, 1988, p. 364).

# ■ Points to Remember ■

1. The constant cognitive mental activity that all engage in, overtly or covertly, is central to living and thus central to clients' concerns. Cognitions do not occur in an independent, happenstance fashion. They are related because they are nested in a cognitive structure, or system.
2. There is a core cognitive structure, but there are substructures, called schemata, within which related cognitions function.
3. Cognitions can be viewed from a rationalist perspective, which sees them as operating in a linear, objective manner to uncover the fixed characteristics of the real world. That view is rejected in this text.
4. Cognitions are flexible, generative, complex, and resilient, employed by each person to fashion and maintain an acceptable explanation of self in the world so that self can be somewhat in control. This stand, accepted in this text, is called either developmentalism or constructivism.
5. Cognitions have been identified as four processes and six kinds of content. The processes are perceptions, analytic thinking, attributing, and imagining. There are parts of some of these processes. Cognitive content comprises concepts, data, self-views and world views, automatic thoughts, rules, and aspirations and goals.

# ■ Counselor Formation Activities ■

1. Ideas—cognitions—do not have a separate existence but are related to other cognitions when any one topic is thought about. Beck labels these related ideas as schemata. Select one relatively discrete topic, such as your views of a particu-

lar race, and identify the separate and distinct cognitions you have about that race, but cognitions that agree with or support one another to constitute a schema.

2. Disequilibria in one's life are certainly useful, if not essential, for producing more mature cognitions. Recall some childhood event that had a pronounced disturbing effect—perhaps some event your parents caused. Can you recall how you viewed life differently after that event? What of recent times? Has some disruptive event, such as an impassioned argument, caused you to see things differently and brought about useful cognitive change? Could a counselor have been an agent to bring about that change?

3. A major goal for you as a counselor is to help clients identify their cognitive distortions and to be able to accept change in them. Do you have or have you had cognitive distortions that enable you to cope with some of life's complexities? You probably cannot identify them, so you will need the help of a trusted friend to give you his or her view.

■                         **Complementary Reading**                         ■

Although this brief chapter adequately introduces you to the significance of cognitive processes in counseling, the importance of mental processes in changing cognitions (using cognitions to change cognitions), changing emotions, and changing behaviors is of such importance that you are urged to promptly complement this chapter with other reading. If time permits perusal of book-length material, you can start with *The Mind* (Restak, 1988) for a general treatment.

Most published material on the topic has grown out of the cognitive revolution in counseling and therapy, which, of course, is germane for counselors. A place to enter that reading are the two chapters on learning and cognitions in:

GARFIELD, S. L., & BERGIN, A. E. (1986). *Handbook of Psychotherapy and Behavior Change*, 3rd ed. New York: Wiley.

I propose that you read Mahoney (1988), from which some material and figures were excerpted for this chapter. Its content may be somewhat advanced but will thereby be challenging.

# 3
PART

# Counseling Procedures and Techniques

## 9

CHAPTER

# Counseling Precepts and Practices

## Overview

Concepts covered in prior chapters and in the two following ones are brought together here as nine counseling precepts, summing up scientific thinking and evidence. These precepts overarch schools of counseling, thereby eliminating their need.

Although these precepts apply to counseling, the question must be asked, Do they not also apply to psychotherapy? There are some differences between counseling and therapy, but because both are based on knowledge about cognition, affect, and action, the precepts apply to therapy as well as to counseling. The difference between these two lies in variables other than their undergirding precepts, and these variables are reexamined briefly.

The topic of counseling schools is addressed again, first by classifying schools into several categories and also by examining some of these schools with regard to the particulars of certain of the nine counseling precepts.

As the first chapter of Part III, this chapter bridges the concepts set out in prior chapters and the applied aspects of counseling in this part. It serves both as a summary of concepts and as an introduction to practice.

## Introduction

It is now appropriate to draw together the results of inquiries into counselor knowledge, skills, and characteristics based on scientific reasoning and empirical evidence. This summary is embodied in nine precepts, which arise partly from seven topics treated in prior chapters and two yet to be covered: the 8th in Chapter 10 and the 9th in Chapter 11. In most instances, the precepts are based on meta-analyses of research and thus represent the widest range of thinking and findings. Because the precepts represent counseling that is not restrained by a commitment to older knowledge or partial thinking, they overarch schools.

# Precepts of Counseling

## 1. Counseling's Epistemology

Science, defined earlier, is the source of a counselor's knowledge. There is a more fundamental epistemic commitment, however, shown by the answer to these questions: Is there an objective world "out there" that can be known (the philosophy of realism)? Alternatively, is reality confined to what each person perceives; that is, is reality only "in the head" (the philosophy of idealism, or phenomenology)? Or is reality to be found in both the objective and subjective worlds?

Although philosophers do not agree about this issue and probably never will, the convincing position to which credible scientists in psychology have arrived, the one basic to counseling, is that *reality lies in both the objective and phenomenal worlds.*

## 2. Nature of Individuals

Inquiry into the nature of humans provides ever-accelerating knowledge and yields these conclusions that are significant to counseling:

1. Although human functioning can be arbitrarily rendered into such useful separate entities as mind, body, emotions, and behavior, in actuality *the human being functions in all instances as a unity, a totality.*

2. Evolving individuals develop over the life span, slowly but continuously redefining themselves as they cope with needs to adjust to changing perceptions of their effectiveness in social systems. To grasp where a client is at any moment in development requires some exploration of both past development and the client's expectations and hopes for the future. *Counseling attends to immediate client concerns from a life-span-development perspective.* Without this context, any one client concern cannot be properly sited on a developmental continuum. Important perspectives on a client's life, such as those of client-in-systems, the nature and integrity of self, and functioning by mental-health criteria, are given their proper dimension when put in the context of life-span development rather than being judged by immediate criteria only.

3. Because each person is a unique system who functions in environments or psychological fields that also are systems, *counseling attends to the contexts within which clients' developmental concerns occur, including the transactions in which clients experience other people.* Counselors therefore are versed in the systems concept and functions as they apply both to individuals and to social structures.

4. An individual operates as an organized being seeking affirmative self-definition and a sense of personal mastery over life, constantly striving to enhance his or her personal and social realities. Each individual is a somewhat steady-state organism, even though slowly evolving at the same time. *Counseling deals with the structure of genetically influenced, relatively fixed mental processes, emotions, and behaviors called personality. This personhood is common in structure but unique to each individual in how it is expressed.*

5. There are two components in the structure of personality, temperament and cognition, each comprising subsets. A subset of cognition is those mostly aware appraisals that individuals make of themselves, called self, a concept that has explanatory power in understanding the nature of each person's organization. Each individual's behaviors are partially under the control of views of the world each holds, another cognitive subset. These life views (as they are called here) are not only maxims about the objective world but also those held by individuals who describe themselves when operating in ecosystem contexts. *Counseling attends to the significance of any of a client's life views, but it will particularly attend to statements that the client uses to describe his or her self, a self embedded in a culture.*

### 3. Mental Health
There are objective criteria by which to evaluate an individual's psychological functioning; these are found within the purview of mental health. Although counselors can be less certain of the characteristics of good mental health in varying subcultures, they probably accept as precepts those general (and somewhat overlapping) mental-health criteria that compose, in existentialist terms, one's being. Counseling's mental-health criteria are

• successful lifelong acquisition of adaptive cognitions, emotions, and behaviors
• client awareness of self and its effect on others
• autonomy
• personal meaning
• centeredness
• purposefulness and efficacy
• competency to cope
• strong bonding with a few and affection for some others
• acceptance of responsibility for the actions one takes

Because counselors direct their functions toward client effectiveness in these areas, they earn designation as existentialists and, at the same time, the accolade of being humanists, whether theistic or secular depending on other components of their life views.

### 4. Affect: Mood and Emotions
All humans can roughly identify others' moods and emotions. Counselors operate beyond this simple ability because of their studied knowledge of the nature of affect and its function in healthy or disruptive living. Counselors will therefore treat client mood and emotion professionally, unlike the traditional counselor, who lacks this ability. *Counseling is based on sensitivity to client moods because they color and affect perceptions by providing the context, or background, for those perceptions. It is also based on sensitivity to emotions, which give force and direction to cognitions and behavior, and it enables clients to modify disruptive emotions so that cognitions and behaviors can be objective and thus favorable to client goals.*

## 5. Behaviors

Any person's existential being at any moment within the context of a social system is a compound of cognitions, affect, and psychomotor actions, or behavior. Just as there is a body of evidential knowledge about affect and cognitions unknown to lay people, so too there is a body of research-supported knowledge that informs counselors about behavior. *Counseling is based on the lawfulness of behavior and employs tested knowledge to modify behavior directly when that accords with client objectives and mental-health criteria.*

## 6. Cognitions

Unlike traditional counselors, professional counselors have a studied knowledge of the nature of cognitive content and processes, such as self-concepts, controlling maxims and other life-view elements that affect emotions and behavior, goals, values, and self-instruction devices that clients employ when faced with developmental challenges. *Counseling attends to the role of various cognitive processes and contents in the control of client affect and behaviors, and it employs them to change emotions and behaviors.*

## 7. Change Techniques

Counselors who are not committed to a school will know and are ready to use a variety of procedures for assisting clients. In contrast, counselors who are committed to a school know only the techniques of that school. Because schoolless counseling is committed to knowledge and skills rooted in science, it is pragmatic. Therefore, *counseling employs any proven technique to replace clients' disabling cognitions, feelings, or actions with enabling ones.*

## 8. Client/Counselor Alliance

*Counseling is conducted in ways sensitive to factors that promote or diminish the essential working relationship on which the success of counseling rests, the alliance, or emotional bond, between counselor and client,* a topic considered further in Chapter 11. This alliance is illustrated by the dictum that counselors do not *do* things to clients but *work with* them.

Without that knowledge and sensitivity, it cannot be taken for granted that anyone completing other parts of a counselor-preparation program will be able to propagate this alliance. For some prospective counselors it will be necessary to monitor their personal qualities to bring under control any characteristics that may be a handicap in creating this bond.

## 9. Communication Skill

Counselors do not speak impulsively; they have been trained in the skills unique to counseling, although new counselors may be somewhat clumsy in applying these skills. Experienced counselors may seem to be speaking spontaneously, but that is because essential communication skills have become "second nature," and their employment is effortless.

Of the numerous technical skills a counselor has, communication skills are basic to the others. Their outcomes can be several: being a skillful listener may be sufficient to bring about attainment of the client's objectives; it is tenable to believe that the positive effect of counseling's unique communication skills contributes to the emotional bond that produces counseling benefit; clients may acquire some of these skills at an aware or unaware level, thus benefiting their interactions in other social systems.

*Counseling communications are not casual, nor do they express counselors' life-view biases. They are consciously based on the communication skills unique to counseling, including competence in reading body language.* For specialty settings, counselors will acquire additional communication skills, such as general group procedures or psychodrama and the use of dolls and other play materials.

## Counseling or Psychotherapy?

The nine precepts apply to counseling, to psychological assistance to normal people with typical developmental needs. Can counseling also be called psychotherapy? Are the terms equivalent in any way?

The root meaning of *therapy* is attention to another's needs, a meaning with a long history in medicine. Well before medicine became a profession, there was lay healing assistance to people experiencing physical and psychological concerns. Because even traditional counselors try to help, that broad definition allows it to be said that they provide therapy. Surely, then, trained, professional counselors give therapeutic assistance. This logic has led some theorists (Rogers, 1942; Patterson, 1980) to assert that counseling and psychotherapy are interchangeable terms. Others contend that therapy applies only to assistance by practitioners with advanced training who serve clients with concerns of a more internalized, more severe, and longer lasting nature.

If a scale is imagined that locates assisting clients with severe psychological difficulties at one end and helping with "normal" concerns at the other, there will be no precise place that divides those two categories, where it can be said, "This is therapy up to this point, and counseling from here on." Because client concerns *are* locatable on a continuum, the undergirding precepts for any part of the continuum must be the same.

This text acknowledges one basis for distinguishing between use of the two terms: the length of formal preparation. The greater the length of academic study and supervised practice, the more qualified a person is to deal with severe psychological needs. This distinction is found between those prepared at the master's-degree level and those at the doctoral level. The position taken here is that in light of common usage among professionals, master's-level counselors do not provide therapy. Counseling psychologists (holders of doctor's degrees) may do so, depending upon the concern addressed.

Claiborn and Lichtenberg (1989) see a distinction, based not upon degree level but upon a theoretical basis. This distinction is rooted in the relationship between practitioner and client, a distinction that they analyze on two dimensions. On one is located the degree of client stability; the other lays out the degree of congruence between the goals of client and counselor. Therapy, according to this analysis, is a process that moves an unstable client from an incongruent relationship to a congruent relationship, even though the client's location on the stability dimension may remain the same—unstable.

Although this matter of a distinction between psychological counseling and psychotherapy is a relatively minor one among professionals and the service-seeking public probably makes no distinction between the labels, prospective professionals need to be aware of the issue and arguments.

## The Nine Precepts versus Counseling Schools

Historians usually identify Freud's theories and practices as the first explanatory basis for giving help to those with psychological disturbances. This system, later modified by others, is generally known as psychoanalysis. Within a few years two major competing explanatory systems outside the psychoanalytic tent emerged, one labeled behaviorism, the other humanism, or humanistic psychology. This latter emphasis developed among certain psychologists who could accept neither the deterministic psychoanalytic view nor the "mechanistic" stance toward humans that they saw characterizing behaviorism—a "pox on both your houses" position.

As we saw earlier, schools of counseling filled a historical need in counseling's early days. This period brought new conceptual emphases to professional awareness, emphases that were given a title by their originators as distinctive kinds of counseling or therapy. A major thrust of this text is that scientific thought and research have been moving at a geometric rate of increase since those early days, providing precepts based on thinking and research that are appropriate for all counselors. Although these precepts incorporate contributions made by some schools, they overarch all schools and, by doing so, surpass the need for adherence to any of them. Indeed, the stand here is that adherence to the theorizing and practices of a more primitive time in counseling acts as a deterrent to its evolution.

### The Three Categories of Counseling Labels

The variety of labels that the counselor-to-be comes across is confusing. Here are a few from among the scores that abound, each a modifier for the unwritten words *counseling* or *therapy:* rehabilitation, reality, person-centered, school, career, family, rational-emotive, and substance-abuse. Because the first step in science is to create an accurate taxonomy of the phenomenon observed, the list above has to be factored into the three separate classes it contains.

One category is that of the institution or agency in which counselors are located. A sweep through the list above shows those to be rehabilitation, school, and family. Another category is a topic emphasis, no matter the agency. In this classification we place career and substance-abuse. The third group includes schools of counseling (purportedly distinctive in theory and techniques), such as person-centered and rational-emotive.

The school-of-counseling category can be further classified into four subsets reflecting different emphases. Some schools emphasize theory more than technical processes, as do existential and person-centered therapies and the several schools subsumed under the title psychoanalytic. Some emphasize technique but do not have theoretical elaboration, such as primal scream therapy. Others emphasize a portion of a theory or one procedure (instead of all proven ones), such as rational-emotive therapy, Gestalt therapy, and transactional analysis. Others can cross the three classes, as does family therapy; it can be an agency, a counseling topic, and a theoretical emphasis.

We can take any labeled agencies, such as rehabilitation or school, and ask, Is there any "kind" of counseling connoted by either label? The answer is negative; there are minor topic differences between agencies, but no school of counseling is appropriate just for rehabilitation agencies or secondary schools. These labels are merely a device to show the type of institutions in which numbers of counselors are employed. The label "rehabilitation" must be used by some agencies, not because they offer distinctive procedures based on theories that differ from other agencies but because federal money is used for the preparation and employment of counselors in rehabilitation agencies. Counselors in both rehabilitation and educational agencies, asked about their commitment to a school of counseling, report differences that depend partly on the authorities they accepted during their training. Graduates of a program that emphasized operant conditioning, for example, would classify themselves as behaviorists, whereas graduates of a program committed to the person-centered perspective would counsel in accord with that perspective.* The proposal here, of course, is that counseling will be the same, regardless of setting, when it is based on the best thinking and practices so far uncovered from a science-oriented epistemology.

Examination of family therapy presents a test of this and several other issues. In a text that presents a number of kinds of counseling, perusal of the chapter on family therapy (Foley, 1984) shows how its content and practices are thought to differ from other schools of counseling. The inference can be made that family therapy operates on a different theoretical base from others schools. That is a regrettably accurate impression because it does reflect the current status.

Just as counseling that specializes in substance abuse or geriatrics is aimed at a special clientele requiring counselors to have supplemental knowledge and some unique techniques, so does counseling that focuses on families require some supplemental preparation, but nonetheless all programs that address a particular clientèle can be based on the same theory and employ common procedures. The second precept implies that fundamental to all counseling, not just to family therapy, is the need for counselors to communicate to clients and carry out with them those practices that acknowledge that clients function as members of systems. Counselors in all settings, no matter with what topics they are dealing, cannot adequately grasp the meaning a person sees for himself or herself without having a feel for that person's functioning as a member of a number of systems.

Another test is provided by attending to mental-health agencies and to the label "mental-health counselor." Under schoolless counseling, practitioners in all settings dealing with all topics will have the same knowledge about the origins of and approaches to thinking, feeling, and behaving that bear on clients' mental health. Although *all* psychological counselors hold to mental-health goals, assess clients' mental health, and engage in developmental procedures to enhance mental

---

*Some experienced counselors may have moved away from their earlier commitments to a school.

health as well as remove obstacles to it, those counselors in agencies labeled as emphasizing mental health may need supplemental knowledge and skills.

## *Need for Supplemental Procedures*

The experience of counselors will continue to inform the profession how much specialty knowledge is required to counsel in a particular agency or a specialized area. Medicine's similarities come to mind, although it can serve only partly as an analogy because bodies are relatively closed systems whereas psychological systems are open.

In medicine's early years most physicians were general practitioners whose ministrations were sought no matter the symptoms. Over time, medical specialties evolved as a result of increased knowledge and specialized skills, but these are extensions of the common knowledge and skills learned by all physicians, no matter (with rare exception) the medical school attended. By taking appropriate additional courses and through practice supervised by specialists, counselors-to-be are prepared for the special clientele to be found in the setting or counseling topic in which the student wishes to practice. In particular settings these clients may be students, prisoners, parish members, or families, to name some. Topics may focus on such normal concerns as psychosexual development, obsessions, interpersonal competencies, parenting, separation anxiety, and careers—a small sampling from the long list of developmental concerns that typical people have. It is appropriate that the same counseling principles and practices apply to all settings and topics.

Group procedures around specific topics of concern enhance the positive outcomes acquired from individual counseling. Counselors specializing in those topics need training in group process beyond that acquired by all counselors, illustrated by counselor-run support groups on topics such as grief, withdrawal anxieties, sexual aberration, disabilities, or felonious behavior. Other clients may require communication or assessment procedures beyond those acquired by all counselors—for example, the use of play materials when working with young children.

Differences in gender, race, and cultures are additional and significant subsets of setting and topic specialties; they require specialized knowledge when the emphasis is on any one of them. A university counseling center represents these specialized needs by providing counselors who reflect the gender, ethnic, and racial differences among the student population. At the same time they correctly do not require that client and counselor be matched on variables such as these. That would remain a matter of client choice.

A master's program common to all counselors-to-be, regardless of topic or agency, will provide starting knowledge and skills required to be effective with clients. If a counselor begins service in an agency serving specialized clients with only that general preparation, he or she will have to count on experience and mentoring to provide the additional knowledge and skills required by that agency. The advantage of a 45-credit or more master's program (or advanced specialist diploma program) that includes the additional preparation necessary to function in a specialized agency is obvious, as, of course, is the advantage of the additional knowledge and skills that result from a doctor's degree, with its intern- and externships.

## *Summary*

Counselors and their practices are sometimes identified by the institution or agency in which they work. Others are labeled by a topic specialty. (A minority are in independent practice.) It is common for counselors also to identify themselves as adherents to a school of counseling (or therapy), regardless of setting or topic specialty. This text's stand eliminates the latter characteristic: all should be prepared similarly without reference to any school.

Even though setting and topic levels are employed, that does not mean that they are based on different counseling practices. The topic of substance abuse can be addressed in a rehabilitation agency by counselors who have had supplemental training about drugs; treatment in that instance does not require going to a substance-abuse agency. Because the population of secondary schools includes every variety of developmental concern common to adolescents and young adults, the label "school counselor" does not provide information about the topic specialties to which a school counselor may be called on to attend. Additionally, as a reminder of the confusion about labels, counseling practices in those two settings and others could appropriately be labeled mental-health counseling. The concern of mental-health counselors with the quality of client being also earns them the mantle of existentialists.

In any setting, as noted earlier, counselors may work on cognitive and behavioral change in groups of individuals having to cope with adjustment concerns related to a specific topic. In educational institutions the topic may be persistent tardiness or absence, extreme shyness or aggressiveness, or racially contentious activities among students, calling for small groups of different races to be led by two or more racially different counselors.

## Concluding Reflections

The nine precepts featured in this chapter summarize current scientific emphases in the major areas with which counseling practice is concerned. They incorporate, as well, a humanistic quality that gives purposes to counseling. Equally important, they constitute a unified approach to examining human development and applying change procedures, a quality that constitutes an overarching of current schools of counseling and thereby obviates the usefulness of those schools.

Seven of the precepts were excerpted from prior chapters, but the eighth and ninth precepts are treated at length in Chapters 10 and 11. As this chapter's function is to provide the basis for counseling practice, those last two precepts were added prior to their full examination so as to have a complete array.

■                              **Points to Remember**                              ■

1. The primary points are the contents of each of the nine precepts set out under the headings:

    (1) counseling's epistemology,
    (2) the nature of individuals,

(3) mental health
(4) affect: mood and emotions
(5) behaviors
(6) cognitions
(7) change techniques
(8) client/counselor alliance
(9) communication skill

2. The names of schools of counseling (therapy) are a mixture of three categories. One of these categories is the type of employing institution (for example, college). Another is the topic addressed (drug abuse), and the third kind is the theory emphasized (Gestalt).
3. Many schools imply, if they do not assert, that they differ from all others, that they are complete in their theory and practices, and that they offer assessment data to substantiate their superiority.
4. Evidence does not support this division of counseling or therapy into schools. To the contrary, the evidence is that counseling principles can and should be the same regardless of setting or topic. Some counseling specialties warrant supplementary training beyond this common core.

## ■ Counselor Formation Activities ■

1. Critically examine the nine precepts given in this chapter. Some of them may differ from your prior assumptions about counseling. With which ones are you in full agreement? Which cause you some questions? What alternative positions regarding those questioned precepts can you offer? Discuss with your small group of fellow students what your questions or reservations are, and your alternative positions. It is assumed that you will also raise those concerns with the course instructor.
2. Are you comfortable with the idea that counseling and therapy are different? If you see them as different, describe that difference to your satisfaction to someone or your small group as if you have been asked by a noncounselor what the difference is.

## 10

**CHAPTER**

# Counseling's Unique Communication Skills

## Overview

From prior chapters you have learned what purposes psychological counselors serve and have noted this text's commitment to an epistemology of science. The physiological and developmental variables affecting a client's feelings, actions, and mental processes have been examined. The benchmarks that establish the psychological geometry of individual functioning have been set up. We are now ready to start the process of entering the subjective and objective realities of any individual, at his or her request, with the aim of enhancing that person's life.

Words are the devices used to bring about this enhancement. The setting is probably a professional-appearing interview room but can be anywhere that client and counselor come together. It is what goes on in client/counselor interviews that identifies counseling and distinguishes it from similar professions.

Counseling centers on a relationship that is unique in clients' lives, the result, primarily, of the distinctive ambience of interviews and communication procedures. This chapter examines these singular devices, organized into a taxonomy of 13 kinds of counselor word use.

Seven topics that address other characteristics of interviews are examined, thereby preparing the way for later chapters to present the cognitive, affective, and behavioral content of counseling to which prior chapters have been leading.

## Introduction

In professions such as accounting, medicine, or law, a person's counseling needs are dealt with objectively, which is what the person to be helped expects and seeks. In those professions it is sufficient to attend only to objective content. Objective content is important in psychological counseling too, but of equal or greater importance is subjective content. Thus, counselors in their interviews pay skillful attention to the subjective aspects of client concerns, to which they have been sensitized by study of a variety of topics relating to development.

The effectiveness of psychological counseling is highly dependent upon how counselors relate to clients and help them deal with their subjective views of the world. These steps in turn contribute to changes in the clients' objective world. The relationship on which these outcomes depend is largely the product of the unique communication skills that counselors use, particularly in early interviews. The communication skills that create the conditions for establishing a therapeutic alliance enable clients (1) to raise to awareness any subliminal aspects of their concerns and (2) to reduce emotions that may prevent them from dealing objectively with their concerns, although negative emotions may sometimes be permitted to run their course to permit cognitive restructuring.

The fact that counselors experience common training in communication arts does not mean that they will counsel similarly. Hypothetically, if a half-dozen trained counselors were picked at random to assist a counterfeit client who was trained to present a difficulty to each counselor with not only the same words but with the same level of affect, there would be noticeable interview differences among those six counselors. This can be assumed because counselors, like other humans, differ in personality variables, such as introversion/extroversion, intellectual acuity, emphatic sensitivity, life views, and creativity—attributes that are compounds of genetics and experience. People drawn to the counseling profession are more alike on some gross measures than those who enter business, science, or the performing arts, but they nonetheless differ noticeably within their own subpopulation. These differences affect their behaviors no matter how similarly they are trained in the communication skills distinctive to psychological counseling.

If counselors in other professions have psychological disorders or if there is some dislike between them and their clients, they can still effectively deal with clients' problems. An alcoholic, child-abusing pediatrician can be an effective and admired doctor with others' children. A surgeon who has a strong dislike for members of a group he or she negatively stereotypes can carry out a perfect coronary bypass operation on a patient who matches that stereotype. A sexually confused financial consultant with severe neurotic symptoms can counsel about a client's investments with a full measure of professional competence and to the client's full satisfaction. These examples are possible because the client's concern is either solely objective or mostly so. The professional outcome is not dependent upon the quality of the interaction between helper and client. In psychological counseling the quality of the relationship between client and counselor is critical and can readily be affected by a counselor's personality, let alone by his or her chronic and gross disorders.

# Barriers to Communication:

## *Habituated Speech Mannerisms Needing Change*

The habituated communication mannerisms that most students bring to counselor-preparation programs are likely to impede counseling success unless they are brought under control. Training is required because the habituated patterns described below are resistant and therefore are little affected by mere explanation of the problem or by a one-time demonstration and opportunity to practice. The amount of time and effort required for their change will vary with individuals, of course, but in any case, some deliberate work will be required.

## *Talking, Not Listening*

Most cultures prize easy speakers. In social gatherings people who participate readily and frequently in conversation are valued, while the quiet person's behavior is considered less desirable. This socially trained proclivity to talk is found in the speech patterns of traditional (untrained) counselors. An eagerness to help and an assumption that such help is given by telling the client what to do typically results in untrained counselors taking over an interview after only a brief statement from the person seeking help. They interrupt, ask questions, mollify ("Everything is going to be all right"), advise, counter client emotion with reasoned arguments, urge a course of action with illustrations of how the helper met a (seemingly) similar difficulty ("If it worked for me, it will work for you"), even scold ("You know better than that! After all your mother has done for you!"). Trained counselors will not use such tactics except rarely, and then deliberately instead of spontaneously.

## *Intolerance of Silence*

The other side of that coin is the typical person's intolerance of silence. At several points I have observed that just listening may result in the relief a client seeks in counseling, a point supported by the reported positive outcomes that result from early interviews, no matter from traditional or professional counseling, or the theory from which the counselor operates. Clients are animated by the experience of meeting a new person, one whom they expect to be of help. Additionally, they receive the counselor's full attention, probably a rare experience. Much or, in some case, all client gain occurs in this first, critical interview.

There may be no need for the counselor to struggle to remain silent at the outset of counseling, because the client will be eager to explain his or her concern.* On the other hand, some clients who expect to be talkative, and even have practiced some imaginary interviews, when actually facing a counselor may be inhibited by shame or other emotions and become reticent.

Later in the first interview or in subsequent interviews, a talkative client may become introspective. Clients may silently cogitate about what they have heard themselves say, such as rules of life to which they subscribe but of whose contradictions they had not been aware. This is clients' working time, just as if they were alone and pondering about their lives. The counselor lets it be their time by being silent for however long it takes.

In social situations, the sudden silences that randomly occur are embarrassing, and several persons start to talk about anything at the same time to relieve this unbearable condition. Impulsive talking in such cases is a behavior that has been

---

*Silence in the first interview is relative because total silence on the counselor's part is rare. There will be the expected "Um-hmmms" and some "I sees" or similar brief oral reinforcers that act as taps to keep the client's talk hoop rolling. They are not seen as breaking silence.

negatively reinforced by the easing of discomfort. In interviews counselors readily practice silence that they would find intolerable in social settings.

## *Impulsive Questioning*

A related habituated speech behavior that most students bring to a counselor-preparation program, one that impedes counseling progress in its early period, is the proclivity to ask questions. At some point questions will be appropriate, even imperative, but their effect at the start of counseling is usually negative. Spontaneous, impulsive questioning at any time, but most particularly at the beginning of counseling, is a behavior to be brought under control, because all communication should be designed to forward counseling objectives, not be "off the top of the head" or designed for counselor satisfaction.

The questions to be avoided are inquiries that can be answered briefly; they typically are about facts that can be brought out later. Ivey (1980) identifies two kinds of questions, closed ones, which are the ones just described, and open ones, which cannot be answered briefly but have the effect of drawing out useful explanatory information from clients, causing them to puzzle about something new or to think about a topic heretofore avoided. This latter speech device will be referred to here as an *invitation,* so that when the word *question* is used, it will refer only to the short-answer kind.

Questions have several undesirable results when counseling is getting under way. They set the tone of counseling as an event in which counselors take charge, and thus they support clients' misapprehensions that counselors, after collecting sufficient information, will, like physicians, either do something to clients or prescribe actions they are to take. Questions prevent clients from thinking in an unstructured way about their concerns; conversely, they direct clients' thinking and therefore determine what clients will say, not what needs to be said, unless the client is unusually assertive and will speak at length despite the counselor's questions. A client's developmental difficulties may include overdependency, and a take-charge counselor will probably worsen, not ease, that client's difficulty. In most instances there are emotional concomitants to portions of clients' concerns; questions hide those by reducing the interview to a cognitive question-and-answer session. It is important that affect associated with clients' concerns be recognized by counselors to let them be assured that clients are also aware of these feelings, which must then be dealt with by both parties.

When treating the topic of questioning in counseling, Cormier and Cormier (1991) offer several quidelines (p. 116):

Questions should not be a counselor's primary response mode.
Questions should center on the client's concerns and what the client has already said, not on what the counselor is curious about.
Ask only one question at a time, and provide sufficient time for the client to reply; pushing for a reply can be threatening.
Improper questioning can create dependency and the aura of the counselor as an expert, thus minimizing the client's responsibility and involvement and creating resentment.
Improper questioning causes the client to feel interrogated, not understood.

There is a counterpart skill a counselor acquires: avoidance of answering clients' questions under a number of conditions, such as those in which a counselor's direct response would draw the counselor into taking sides (which some clients will try) when the situation requires the counselor to be neutral. As an example, assume that a client is describing an unsatisfactory relationship with someone and then asks the counselor, "She had no right to do those things—to behave like a scumbag to me, did she?" Later we will look at a skill to avoid answering that kind of question while at the same time dealing with clients' concerns to their satisfaction.

Counselor training replaces this eagerness to speak (and its counterpart, intolerance of silence) and inappropriate (impulsive) questioning with useful communication skills. Although new students have shown frustration in mock counseling interviews when prohibited from asking questions, they accept the notion that the ban is intended not only to supplant questioning with other communication devices but also to bring about a disciplined cognitive process that eliminates the need for impulsive questions.

Training in other professions that provide counseling (law, accounting) does not include efforts to alter these behaviors, because they are not inappropriate in those professions. Their practitioners are quick to be orally active right from the start of an interview. Even clinical psychologists, when their training programs emphasize diagnosis and treatment, do not receive training in communication skills essential to counseling.

## Counseling's Unique Verbal Skills

Silence is not necessarily a sign of listening. Hearing facts, and maybe even making notes of them, does not mean listening in the counseling sense. Listening is being sensitive to slight tonal modifications that may indicate affect of which the client is unaware or unready to talk about. Listening means accurately grasping the client's subjective world while concurrently searching one's knowledge of development for explanatory cues and thoughts of how to bring about client change.

The unique listening and response behaviors of counselors wed the counselor and client in a relationship of collaboration and trust. This relationship requires that the counselor not only be silent when the client is speaking easily but also nurture periods of silence. Different terms have been used to describe these communication behaviors. Ivey (1980) speaks of attending behaviors and intentional listening. The Cormiers (1985) use the latter phrase but also speak of effective listening. Still others (Egan, 1982) use the term *active listening*. Because all these terms imply that counselors listen intensively and respond in distinctive ways, they will be employed here interchangeably. Each profession and trade has its own unique tools; counselors' words are their basic tools, but uniform labeling of counselors' responses has not yet been attained.

As a rule, counselors do not just talk; the content of what they say is deliberate, based on a running assessment of a client's report of cognitions, feelings, and behaviors and on the potential effect of responses they might make. With practice these thoughtful responses to clients' statements flow effortlessly, although new counselors must expect that at first their responses may be slow in forthcoming and halting in presentation as they seek out the principles by which to guide each response and the words to employ. Experienced drivers shift gears fluently; new drivers grind (and swear) and stall. The deliberate care with which counselors' responses will be chosen is a far more demanding skill than shifting a car's gears.

Over 40 years ago, Robinson (1950) published the first taxonomy of counselor responses, or leads, as he called them. They were based on an extensive study of how counselors responded to clients, a study that remains essentially valid although additional responses have been identified since then.

To explain what he connoted with the word *lead,* Robinson used the football pass as analogy. Just as the quarterback does not throw the ball to where the receiver is but to where he will be, counselors employ responses to lead clients along in their thinking to where they want to be. My figure is a pair of ladder uprights without rungs. Counselors' responses are somewhat like the placement of rungs in the uprights, requiring psychological reach. Sometimes that reach will be short; at other times the counselor places a rung that requires the client to reach far.

Robinson identified 14 leads, running from the least to the most leading. In the least-leading ones, counselors provide minimal direction to interviews or thrusts for client change. Leads progress with an increasing degree of counselor direction up to the most leading. Robinson's leads, starting with the least leading at the top of the left column, are:

| | |
|---|---|
| silence | tentative analysis |
| acceptance | interpretation |
| restatement | urging |
| clarification | introducing unrelated topics |
| summary clarification | assurance |
| approval | depth interpretation |
| general lead | rejection |

Contemporaneously, Rogers (1942, 1951) proposed general principles for the conduct of interviews in which counselors were to be trained, but he did so without stating a taxonomy; counselors' words would naturally flow from their adherence to the principles he offered. Reflection of feeling was given as the major way in which counselors were to respond.

In addition to identifying a taxonomy of counselor leads, Robinson's research showed the need for counselors to be trained to identify and deal with the essential substance of what clients were talking about. For this skill Robinson used the phrase, identifying the core of the client's remarks. It was found that counselors often could not identify the essence of what the client was saying without training in that skill. When clients spoke at length, stating several related or illustrative topics, a counselor might miss the gist of what the client was saying, a circumstance that led to the error of responding only to the last topic mentioned, not to the content the client was really talking about. For example (CL = client, CO = counselor):

**CL:** I always felt remote from my father—I guess I never saw him as a father the way my friends did theirs. He was never around, or if he was, he was more interested in his hobby than us kids—even Ma. Jim—he was my best friend—he had a great dad. I wanted my father to be like him. He [CL's father] would be away on his job for long periods—a week, sometimes longer, but when he came home he'd go right to the workshop out back to work on that stupid hobby of his.

**CO:** What was that hobby?

Had the counselor grasped the core of the client's remarks, the lead would have been something like this (paraphrasing and reflection of feeling):

**CO:** You really missed having the kind of father you dreamed of and your friend Jim had.

Note the absence of a question mark after the revised lead; that makes it clear that the counselor was making a statement, in which the voice drops at the end. Note also that the incorrect counselor response not only missed the core of the client's remarks, attending only to the final item mentioned by the client, but also was a question. Having missed the substance of the client's remarks, the counselor might have used another lead instead of a question, such as invitation. That lead might have been "Tell me more about his hobby, Jack," appropriate only as an attempt to restore counseling communication.

Had the client replied, "Building model ships," what would the counselor have said next? The counselor has taken the initiative away from the client, has missed the gist of what the client was saying, and has put himself or herself into an embarrassing box. Were this an experienced counselor whose attention had briefly wandered, resulting in missing the point and in asking a question, the counselor would see the error and might return to professional communication by saying, "Well, of course, his hobby is not of importance right now. What *is* important is that you really missed . . ."

Ivey (1980) has analyzed counseling into its small elements, called microskills, in which counselors-to-be would be trained. Ivey offers this taxonomy of counselor responses, each of which is a microskill (p. 71):

| | |
|---|---|
| closed question | directive |
| open question | influencing summary |
| minimal encourager | interpretation |
| paraphrase | self-disclosure |
| reflection of feeling | direct mutual communication |
| summary | expression of content |
| | expression of feeling |

This list includes some responses that Rogers considered essential, although he did not give them specific labels. Others in the list are discordant with Rogers's theoretical position. The taxonomy proposed by Cormier and Cormier (1991), in like fashion, contains some responses similar to Robinson's leads and some that are in accord with Rogers's general principles, as well as some that do not fit with Rogers's theoretical stance. Cormier and Cormier provide two categories of counselor response:

| *Listening Responses* | *Action Responses* |
|---|---|
| clarification | probes, comprising open questions |
| paraphrase | and closed questions |
| reflection of feelings | confrontation |
| summarization | interpretation |
| | information giving |

My experience leads me to a taxonomy that differs somewhat from those by adding a few terms and eliminating others. These are not essential differences; what is important is that you become aware that counselors do not just say what comes to mind. They use words with deliberation, based on clients' stated concerns; what has transpired in interviews so far; what the client has just said and how it was said; the client's objectives; and an analysis of the fit between the client's development, cognitions, affective state, and reported behaviors, on the one hand, and mentally healthful outcomes on the other. And, of course, on the immediate objectives the counselor is working to achieve.

This intentionality is informed by counselors' knowledge of how it is that people come to think, feel, and act as they do and how change can be nurtured in these functions. They know that finely tuned communication procedures contribute to client change and, particularly, how necessary such careful speech is at the start of counseling. Of most importance, they are skilled in these procedures, these ways of speaking, which are the result of research and are not tied to any school of counseling.

## Taxonomy of Counselor Responses

Some cautions must be stated before specific oral behaviors are examined. On the one hand, counselors will be aware that there is a typical way in which interviews develop and thus an expected way in which they will first employ responses. Counselors must be cautious about ritualistic behaviors, however. Counselors may unintentionally seek to have the progress of each series of interviews conform to an average. Similarly, there are preferred ways for responding to clients' oral and nonoral behaviors, but again the danger is that these will be employed ritually. It is relevant to a counselor's professional sense of situation to know when to employ any of the following leads and to orchestrate their use in a way designed to bring about desired results.

I have said several times that questions are inappropriate, at least in the first part of a first interview. This view assumes that necessary client data have been acquired by a receptionist or intake interviewer. Avoidance of questioning is defensible in general, but if it is viewed as an absolute prohibition, it is not only a ritualistic prohibition but also cannot be defended by any empirical or logical evidence. Counselors have been trained how and when to ask questions based partly on principles and partly on their clinical sense of progress in counseling.

The 13 leads below are listed in order of the likelihood of their use in the first part of a first interview, the least leading response given first. The assumption is that the counselor has studied necessary data about the client and that the client has been introduced and welcomed into the counseling room, has been seated, and has been invited to tell what it is that concerns him or her, or how the counselor might be of help. The phrasing used in those moments is whatever the counselor feels comfortable with.

Each specific lead, or counselor response, below is followed by noting whether the Cormiers ("C") or Ivey ("I") propose either an identical or a similar response; the absence of reference to either or both names shows that neither proposes a similar lead:

1. simple reinforcers (I—minimal encouragers)
2. invitation (C—probes, which can be direct questions)
3. restatement
4. paraphrasing (C—same; I—same)
5. reflection of feeling (C—same; I—same)
6. clarification (C—same)
7. summary (C—summarization; I—summary)
8. conjecture, or hypothesis
9. approval
10. parrying clients' questions
11. confrontation (C—same)
12. emotion management
13. information giving, interpretation (C—same), and planning

## 1. Simple Reinforcers

Simple reinforcers are any sounds or phrases that abet the client's speaking. The most common are "Um-hmm" (likely with small head nods) and "I see." If counselors have three or four phrases in their repertoire, they can avoid distracting the client by repetitive words or frequent use of simple reinforcers. Some clients (and practicum supervisors!) find an almost incessant "Um-hmmm" or "I see" to be irritatingly distracting.

## 2. Invitation

By whatever name this lead is called, it is a most useful tool. At the start of counseling a client may be expected to describe concerns and their context in a general, nondetailed way. If the counselor deems it important that details be explored, an invitation can be offered, like "Can you tell me more about that" or "Why don't you continue; that's an important point." There will be times when a counselor considers it best to have a topic described in detail but thinks that the present is not the best time. In that case, a mental or unobtrusively written note is made. (The client is aware of the latter.) At some later time the counselor might say, "Awhile back you mentioned . . . but I wasn't sure what you meant. Can you clarify that a bit for me." These invitations are marked by a dropping inflection; a rising inflection would turn them into questions.

Sometimes the same effect is achieved by repeating a single word or very short phrase with rising inflection. For example, were a university student, in speaking about academic difficulties, to say of a professor "He's the most vindictive person I've ever met," the counselor might elicit clarification by saying "Vindictive?" Some speak of this device as a tack.

### 3. Restatement

The occasional verbatim repeating of some brief statement by the client is rare after counseling's earliest hour, but it may serve early on to convey to the client that the counselor is attending.

### 4. Paraphrasing

A step beyond restatement is paraphrasing. The counselor takes a longer statement by the client and puts it into the counselor's own words, as shown in this illustration: an adolescent has been describing difficulties at home and says:

> **CL:** My stepmother has her problems too, I know, so I see why she's rough on me at times, but my Dad, well, he don't have any problems—but he sets such dumb rules and keeps changing them. I can never be sure what he wants, what he's going to yell at me for. I get mad as hell at his old-time views—we argue all the time. Particularly on weekends. [pause]
>
> **CO:** Your Dad has rules you think are old-fashioned that he keeps changing. Because you don't know what he wants, you get upset and argue a lot with him.

### 5. Reflection of Feeling

The placement of reflection here does not mean that it is used only after the first four; these lower numbered leads can be used at any point when the counselor judges their use to be appropriate. It may be the counselor's first statement, as "I sense an unhappy person sitting there."

Reflection of feeling is vital in creating the therapeutic alliance on which counseling success largely rests, but there is the danger of ritually employing some standard phrasing such as "You feel . . ." Clients are quick to note such formalism, and some report skepticism about the counselor's competence. One was so piqued by hearing that phrase frequently used as to burst out with, "Why do you keep saying 'You feel' so much?!"

There are easily recalled alternative phrases for empathically acknowledging clients' affective states, such as "I can understand that what she said made you angry," "You're feeling good right now for having done that," "It seems to me that not having finished that report has made your insecurities come back when you thought they were gone—that you're feeling some panic," or "You're really pleased with that—it shows in your voice and face. I'd feel pleased too if it happened to me."

### 6. Clarification

As paraphrasing builds on restatement, clarification builds on paraphrasing, but with an important difference. The first two leads are not intended to move the client to a higher rung on the insight ladder and thus are commonly used in counseling's earlier moments. As the client develops confidence in what is happening and as the counselor senses that the client is ready to accept more leading kinds of responses, clarification may be among the first to be employed. It is intended to add new material to the interview, something not raised by the client.

In this lead, the counselor puts together ideas that go beyond those stated by the client, ideas shading upon interpretation. The function of this lead, in addition to the hoop-tapping effect of the first leads listed, is to bring clients to face and comprehend the significance of details and experiences that have recently been related by tying them together in a way they may not have seen. This lead may sound like this: "You've been describing your mixed—your off-again on-again—relationship with Betty and how frustrating that's been for you. I think I'm seeing some relationship, umm, some connection between that kind of relationship and what you said earlier about the ideals you hold about what a woman should be like."

## 7. *Summary*

A step beyond clarification is summary. The degree of counselor leading ranges from none at all, in restatement, to a small amount, in paraphrasing, to even more, in clarification, and now more significantly, in summary. The counselor's net is cast wide in a summary, drawing together sequentially several discussion topics that have been covered; thus, this lead is likely to be found near the end of an interview. It is a powerful lead; its use frequently provides clients with insight and a grasp of the connections of parts of their concern they have missed. Because it is a leap on the counselor's part, it may err in spots. For that reason experienced counselors use refutable phrasing in introducing this and other leads with which they are moving somewhat ahead of what the client said. Such phrases are "It seems to me . . .," "I wonder if . . .," or any other tentative phrasing that makes it easy for the client to reject an idea without rejecting the person putting it forth. In a social situation peers are quick to say, "You're wrong about that." The counseling relationship in its earliest stages is far from social. The client may be in a delicate psychological balance and thus be easily put off by what is perceived as a counselor's know-it-all attitude and not return. A condition of this kind is rather easily sensed, so a counselor can assess the degree of bluntness and oral initiative the client can tolerate. When unsure, the counselor treads softly and employs tentative phrasing.

## 8. *Conjecture, or Hypothesis*

Conjecture is a relabeling of Robinson's term *tentative analysis*. I have found that the word *analysis* confuses some students: "Are we supposed to be (psycho) analyzing clients?" Moreover, conjecture is what the counselor does: "I'm led to think that your insistence that [your 14-year old son] go heavily into sports may reflect a fear that if he continues to concentrate on art, he may become homosexual." This conjecture reflects a father's fears that the counselor had inferred earlier. To offer a conjecture, or hypothesis, is to state a lead of a greater reach than that occurring in clarification.

## 9. *Approval*

Simple reinforcers are a weak form of approval, saying, in effect, "When you talk, I reward you by giving my complete attention to you." The effect is the reinforcement of the client's speaking behaviors. Approval serves the same function: reinforcement of something reported by the client. If the client recounts having taken a new and desirable action or having acquired a new, desirable cognition, the counselor will wish to strengthen the likelihood that the new action or cognition will be permanent. Approval contributes to that reinforcement:

> **CL:** I tried that relaxation exercise you told me about, and it really works! I've been using it regularly at work, and I can just feel the tension leaving.
> **CO:** That's great, Nancy. I'm delighted to hear that you're able to do that.

## 10. Parrying Clients' Questions

Counselors will avoid answering some kinds of questions, such as those that try to euchre them into making a favorable judgment about the rightness of a client's viewpoint in a dispute. Clients may put this kind of question as a test of counselor loyalty but also to gain the support that will come from the counselor's (expected) agreement with the client's evaluation.

At times, particularly when strong emotion is expressed, the client may be engaging in rhetoric, not really asking a question. A characteristic of a question is that an answer clearly is possible and sought. Rhetorical questions may be answerable, but a response is not necessarily expected. The orator who, in a political frenzy, asks a crowd, "What party is best for our country in these perilous days?" expects no answer, although hearers are subliminally supposed to think, "Your party." Many times, when offering what sounds like a question, clients are expressing emotions in question syntax—rhetorical questions: "How long am I going to have to put up with her [the employer's] nasty tongue?" The preferred counselor response is silence—waiting for the client to continue. That silence is couched, however, in facial and body postures and simple reinforcers that communicate full attention to what the client is saying.

At other times the counselor can sense that the client is asking a genuine, not rhetorical, question but still one that should not be directly answered. The first parry to try is to focus on the emotional content, as in "Just thinking about that now makes you quite angry." But what if, as new students often ask, the client persists and practically demands an answer? The honesty with which the client is approached in all matters, the trust to be built, provides the principle on which the counselor's response is based. That response may be a compounding of reflection of feeling and clarification, evenly made: "Juan, it's clear that you see that you've been wronged, and I understand your anger, your feeling alone—your friends all siding with Rosita. I don't have an answer to your question, but I want you to know that I understand why you're upset. I want you to see that I want to help you, and I'm confident I can." This probably provides the client with the support he was seeking and confirms his good standing with the counselor, which he was doubting.

It is in treating the matter of questions that the changing nature of the client/counselor relationship is significant. As in any other new relationship, when one of the two participants is eager to develop that relationship, the first moments can be delicate, with sensitive probing about the other's values, preferences, and so on. The individual eager to advance a social relationship would not say to a new acquaintance with whom a friendship is desirable, "You voted for *her!* I think she's a disaster" but might say in a conversational tone, "Sometime I'd like to hear what you see as her qualifications." At a later time, with the relationship on solid foundations, blunt disagreements can be expressed with no likelihood of harming the relationship.

In like fashion the first minutes or hours of counseling can be decisive; a relationship may have to be delicately nursed. If counseling should run into three or more interviews and the counselor senses that a solid working relationship has been attained, leads will be less studied and no longer tentatively phrased. Instead of a counselor using the delicacies employed in early invitations, "I wonder if you could explain that a bit further," the invitation might have the bluntness of "I don't get that, Jan; what do you mean?" So also questions, avoided assiduously (and with difficulty) in the early moments, may now be posed at any time. Even so, these should not be asked impulsively but posed when there is need for information that will help the client move on, such as clarifying self-views or how the client functions in situations. Clients' questions also now may be directly answered, but in a measured manner, not with the abandon and bluntness that may occur in social situations.

## *11. Confrontation*

Although the word *confrontation* is open to misunderstanding because of its meaning when used socially, it will be employed here because it has become common in counseling literature. In social use it typically connotes an oppositional, face-to-face dispute: two assertive persons arguing, perhaps peers or a parent with an adolescent child. In counseling there are moments when client growth is contingent upon becoming aware of contradictions, such as the expression of contradictory rules of life or other conflicting cognitions. The counselor confronts the client with these discordances, but the confrontation is not personal as in the disputatious social sense. Social confrontation is between antagonists; the counselor is the client's protagonist, working side by side to eliminate a concern, and thus cannot act antagonistically.

The speech employed by the counselor may include blunt words, but the voice tone suggests that "I'm here to help you," not the tone of "Give me an accounting for this untenable contradiction." In a case where a client may be indecisive about an action that needs to be taken, the counselor's phrasing may be: "I sense a contradiction, Lynn. Awhile back you said that you could never do anything to hurt your parents, to go against their values, but now you say that you're going to move in with Dave. Don't those two contradictory statements pose some problems for you?" The counselor neither approves nor disapproves, no matter how much the client appears to seek exculpation for what he or she sees as misdeeds. The counselor's function is to cause the client to become aware of contradictions and, further, to deal with them, resolutely if possible and painfully if need be. It is the client's problem; the counselor can provide great help, but it is the client who must act, with counselor support.

## *12. Emotion Management*

There is justification in seeing emotion management more as a process than a lead. That may be said of No. 13 too. One justification for mentioning emotion management as a lead is to convey that counelors deal with client emotion in more ways than reflection of feeling. Reflection is employed early in a series of interviews, but it can be used at any time when the counselor judges it appropriate. At other times the counselor may deliberately provoke an emotion for therapeutic effect, thus managing the emotion. Other examples will be briefly explored in Chapter 13.

### 13. Information Giving, Interpretation, and Planning

In advanced stages of counseling the communication tone will often be noticeably cognitive and counselor-dominated: (1) questions are asked and answered, (2) the counselor expresses his or her views about what is happening in the client's life (interpreting) and discusses these views with the client, and (3) the counselor proposes steps the client can take to achieve his or her objectives and suggests how to implement those steps. It may be that these pronouncedly leading activities can be reached only because earlier, gentler responses led up to this point, although some client needs may be handled in a cognitive manner right from the start—career concerns, for example.

In this counselor-dominant lead we can discern some of the difference in interview behaviors between professional and untrained counselors. The latter can be expected to listen briefly and then move directly into explanation, followed likely by prescription. People practicing traditional counseling would not have learned why other steps are usually necessary before undertaking these advanced steps. Professional counselors not only know the purposes of the least leading responses but also have had the practice time required to acquire skill in these steps.

In some client concerns that are highly cognitive, however, such as those requiring decisions of immediate importance, this step may be reached in the early part of the first interview. Judgment by the counselor of what is happening in the interview determines that, not ritual.

One form of information needed by some clients relates to careers, information that taps into a massive pool of data about occupations and the education and training required for them, as well as data acquired about the client, such as through psychological assessments.

Counselors cannot be expected to be a reliable source of occupational information. Few counselors have acquired or retain much career information, because there is no need. (Counselors in employment services may retain a lot of information because their specialty provides occasion to acquire it.) Additionally, there are superior printed, audiovisual, and personal information sources available. Career information is a common need in educational and some other agencies, and therefore group activities to build information-seeking behaviors are appropriate; information seeking is a task for which individuals are responsible. If those agencies fail to equip prospective clients with information-seeking skills, they are pushing a burden onto counseling that will take time from a counselor's more important functions and face the counselor with a demand that cannot adequately be met. Not providing experiences that build information-seeking behaviors will also deny the agency's charges an opportunity to acquire lifelong skills that will reduce their dependency on counseling. Secondary schools with adequately staffed guidance programs have professionals other than counselors who, as information specialists, are rich sources of information and who lead groups of students in acquiring information-seeking behaviors.

Counselors employ the leads of clarification, summary, and some hypothesizing in early parts of interviews, but only to the degree that these stimulate further self-exploration by the client. With a solid working alliance established by the advanced stages of interviewing, the counselor may present to the client a synthesis (interpretation) of the intertwining of cognitive, affective, and behavioral elements of the client's life and the effect they have.

Clients cycle in and out of interviews, with the interviews being only brief periods in their lives. It is in their daily lives that clients have to practice new cognitions, changed affect, or new or altered behaviors. These activities must be planned and their effectiveness assessed. Although this planning is not deferred to the final interview—it can start in the first interview—in the early periods of counseling the plans are probably simple relative to the kind of complex plans of major significance that can be proposed in later interviews.

To think of leads as the colors on the palette of the artist/counselor is to suggest that the art of counseling is solely the expression of the counselor's subjective being, as it is for the painter or sculptor. Counseling is an art, as, to a lesser degree, is medicine. However, art in these instances is not intended to express the practitioner's subjective world, but primarily to establish conditions that are judged to best serve the interests of those who come for assistance. The use of any particular lead at any particular time is a judgment call by the counselor/artist, informed partly by conjecture and partly by evidence (these sum to theory).

## One School's Classification of Communication

Some schools of counseling or therapy do not analyze communications or present a taxonomy because their theoretical substratum does not require it. One school does present an analysis—one quite different from that given in this text. We look briefly at that analysis to illustrate how differences in communication among schools can vary with the theoretical premises on which a school or theory is based.

Berne (1961) set out a communication schema for the school he originated called transactional analysis. The core of the school's theory is the psychoanalytic tenet of ego states, of which Berne identifies three: Parent, Adult, and Child. These three states, with two subsets each for the parent and child ego states, account for the way persons interact from time to time with other persons, and therefore the communications employed. At times this calls for confrontation. As with other schools, no systematic examination of this school is undertaken here. Transactional Analysis provides fetching terms to describe interfacing behaviors, such as strokes, games, and scripts, and a fresh way of examining transactions. Although Transactional Analysis in its full form is not supported by evidence that it approximates a valid explanation of human behavior, certain of its propositions are imaginative and useful. On the other hand, its analysis of oral transactions into three major plus two minor categories is an oversimplification. Evidence suggests that transactions are more complex, and communications less simple. During counseling a client at times may be as dependent, manic, and naive as a child, at times calm and rational like a mature adult able to objectively acknowledge and deal with his or her faults, or at times judgmental about others. There is no advantage in identifying these fleeting changes as particular ego states; a counselor can handle each change with an appropriate lead as the shifts occur. If an adult client describes his or her concern as being locked into unwanted dependency actions related to a parent, for example, any number of ways to assist the client in easing this relationship without harming client or parent are available. No gain has been demonstrated by labeling the client's or parent's behaviors, including communication mannerisms, as either Parent, Adult, or Child.

## Communication Skills Are Not Ends in Themselves

Persons come for counseling about a variety of concerns, such as relationships that are not fulfilling or are disturbing, inadequate self views, undesirable behaviors (or lack of desired ones), planning a future, or correcting development that otherwise is not proceeding in a desired manner. Additionally they may

- seek validation for their thinking or behavior,
- want to have the counselor make difficult decisions for them,
- just want to get some information,
- look for advice, such as how to deal with a difficult mother-in-law or obstreperous children,
- long to be prodded into taking a long-delayed course of action,
- want to be psychologically punished by the counselor to relieve guilt.

They may not be aware of why they have sought counseling, knowing only that "something isn't right." They may see the origin of their concerns lying largely in situations, including other persons, or may attribute their concerns to defects of character or to incompetencies, perhaps to both the situation and self. As the client deals with these concerns, emotions may be cued off as well as cognitions and recollections of behaviors. These will form the unpredictable nature of client communication. The client speaks spontaneously; the counselor responds with skilled deliberation. One important consequence will be the gaining of self-knowledge, the acquiring of insight.

### *Insight Is Not Enough*

The insights acquired through counseling can bring about some improvement, and insight counseling has long been praised. Insight cannot be counted on to be sufficient, however. An oft-repeated anecdote carries a good message: clients concerned about their alcoholism gain insight through counseling into the kind of person they are and the reason why they are alcoholic. At the end of the counseling they are now insightful alcoholics. The obvious message is that counseling cannot end unless clients are thinking and acting differently and experiencing emotions constructively, outcomes partly facilitated by insight. Counseling is effective when clients no longer experience the concerns that brought them to counseling and are able to continue development in a constructive, mentally healthful way. This outcome typically requires changes in cognitions, emotional responses, and behaviors, usually compounded into a single dynamic within which, nonetheless, the function of these three elements can be separately identified. These changes occur not because a counselor tells a client that those kinds of changes are needed but as a result of the change efforts jointly engaged in by client and counselor, a pronounced cognitive activity toward which earlier leads were employed.

## *Attentive Listening Is Not Enough*

Carl Rogers was the major force in counseling for decades, a phenomenologist whose counseling focused on client feelings and self-concepts. Rogers proposed two essentials for effective counseling. One of these comprises three necessary counselor characteristics: (1) authenticity, (2) congruency, because counselors' actual and ideal selves must match, and (3) the capacity to experience and demonstrate unconditional positive regard for clients. The second essential involves the nature of interviews. In successful interviews, clients can sense those counselor qualities, and counselors demonstrate their empathy with clients by reflecting clients' feelings.

Clients experiencing these two essentials, Rogers maintained, will be able to face up to the incongruities between their ideal and real selves. Through this confrontation, a congruency will emerge, and clients' difficulties will be resolved. The purpose of person-centered counseling is to bring about this congruency by reflecting clients' feelings, a reactive stance to clients' statements.

Science-oriented studies over the years have demonstrated the limitations of Rogers's ideas by showing that beyond clients' perceived self-concepts there are other cognitive as well as behavioral variables that influence their coping competencies. Unlike people committed solely to phenomenology, science-oriented counselors acknowledge that clients must relate to the real world not just in accord with their perceptions but with how it actually is. It may be important at times to lead clients to achieve agreement between the concept of their actual self and that of their ideal self. It is always important to enable them to have their perceptions of the objective world match its reality.

These and other determining variables have been examined in earlier chapters. To acknowledge their authenticity is to hold that employment of an array of communication skills cannot be an end in itself. Those skills create a climate that retains clients in counseling by fostering a therapeutic alliance, which then leads to changes in specific thoughts, emotions, and behaviors (usually inextricable mixes of these) required to help clients attain their objectives.

More than active attending skills and empathy is required to reach those objectives. There is a need to seek out the broad sweep of client development to permit counselors to join clients in "their experience of *making* meaning rather than to . . . join their *made* meaning," Kegan's felicitous phrase (1982, p. 277; emphasis added). Counselors work *proactively* to help clients resolve developmental difficulties, but they are equally interested in what Kegan calls the client's evolutionary self, the self in continuous development, or construction. Development enhancement is a responsibility of counselors in educational institutions, and it is carried out by meeting with students in groups to lead them in acquiring developmentally useful thoughts and behavior skills.

Counselors employ minimally leading responses when and for as long as they judge there is a need. More leading responses will be used as soon as counselors sense that a less tender, less protective, more proactive manner of interacting is best—when the time has arrived to lead clients in making specific changes.

## Concluding Reflections

Part I put primary attention on counselors, while Part II was focused more on clients. Part III is attending to the practice of counseling.

This chapter's examination of communication brought attention again to the importance Carl Rogers gave to the characteristics of counselor authenticity and genuineness in the success of counseling. The unique communication procedures of counseling would enable clients to sense these characteristics, while their existence would contribute to the trustful alliance between counselor and client. Even though present-day knowledge of counseling practices informs us of the influence of other variables needed to reach counseling objectives, the important influence of those two counselor traits has not been challenged.

No matter how much counselors are authentic, genuine, and skilled in communications, of equal importance are their abilities to cope with the vicissitudes that naturally assail them, to resolve challenges to their own being. The first rule of medicine is to do no harm to the patient; that also has to be the psychological counselor's first rule. It surely means that counselors facing disruptive events in their own lives will forgo trying to help others until there is a resolution of those difficulties. This precaution is necessary to prevent their own concerns being worked out on clients. The importance of counseling's unique communication skills for the success of counseling, as well as the importance of other technical competencies, is matched by the importance of counselors' characteristics.

The presentation of communication skills here is primitive because it is introductory. If only one message is learned it should be that counselors do not speak off the top of their heads—impulsively, that is. When counselors engage clients, it is with a broad perspective on human existence and considerable knowledge about the intertwined operations of thinking, affect, and behavior. When counselors and clients have moved out of the introductory moments, verbal communication is creative and includes manners of speaking that go beyond the classification system presented in this chapter. Some of that will become more apparent in Chapter 13.

## ■          Points to Remember          ■

1. Clients come to talk about their concerns. Counselors respond thoughtfully and carefully (even if quickly) to clients' statements. To be able to do this, they acquire skill in counseling communication devices.

2. Two social behaviors, eagerness to talk and spontaneously asking questions, are potentially harmful to counseling communication.
3. Counselors' use of words has been studied for years and has been differently analyzed into hierarchies or classes. The hierarchy of 13 responses offered here is:

| | |
|---|---|
| simple reinforcers | summary |
| invitation | conjecture, or hypothesis |
| restatement | approval |
| paraphrasing | parrying clients' questions |
| reflection of feeling | confrontation |
| clarification | emotion management |
| | information giving, |
| | interpretation, and planning |

4. Counselors and clients alike communicate nonverbally through facial features, postures, and gestures.

■                        **Counselor Formation Activity**                        ■

With two other students, form a practice group. The group will carry out a series of brief exercises in which group members will rotate the position of simulated client, simulated counselor, and observer. The key part is played by each as simulated client because it is imperative to make each exercise as realistic as possible, to "be" the person portrayed. There likely will be considerable self-consciousness to overcome at first, something students with acting experience will be able to do quickly.

The student simulating the client can fill that role by recalling a developmentally disrupting condition from some time past, no longer an active concern. Alternatively, the simulating client can present a concern currently experienced by someone known to that student. The other group members are not to know whether this has been a real problem of the student client's past, the concern of another person, or one created by the client.

Each experience may begin with the student counselor greeting the client at the entrance of the room and becoming established in a counseling setting. Alternatively, the exercises can be carried out while seated only, without the greeting at the door. The function of the exercise is to provide the simulated counselor an opportunity to practice starting an interview with invitation and other minimal leads, listening, not interrupting, and showing empathic understanding of the client. Group members will determine appropriate length for each exercise, but fifteen minutes is typical.

The observer records the details of the interview on a simply prepared sheet on which can be noted the number of simple reinforcers employed as well as other leads, expecting that only the least-leading ones will be employed in a fifteen-minute segment. The observer also notes instances wherein, in the observer's judgment, the counselor could just as well have listened instead of speaking. The observer will assess the proportion of time used in client and counselor speaking, with the ideal being minimal talking by the counselor. The observer also will note (1) any interruptions by the counselor when the client is speaking (none should occur), and the content of such interruptions, and (2) questions the counselor asks (there should be none, but do not count invitations as questions).

After each segment the simulated client evaluates the experience, the student observer reports, and the student counselor comments.

With time and a number of efforts given to this experience, and assuming realization of the necessity for this practice, self-consciousness will ebb and each will be able to enter into the simulated reality. A classroom demonstration and trial with several student triads will facilitate student practice on their own in the small groups. Careful exploitation of these experiences will provide maximum opportunity to exchange undesirable communication habits for desirable ones, and to gain comfort in interviewing by acquiring counseling's unique communication skills.

■                        **Complementary Reading**                        ■

Another analysis of communication in counseling, with a tone that is somewhat more Rogerian than found in this chapter but deserving examination, is provided by Egan (1982), Chapters 5 and 6. Ivey's (1980) analysis of communication was cited in the text. See his Chapters 3 and, especially, 5.

## 11

**CHAPTER**

# Other Counseling Issues

## Overview

The manner in which counselors communicate with clients, as we have seen, is central to attaining the objectives of counseling. Although that statement defines other interview elements as being somewhat peripheral contributors to counseling's success, the sum of these other elements can have an effect on the quality of the relationship between client and counselor. Some of these lesser but still important matters, questions often raised by students, are considered here.

We will then give our attention to the topic of the effectiveness of counseling. Pursuit of this topic requires a brief consideration of schools of counseling, because the history of the research on counseling's effectiveness has centered on the claims made by different schools. A meta-analysis summarized in this chapter examines those claims and finds no defense for them. Instead, that analysis finds, the effectiveness of counseling lies in the quality of the emotional bond, or therapeutic alliance, between clients and counselors. This finding does not mean that other issues are unimportant. We will note that the quality of that alliance depends to a significant degree on the effectiveness of techniques, but there is no credibility to the notion that the package of limited techniques that characterizes any one school is more effective than that of other schools.

## Elements of the Interview

### *Meeting Clients: Where and How*

Counseling can occur and be effective in a variety of settings—*al fresco* in camps, for example. However, it is preferably conducted in a professional-looking room that provides privacy. Other surface elements are equally professional, shown in the way appointments are made, how clients are greeted, the attire of the counselor, the appearance of the room, how interviews are begun and ended, and how payments (if any) are handled.

The room will be pleasantly and neutrally furnished, with chairs comfortable enough not to be distracting for at least 50 minutes. The neutrality is maintained more by what is not present than by what is. There will be no polemical posters, for example, unless the counseling is conducted by a distinctly protagonistic agency, such as a prolife, homophilic, or religious body.

In the absence of a separate room, requiring interviews to be held in a counselor's office, a spot is set up for the purpose away from the desk. Some clients sitting at the side of a cluttered desk report feeling that they are interrupting a very busy counselor. The worst of all arrangements is for counselors to sit on one side of a desk full of working papers, distancing themselves from clients on the other side of the desk. Phone interruptions are prevented by turning off the ringer if no one can intercept calls. Ignoring a ringing phone is greatly distracting to some clients. If there is no receptionist who can prevent intrusion into the counseling room, a Do Not Disturb sign on the door serves the purpose.

New counselors are advised to sit at an angle to the client to avoid face-to-face (confrontational) seating. The counselor sits alertly, leaning a bit toward the client, and maintains eye contact to a degree that is comfortable for the client. On the counselor's part this should be substantial to convey attentive listening but continuous only if that is the level set by the client.

Attention to clients' faces permits sensing the presence of affect and of changes in it. The clients' eyes are useful for this, but even the mouth and nostrils are revealing. Recent developments in *neurolinguistics* provide potential new sources of information about clients' states. One group of research shows that the counselor can identify clients' mental processes by where they direct their eyes: to the upper, middle, or lower right or left. It is believed that deployment of one's eyes in those directions corresponds to parts of the brain being searched, each hemisphere giving different information.

The general principle: do whatever conveys to the client that he or she is the one important person in the counselor's life during interview time. The atmosphere is a balance between intensive attention and ease. Although the counselor may remain in one position throughout early interviews, when a working alliance is established, the counselor's posture and actions will be more spontaneous. This may include moving about occasionally, such as looking out a window while pondering, or consulting a professional book. New counselors will attend to the professional tone of first interviews, restraining for a while such idiosyncratic behaviors that may distract new clients. Those natural, more spontaneous behaviors will have a place after a comfortable working relationship has been established.

## What's in a Name?

Is there a best way for counselors to address clients? If counselors address clients by given names, are clients to address counselors similarly? If counselors are to be addressed by an honorific (Dr., Mrs., Mr.), are clients similarly addressed? Some considerations follow, but they must be tempered by the fact of regional, even local, differences in practices.

If a fee is charged, the client is, in one sense, an employer. The client may address a plumber or car mechanic by first name, an accepted custom, but expect to be addressed by an honorific, except in parts of the South. Because the client employs you, will you be addressed by your first name while you address the client by an honorific? No, because yours will not be a typical employer/employee relationship. A plumber is employed to make repairs as directed, with the status of employer and employee established by custom, no matter the likelihood that the plumber earns more than the employer. It is a culturally determined superior/ inferior relationship, even if a friendly one.

The relationship between counselor and client is professional. Among most professions the superior/inferior relationship is the opposite of a trade relationship. In the culture of physicians, the professional relationship is occasionally demonstrated by the physician's use of the patient's given name, sometimes right from the first, regardless of the patient's age or other statuses; but at the same time the physician expects to be addressed as "Doctor." Is this the appropriate stance of counselors relative to clients? Probably not. The counseling relationship is the determining force in this matter. It is not a relationship of friends, with use of first names expected for that reason. Nor is it the relationship a client would have with other professionals involving objective data, such as parts of the body, in the case of physicians and dentists, or legal concerns. Psychological counseling, in contrast, is a relationship of trust between a professional person helping another person resolve a highly subjective, value-laden, potentially emotionally intense concern. This relationship involves, ultimately, the quality of the client's life.

Each counselor's social background and experiences will bear on this matter. Some counselors elect to address a client with a given name from the first moments but say nothing to the client about how the counselor is to be addressed. Others also use the given name from the outset and direct clients to use the counselor's given name without asking clients if that is agreeable. In public schools, where professional employees are expected to be addressed by an honorific but students are addressed by first or family name, this is not an issue. Nor is it in agencies where the use of given names by counselor and client is agency policy. In colleges the issue is less culturally determined, and all varieties above may be found. My preference, in settings where name use is not institutionalized, is to ask clients if I may use their given name, at the same time inviting, not directing, them to address me by given name. The invitation aspect is of some importance. Some people are accustomed to addressing adults in educational institutions or professionals in any setting by only an honorific and prefer to continue that custom. It would be inappropriate to require clients to use a given name when they prefer not to do so. The relationship may be by crude cultural measurements a superior/inferior one, but the actual working relationship may not convey that kind of status. An effective therapeutic alliance is not built on staking out positions of superiority or inferiority.

## *Note Taking, Recording, and Record Keeping*

Taking of notes during inverviews is defensible for later reminding the counselor of an important point made by the client that cannot be immediately pursued. Depending upon the quality of interview records to be kept, notes will ensure the inclusion of items that might otherwise be forgotten after the interview.

Some counselors are convinced that taking any note is a distraction to both counselor and client. Others see an advantage in the message given to clients that what they are saying is important enough to merit notes. My preference is for counselors to be ready to make an unobtrusive note, having explained the reason beforehand, and to invite clients also to make a note for similar purposes. A pad and pen are placed by the client.

Audio recording is an alternative, one that requires clients' approval, preferably in writing. The major disadvantage is the need to spend considerable time in replaying just to find one or a few points that need recollection. Audio tapes can be used to benefit clients by having them listen to one or more interviews. Some clients have reported gaining considerable insight. Another advantage is their occasional use by counselors to monitor their interview competencies.

A professional practitioner makes and retains client or patient records. The content of medical and legal records is obvious, and some counseling records are also uncomplicated and clear, such as protocols of psychological tests and measures. The nature of interview records poses problems, such as how much to record so as to permit a grasp of the subjective and objective variables and their combinations when a counselor reviews records before the next interview. The confidentiality of such highly personal data is critical and is an issue in what records of interviews are kept. A counselor's interests in a malpractice lawsuit are ill served if the counselor cannot support his or her defense with evidence from professional records.

Because most counselors are agency employees, the issue is mostly resolved by agency policy. For the counselor who also engages in some independent practice, the issues are different.

### *Closing the First Interview and Starting the Second*

Part of the professional tone of counseling is that it typically occurs at an assigned time. In schools that is usually a class period. In other agencies or in independent practice, an hour has become the customary time block, of which 50 minutes are for being with a client. Conditions may permit or require counselors to go beyond 50 minutes at times. In any case, counselors start at some point to wind down interviews to allow time for summary and plans for the next session. In order to be aware of the time without putting pressure on clients by glancing at your watch, a clock can be placed on a bookcase or table behind the client's chair.

A counselor, with ten or so minutes left, will say at the end of a discussion unit something like: "Our time will soon be up, Barry, and I think it will be helpful to tie together what happened here today. What seemed important to you?" The client and counselor can together summarize the session, effectively bringing the interview to a close. If halfway through an interview a client becomes emotionally distressed, the counselor must judge whether to start then to slowly ease the client out of the distress so as to be ready for the next client or to relinquish an expectancy that the interview will be ended on time. As no two interviews are similar, no two closings can be. Counselors quickly acquire deftness in managing to close interviews in a professional manner.

Before the next session the counselor will review a client's records so that the interview can smoothly take up where the prior one left off. It will be the counselor's own doing if he or she cannot remember data deemed critical by the client if asked to do so.

Although counselors will have studied the prior week's session before the next one, interviews do not start with the counselor talking about the previous one. Considerable change in the client should have occurred in the intervening period, and therefore the counselor opens the interview, if the client does not, by saying something like this: "I recall events from last week's session, Barry, but a number of things may have happened to you about [the client's concern] since then. Can you tell me how things seem to you now." There are numerous alternative openings, if the client does not open. For one, the counselor may reflect change in affect: "Last week you seemed to me to be a worried, distracted, unsure person. Today you seem calm and confident." Just to say that much is enough to stimulate the client to lead interview developments for a time. If in reply to the first of these openers ("how things seem different") the client seems somewhat apathetic and replies, with a shrug, "Oh, I don't know; I guess it's about the same; I just don't know what to talk about today," the counselor can recall a central topic from his or her review of notes of the prior week's interview. The counselor then might say, "Last week [naming the event] seemed important to you. How does that seem now, Barry." (The dropping voice marks this as an invitation.) It is the client's counseling session; let him take as much responsibility for it as possible.

## Identifying Counseling Objectives

I have referred to three kinds of counseling objectives. The important ones for clients are the changes that they want counseling to bring. These changes have been labeled intermediate objectives. Immediate objectives are set by the counselor: specific changes usually associated with specific change strategies. There may be a half-dozen of these over time with one client. The sum effect of achieving each of these immediate objectives is the reaching of the client's (intermediate) objective(s).

Beyond these are the unexpressed, and indeed possibly unaware, views that constitute counselors' ultimate objectives for clients. In this section, the term *objectives* refers to relatively clear outcomes that *clients* want and thus are intermediate objectives under the classification described.

People seek help from trained counselors when forced to acknowledge that they do not have the resources within themselves to make changes they desire and that counseling with untrained persons (best friend, neighbor, and perhaps minister) has not helped.

Sometimes clients' purposes are not fully known to them, as in the case of one who tries to displace guilt onto the counselor or one needing an authority (like Daddy) who will tell him or her to "get on with it." In most cases, however, clients are fully or mostly aware of what their concerns are and as self-directing individuals are ready to tackle them. They are also able to define their counseling objectives in rough terms: control temper, become more assertive, resolve long-lasting ill feelings with another person, acquire friends, either be confident about or change a career direction, stop a marriage from falling apart, correct a child's wild, undisciplined behaviors, and on and on.

Sometimes clients can say only that their persistent unhappiness means that something is not right about their lives but at the time cannot specify what is causing their anomie, acedia, or general discontent, vague complaints that are maximum challenges to the conceptual and practice skills of the psychological counselor. Even here an objective can be stated, even if it does not specify the directions to take. The objective of a person experiencing apathy is to become enthusiastic about life. Not much to go on, but it is a start.

When specific goals can be set, they are as if in reply to questions such as "What kind of changes would you like to make in your life?" or "What changes do you look forward to at the end of counseling?" It may be the counselor who first states (as a hypothesis) a client's objective: "As I've been listening, Audrey, it seems to me that you'd like [states one objective]."

Client objectives may be stated as changes in mental processes, feelings, or behaviors or, more likely, those in combination. One facet of the totally functioning person may be employed to assist change in another facet, such as emotion to bring about cognitive restructuring, or cognitions to facilitate behavior change. Whatever the objectives, they may become clear only in some later interview, but whenever they are set, any is open to change as clients change, as, for example, alterations of perceptions of self-in-world would naturally come about in many cases, in and out of counseling sessions.

### Psychological Measurement

The complex, technical topic of psychological measurement requires treatment beyond the scope of this text. This portion of the topic touches only on the connection of such measures to interviews.

Ideally, counselors administer all psychological measures to their clients to permit observation while the clients are engaged in the testing process, because clients' approaches and reactions to testing sometimes reveal valuable information about them. That ideal usually is not possible, because counselor interview loads are too demanding, counselors may be unfamiliar with the instruments, and the occasional bit of information gleaned does not justify commitment of the time.

Some counselors administer a certain few tests, particularly individual intelligence tests, but send clients to psychometrists for other measurement. Larger agencies employ psychometrists who do the testing for the agency's counselors, but counselors in independent practice may be forced to become proficient in a number of measures. Some instruments can be taken away by clients to be completed before the next interview. In that case, counselors should get clients started on each instrument, both to make sure they know what is called for (how to "do" the test) and to get them started on a task that otherwise may not be done or be done shabbily at the last minute.

### Planning for and Assisting Changes

Counseling is intended to bring about some change a client wishes to make, a change that will be legal and agreed to by the counselor and be in accord with the counselor's moral code. Changes will comport with the criteria of good development—that is to say, with mental-health criteria. The changes may be solely cognitive, as is often the case with clients who ask for help with career plans. Such planning is often long and complex and involves numerous steps the client must take under counselor leadership. However, concerns that are solely cognitive are rare. Most will be colored by affect and include unproductive behavior patterns, requiring counselors to attend to concerns that are a mix of the three facets.

Although the objectives that clients wish to reach usually require employment of one or more specific cognitive, emotional, or behavioral techniques, it must be recalled that sometimes just "talking to" a counselor before any specific change technique could be employed results in clients' concluding that their concerns have gone. Although this process has an air of mystery about it, such change without effort may be accounted for as a rapid cognitive restructuring that permits the client to reconceptualize troublesome social systems and to have changed perceptions of such systems. I have found this to be an event experienced by more intelligent clients. They have had no prior reason to make the kind of examination of self-in-system that occurs when they now try to explain matters to a counselor. And it is more than just thinking about self-in-system. The process of speaking and, thus, of hearing oneself appears to be critical, a step facilitated by the counselor's listening skills such as simple reinforcements. The counselor can "see" the cognitive restructuring occur during the client's speaking. The clues are those pauses in which the client makes such comments as "Now that I come to think about it . . .," "Hmmmmm—I hadn't thought about that before," or "You know, I can see now that I've been taking the wrong approach." Before counseling has arrived at a point where the counselor could begin to identify specific interventions that might be appropriate, the client may announce, "Well, I think I have that problem licked" and terminate counseling.

Another, more complex hypothesis to account for this spontaneous disappearance of clients' concerns is that some clients are so bereft of experiences with a calm, caring, objective, nonjudgmental person that counseling may cause the release of hormones that activate certain energies. These, then, may assuage the emotional traumas that have been inhibiting client effectiveness, therefore letting clients gain sufficient coping confidence to handle their concerns with no further help. This may also explain the beneficial effects that are sometimes the outcome of traditional counseling. There is a lower expectation of this spontaneous outcome in traditional than in professional counseling because professional counselors will avoid the errors of commission and omission that untrained counselors are likely to commit.

The effectiveness of counseling typically depends upon two essentials: the working alliance established and the techniques employed to bring about the changes the client wishes. The alliance depends largely on counselors' communication skills, including management of interviews, and on the employment of techniques based upon the quality of counselors' assessment of clients' cognitions, emotions, and behaviors.

## *Ending Counseling*

Counseling ends when clients and counselors agree that such a step is appropriate. Clients will judge that they can cope with the concerns that brought them to counseling, and counselors will be comfortable that clients are able to continue development in a constructive way with minimal mental-health im-balances. Clients' concerns are typically worked out in two arenas: in consulting rooms with counselors' help and in the social contexts-as-systems in which clients conduct daily affairs. Interviews, in addition to providing an opportunity for change in client cognitions and emotions, are rehearsal sites for the activities that are then played "for real" outside the interview. Clients' judgments that they are now able to cope come to a large degree from the confirmation of their effectiveness provided by their experiences in the "real" world.

Clients may suggest termination after one or two interviews or may wait until months of interviews have passed. The ending of counseling is first the client's option, but it is professionally sounder when it results from an agreement between client and counselor. Counselors must be ready to accept the fact that clients sometimes just do not show up again or telephone. Depending upon the counselors' judgments about those clients' state, they may write or call to inquire about the loss of communication or even to suggest picking up again if assessment of client concerns warrants.

In the normal termination of counseling, proposed either by client or counselor, there may be a brief review of the client's achievements and of actions in the real world that the client should continue. If a counselor thinks that a client's proposal to terminate has been made before the client's concern has been resolved, the counselor will give that opinion to the client but accept the client's judgment. In any case, the counselor invites the client to return whenever the need arises. Counselors know that sometimes clients end counseling, with counselor concurrence, feeling confident that a developmental concern they brought to counseling is behind them, but counselors know, too, that regression may occur. In such cases, clients' prior experiences in having achieved goals for at least a while is evidence to them that it can be done again. Counselors, when meeting clients who have returned because of such regression, remind them that they can achieve objectives, that regression is not uncommon, and that their self-recrimination, if that is occurring, is not productive. What is useful is for them to identify causes for the regression and to repeat the steps they learned earlier in order to regain lost ground.

# Why Is Counseling Effective?

The ultimate measure of counseling effectiveness is provided by clients: have they successfully reached their objectives—are they developing now in more mentally healthful ways? Inspection of traditional counseling shows that objectives are sometimes attained, particularly short-term, clearly identified ones. Professional counseling shows successful attainment of goals too, usually involving more complex, longer-lasting concerns than those helped by traditional counseling. But desirable client outcomes are insufficient data to measure effectiveness. It is necessary to know what counselor practices or conditions bear on the attainment of clients' objectives.

Outcomes attributable to the limited procedures of particular schools have been studied occasionally over many years with no clear conclusions. In a recent meta-analysis of research centering on the counseling practices associated with particular schools, Stiles, Shapiro, and Elliot (1986) conclude:

> Despite clear demonstration by process researchers of systematic differences in therapists' techniques, most reviews of psychotherapy outcome research show little or no differential effectiveness of different psychotherapies. . . . The outcomes of different psychotherapies . . . are equivalent [pp. 165–166].

Although they refer only to psychotherapy, inspection shows that their findings relate also to concepts and practices that others call counseling.

They conclude, additionally, that "it seems implausible that the obtained lack of differential effectiveness could be attributed to a lack of real technical diversity" (p. 167). There is no evidence that practitioners of one school, employing the techniques thought to be unique to that school, are more effective than practitioners of other schools using their particular techniques. The assumption must follow that other variables are affecting the outcome. It has already been noted that two factors have an effect on outcome. The lore has it that if a person seeks professional assistance, 50% of the eventually successful outcome has been reached just by taking that step. The other anecdotal but extensive evidence, examined above, shows that in some cases just listening to a client creates (releases?) possibilities for clients to move on effectively without any technical intervention by the counselor. Stiles and his colleagues locate another factor that is significant, the therapeutic alliance, which will be examined shortly.

It is difficult to compare effectiveness studies using objective data because of the lack of agreed-upon criteria of mentally healthful behavior, even though that is the ultimate goal counselors hold out for their clients. There is agreement among theorists and practitioners about the narrow range of thoughts, affect, and actions that are to be classified as undesirable, as mentally unhealthful—the narrow end of a figurative funnel. At the wider end is found a broad range of cognitions, affect, and behaviors, some of which would be viewed as acceptable by some people but unacceptable by others. Others regard eccentricity or idiosyncrasy as acceptable, mentally healthful developmental goals (Benjamin, 1949). In sum, there is ready agreement about what constitutes undesirable mental health but disagreement about mentally healthful thoughts and behaviors.

Stiles and his associates (1986) concur that "normal behavior varies widely, especially when considered across roles and cultures" (p. 171), a fact that affects research outcomes. For example, a study on effectiveness may use as a dependent variable the quantity and quality of clients' expression of emotion, with more emotional openness judged desirable. There are apparently innate gender differences affecting openness, but additionally, "If . . . a therapy promotes free expression of emotion, and this outcome is seen as positive by some cultures, subcultures, or individuals but neutral or negative by others, the client showing large increases in emotional expression will not necessarily be judged as 'highly improved'" (p. 171).

In medicine there is a commonly agreed-upon model of health, in contrast to the heterogeneity surrounding psychological normality. In areas of cognitions, affect, and behavior there can be several models of what is mentally healthful. Thus, "if psychological health is pluralistic, the psychological treatments may appropriately be so too" (p. 171).

## The Basis of Effectiveness: The Client/Practitioner Alliance

If the effectiveness of counseling is not attributable to the practices of differing schools, what *does* make it effective? Meta-analysis leads Stiles and his colleagues to conclude that the once favorably received hypothesis that therapeutic success lies only in therapists' personal qualities is now less commonly held. There is research evidence now, the authors conclude, that the core element common to the effectiveness of all schools is found in *"clients' behavior or attitudes or in the alliance between therapist and client"* (p. 175; emphasis added). This alliance is spoken of by others as an emotional bond but spoken of even more commonly as the counseling relationship.

Were there unaminous evidence to support that conclusion, it would not follow that counselors-to-be should ignore specific techniques; evidence makes clear that the therapeutic alliance, or counseling relationship, and clients' attitudes toward counseling are dependent on techniques. It is not the conclusion of Stiles and his associates that techniques are ineffective; it is that sets of techniques particular to the theoretical claims of any one school do not make the outcomes of that school's *package* of techniques more effective than another school's package.

Numerous techniques can be used to alleviate concerns. A counselor selects a particular technique for a particular purpose rather than ritually employing a limited package of techniques or only a single technique because his or her commitment to a school dictates it. The subsequent success the client experiences as a result of technical sophistication affects the client's expectancy of positive outcomes from counseling:

> Once a success of any sort has been achieved, clients in any therapy may be pulled along by their own expectations of future change. . . . The varied techniques . . . [may be] no more than diverse means to a common end, namely the enhancement of clients' self-efficacy beliefs [Stiles et al., 1986, p. 173].

Such self-efficacy is proposed by Masterpasqua (1989) as central to effectiveness in general, therefore earning the right not just to be the focus of clinical interventions but also to serve as a basis for those development-enhancing and preventive activities that are also important functions of psychological counseling. The context of Masterpasqua's position is developmental, and as such he subscribes to the proposition of Dixon and Lerner (1989) that three evolutionary themes are coming to dominate perspectives on development. These are "(a) emphasis on the individual's history, (b) the importance of context (ecology), and (c) emphasis on the adaptive nature of development" (p. 1366), the latter being the emphasis that Masterpasqua particularizes. He proposes that people's abilities to adjust "must continually be fed by a lifelong acquisition of adaptive behaviors, cognitions, and relations." These elements provide the competence to meet challenges of living, and "competence can be defined as adaptive cognitive, emotional, behavioral, and social attributes, complemented by the person's implicit or explicit beliefs . . . about his or her access to and ability to implement those attributes" (p. 1366)—that is, to be self-efficacious.

Counselors-to-be can readily learn specific techniques that encourage client activity and induce expectancy of counseling success; it is more difficult to become skillful in determining when and for what specific purposes those techniques are appropriate. Some procedures, such as those for creating and maintaining a counseling alliance, cannot readily be acquired, and certainly not through a didactic approach only. This is understandable in light of the description of that alliance as *an emotional bond and mutual involvement between therapist and client.* Those qualities of a counselor's personality that affect the formation of a relationship, or therapeutic bond, must be acquired or enhanced during training through group experiences designed for that purpose. Recall the new counselor described in Chapter 4, the one whose untenable views of women did not surface and thus could not be challenged in his counselor-preparation program until it was almost "too late," during supervised practice. Without change it was highly probable that no emotional bond could develop between him and a female client.

Stiles and his associates (1986) propose that "competent therapists of all persuasions are able to establish an emotional bond and a sense of mutual collaboration with respective clients, and . . . this relationship carries most of the therapeutic weight" (p. 173). Unfortunately, some schools not only do not attend to emotional bonds between counselor and client but discredit them.

Claiborn and Lichtenberg (1989) have presented a studied analysis of the counseling relationship. They note that any relationship, informal or formal, is a process of negotiating the rules of the interaction between the two persons. Because counseling has general goals to be reached, and later specific ones, the relationship between counselor and client must have certain characteristics and must avoid other ones. The relationship must be professional (Let's get on with the work to be done), socially impersonal, empathic, and focused on change. The client may have aware or unaware reasons to establish a casual, more social relationship, but the counselor must keep the relationship away from having an "anything you'd like to do" ambience.

In some counseling approaches, Claiborn and Lichtenberg observe, although the relationship is valued as the context that facilitates client receptivity, disclosure, exploration, and risk taking, it is viewed as insufficient to result in change. The counselor, those approaches hold, must "*do* something" (p. 392). Claiborn and Lichtenberg see a more radical view of the role of the relationship however: it "is not simply the context of interventions, it *is* the intervention" (p. 392).

This view appears to be in accord with that reached by Stiles and his colleagues in their finding that the relationship carries the most weight in reaching positive outcomes. Acceptance of this conclusion pushes us to ask what, then, justifies the variety of "persuasions"—of schools of counseling? In any case, of the two persons who make up the counseling relationship, it is "the client's contribution to and perception of the therapeutic alliance, rather than the therapist's, [that] best predicts successful outcome" (p. 173).

## Concluding Reflections

This chapter rounds out the characteristics of counseling interviews, letting our attention move next to cognitive, emotional, and behavioral techniques that counselors employ to help clients achieve their objectives. It also marks the end of arguments that psychological counseling should be rooted in the best of scientific thought and evidence and, as a result, should forgo the concept of schools of counseling. The last of those arguments was found in the evidence that the package of techniques carried out by adherents of any one school of counseling demonstrated no more effectiveness than that of other schools.

The emphasis here is on the lack of evidence of the efficaciousness of the *package* of techniques attributed to any one school. Evidence remains that particular techniques have made contributions to client objectives. In recognition of that sureness, the emphasis in the next two chapters is on procedures and techniques that counselors employ, but within the context of the working alliance, or relationship. It will be noted that clinical psychologists employ these techniques too. The difference between the two classes of practitioners lies only fractionally in the techniques employed. It lies predominantly in the clientele served: on the one hand, normal people with typical developmental needs and problems and on the other, people with abnormal and complex psychological difficulties requiring personality restructuring and skill in some advanced techniques not required of counselors. Is there only a narrow line between these two classes of clients, or is there a discernible gap? Neither—the two classes overlap. How far counselors reach into that overlap area is limited only by their native competencies as polished by training and experience and by their ethical commitments.

# ■      Points to Remember      ■

1. Some interview characteristics, although not as important as how counselors communicate with clients, are variables in the success of counseling:

    a. Private room, with no interruption from outside.
    b. Nonconfrontational seating, not at desk.
    c. Full attention given to client; no distracting counselor behaviors.
    d. Addressing client by name he or she prefers, and vice-versa.
    e. Records must be kept; some note-taking during interviews is permissible if it does not distract; tape or video recording if counselor choses and client permits.
    f. Second and subsequent interviews usually begin with finding out what relevant events have occurred in client's life since last interview.
    g. Usually clients' concerns can be translated into specific outcomes to which counseling can be aimed, but clients must not be forced to state objectives.
    h. Standardized psychological assessment devices are employed as the need arises; a number of factors determine how this will be done.
    i. The counselor will use specific cognitive, emotional, and behavioral techniques.
    j. Counseling is terminated by agreement between client and counselor.

2. The effectiveness of the techniques that contribute greatly to the attainment of counseling objectives derives from the quality of the working alliance between client and counselor.

# Counselor Formation Activities

The reflections at the chapter's end noted that this chapter had completed the examination of scholarly issues related to counseling. The remaining chapters focus on technical and professional topics. A major scholarly issue throughout has been the stand that schools of counseling or therapy as cohesive, closed packages of theory and practices no longer serve the useful purpose they once did. Scientific thought and evidence now sufficiently inform the art of counseling.

Chapters 2 and 3 led you to examine your epistemic tenets so as to be more able to evaluate propositions with which you are faced, including those offered in this volume, at whatever level of development those epistemic criteria may currently be. You have also been urged to complement the brief excerpts about some schools provided in this text by perusal of material in which the several schools stake out their claims for allegiance.

The time has come for you to draw some tentative lines that mark the shape of your thinking on this matter: to note some epistemic conclusion you have reached and what you think, and why, about a number of the separate schools of counseling or therapy you have examined. Upon conclusion of that task, gather with the small number of fellow students with whom you have been meeting during study of this text to share ideas, thereby testing for agreements and disagreements. The result will be further scholarly growth and further confidence in the important profession for which you are preparing.

The activities of Part III are the application of principles covered in Parts I and II. Said differently, Parts I and II lead up to Part III because it is in these chapters that prospective counselors find the answer to the question raised in Chapter 2 (in slightly different words), "As a counselor, what practices will I follow to help clients?" Your supervised practicum will put a polish on skills, but the basic skills must be acquired earlier. The Counselor Formation Activities of Part III are essential because they provide an opportunity to acquire an introductory level of skill in the techniques that are distinctive to counseling.

Detailed activities are not given for this chapter; the details are in the chapter's contents. The general direction is that you retain the small groups set up for other chapters' activities (or form new ones)—preferably three-person groups—and take turns creating counseling situations and practicing each technique. Three-person groups, as in the activities for Chapter 10, permit each student to alternate among the roles of counselor, client, and observer/evaluator. After reasonable skill is attained for each technique, the practice can be extended to creating counseling situations for which two or more techniques are employed.

# Complementary Reading

Assessment, measurement, or testing is a complex, technical aspect of counseling, and is therefore beyond the scope of this text. Measurement devices were mentioned in a few places, and this chapter places the need for assessment among other events and conditions that occur in counseling.

Before you undertake formal study of the topic, introduce yourself to it by examination of Hood and Johnson (1991). For a more complete treatment, examine this classic text: A. Anastasi. (1988). *Psychological Testing* (6th ed.). New York: Macmillan.

You are urged to read in full two of the journal articles cited in this chapter. The treatment by Stiles and his associates (1986) of the effectiveness of counseling and the report by Claiborn and Lichtenberg (1989) on the counseling relationship provide information essential for all counselors.

## 12

### CHAPTER

# Techniques for Helping Clients

## Overview

Thoughts, feelings, and behaviors can change over a lifetime, justifying counseling older people as well as younger, although the greatest potential for change is with the younger. Some changes result from bodily modifications that are relatively slow, the processes of physical development that occur over a span of years. Other changes from physical causes may be abrupt, such as the radical ones that appear as a result of a brain tumor.

The chance social experiences that people have with individuals and groups result in changes in the ways thoughts, feelings, and behaviors are expressed. Other changes are deliberately brought about by planned societal activities, as found in the systematic cognitive and behavioral changes induced by schooling. Deliberate changes also come about when one person attends to the unique needs of another, as in tutoring in an academic subject, trade, musical instrument, or sport. Significant changes happen when a counselor facilitates new patterns of thought, feeling, and action in an individual who has sought help in coping with a psychological concern. Although help may just involve casual but serious conversation, counselors usually employ tested techniques to deliberately facilitate particular changes or artfully craft new techniques for that purpose during interviews.

This chapter introduces a sample of such techniques for focusing on the cognitive, emotional, or behavioral aspects of clients' lives. Usually, each of these aspects is meshed with one or both of the others, a fact of which counselors are aware even while they may be emphasizing just one of them.

Finally, the chapter presents a sampling of the concerns of the clients and the procedures employed by counselors, showing how a varied mix of techniques acknowledges the functioning of people as unified beings.

# Introduction

Psychological counselors teach people—notably, in groups—how to lead effective lives by mastering the continuing challenges of development. When that development is disrupted by particular concerns, counselors help alleviate those problems. In attending to these specific concerns, they not only make certain that clients acquire the knowledge and skills to prevent or overcome similar problems in the future but also help clients increase their general psychological effectiveness (Dobson, 1988).

Counselors acknowledge the functioning of individuals as psychobiological entities—as inseparable wholes—although they can only partially comprehend clients' unified states. After all, people's beings are not fully accessible even to themselves, so counselors can expect to reach only partial comprehension of clients as entities.

Figure 6-1 portrayed the idea that an understanding of the unitary person can begin with examination of one of the three overlapping facets that make up human functions: cognitions, emotions, and behaviors. Even though counseling procedures initially address one of these facets, counselors remain aware that the division of human functioning into seemingly separate elements, although useful, is artificial. The initial counseling emphasis will be on one facet, but some attention to the other two facets will have to be given.

Clients often describe their concerns as if they were solely behavioral, cognitive, or, less commonly, emotional. If clients identify their concern as cognitive (not with that label but by how they describe what they are concerned about), counseling procedures start by focusing on cognitions. The same is true for emotions or behaviors.

We will first examine counseling techniques that are dominantly cognitive and then address techniques attending to emotional and behavioral aspects of clients' concerns. Before examining cognitive techniques, we will briefly review the principles underlying them.

# Cognitive Principles

Cognitive principles were examined in Chapter 8 and summarized in that chapter's Points to Remember. They are paraphrased here, together with some principles covered in Chapters 9 and 10.

1. Life is marked by a balance between stability and change. The contents and processes of a person's cognitions usually change slowly as a result of physical maturation and experience. Abrupt changes in systems sometimes require abrupt changes in clients. Emotions and behavior patterns, with their cognitive correlates, also change as development occurs.
2. Cognitions are not a jumble of independent mental elements fired off haphazardly in the brain. Each cognition is nested in a structure, or system, that gives people their continuity and acts as psychological ballast to maintain them as totally functioning humans. Cognitive content comprises six somewhat overlapping elements that function in four processes, which also overlap.

3. An individual's cognitive system, or structure—flexible, generative, complex, and resilient—organizes data about self and world, which enables the person to cope satisfactorily with self-in-world.
4. When that coping is unsatisfactory, cognitive restructuring—altering thought structure and content—may be needed for the client to create more adaptive personal and social realities and to eliminate cognitions that prevent desirable outcomes.
5. Cognitions are a variable in the control of the physiological aspects of the totally functioning person.
6. Clients' views of selves in general and of selves in specific situations are central to the cognitive control of their behavior and emotions. Among other significant but overlapping cognitive categories are clients' values, aspirations, rules by which they perceive their behaviors to be controlled, and rules by which they believe the world operates—their life views.
7. Clients' cognitions about the objective world are formed by their perceptions, by their reasoning and abilities, and by their success or failure in managing emotions and behaviors by cognitive means.

### Cognitions: Powerful but Changeable

Cognitions have a powerful control over behavior. That power is related to the emotional intensity with which any cognition is coupled. An intense level of feeling associated with a cognition creates conviction, a state of the individual being absolutely certain about the validity of that cognition, even when confronted by contrary evidence. A positive effect of strong conviction is illustrated by placebos. To determine the effectiveness of medical drugs, randomly selected subjects are then randomly divided into three groups. One receives the drug, another an inert substance, called a placebo, and the third no treatment. If the experimental drug were to result in a cure rate for 75% of the subjects as against 5% for the control subjects and 20% for those who had taken the placebo, the effectiveness of the drug would be demonstrated. The results would also show that some people who had taken the placebo were cured, but the cure could not be attributed either to chance or to the inert substance of which the placebo was made. Cures associated with taking a placebo can safely be described as psychogenic, or caused by the subjects' being convinced that a cure would occur. The annals of medicine report almost incredible physiological changes that can be accounted for only partly by medical approaches.

Similar outcomes have occurred in the spiritual domain, attributable to self-induced (cognitive) convictions. Seemingly impossible physical phenomena that occur among some intensely spiritual people can be explained only as psychological events. Of similar origin are dramatic behavior changes shown by people who have undergone religious experiences of great intensity—peak emotional experiences that change the structure of cognitions.

*Biofeedback* provides evidence of the power of that cognition called intentionality, or will, in controlling behavior. Biofeedback provides instantaneous knowledge about one or more involuntary body functions. The process is demonstrated in hospitals with patients connected to an instrument that continuously records such as data as temperature, pulse rate, and blood pressure. Unlike hospital patients, who do not see the instrument, psychological clients are asked to study the displayed data, thus providing them with feedback. The power of cognitions is demonstrated by positive changes in some targeted biological processes as a result of clients' concentrating on bringing about that kind of change. Although this willing is directed at a change in symptoms, the will is actually that an organ is to function differently. There are numerous demonstrations of the effectiveness of this form of cognitive power, one being patients' control of cardiac arrhythmias while observing data from an electrocardiogram.

This power of cognitive control over physiology has long been recognized— the power of an intense desire to change coupled with a conviction that change will occur. For whatever else the 19th-century French psychiatrist Emile Coué may be remembered, his confidence in this power of people to control change by cognitions is found in his directive to patients frequently to recite, "Day by day in every way I am getting better and better."

Most people know that behavior and emotions have some cognitive correlates, but they are understandably unaware of the principles that explain the origin and maintenance of emotions and behaviors and the procedures required to change them. They therefore believe that cognitions are powerful enough to be the sole way to change emotions and behavior. Others believe that reasoning is all that is needed to bring about behavior changes. For a hypothetical example, we assume that a single mother, who has told her 15-year-old son countless times to pay more attention to his studies, to show more interest in girls, or to help with chores around the house, asks her brother to "have a talk with" her son. The mother surmises that forceful telling by a respected uncle will bring the change desired. Perhaps his uncle's traditional counseling could help a bit with the concerns about study and chores (though not with his social life), but this probably would be with only temporary effect.

### *Emotions and Cognitions*

Three-year-old Patsy fears certain areas of her large, old house, particularly after dark. One evening her father parades her around the house, pointing out that she has no reason to be frightened. The only way he knows to deal with Patsy's fears is by reasoning in a calm, rational manner, a view that appears to be verified by her lack of fear during the time she is going around the darkening house with him. When in an hour she shows her usual bedtime fears, her exasperated father can only attribute them to some deeper factor: "Something's wrong with her; I've *explained* to her there's no reason to be afraid, but she still is."

The cognitive efforts to change emotions or behaviors in these instances are typical folk behaviors. The belief that words alone can produce the desired changes in those instances is not well supported. Proven specific cognitive approaches could be of help in both instances, but they would have to be complemented with noncognitive procedures.

Patsy's emotion was chronic. She was unable to identify cognitive origins of her fear, not only because she was so young but also because the emotion resulted from respondent conditioning. No identifiable cognitive variables were associated with its origin. Her parents, when later consulting with a counselor about her fears, came to suspect that her grandmother might have been responsible. She was a baby-sitter many months back, and her tendency to use mild doses of fear to control children had been noticed but thought unimportant. Patsy was unclear about events but did say that Grandma had told her scary stories. Whatever the origin of the fear, cognitive procedures can help reduce or eliminate the emotion, but not to the exclusion of behavioral procedures.

A sudden and profound negative emotion can permanently alter cognitions, as demonstrated by reports of rapid cognitive maturation and subsequent radical behavior changes of adolescent children after a severely traumatic event, such as the accidental death of one or both parents or the murder of a friend. Scaling downward in severity, we can find other cognitive change resulting from fear, as when some miscreant pupils are sent "to the principal," where they are expected to be "talked to." Whether fear will be aroused in any one pupil depends to a large degree on whether the child has been socialized to respect authority and whether the principal is the kind who represents authority, however benign. Other variables can also contribute to the amount of fear aroused. Indeed, some students' cognitive structures and negative behaviors might be enhanced by their being directed to report to a principal, just as a prison sentence meted out to certain late adolescents and young adults serves as a rite of passage that gives them welcome status among certain peers.

Emotion is but one source of cognitive change. Thought content and processes can be altered with counselor help without being accompanied by noticeable emotional experiences, although emotional distress may prepare clients for cognitive change. For example, a person may experience intense frustration because of an inability to carry out a cognitive task. With cognitive instruction the person becomes able to carry out the task, and the emotion rapidly subsides. The cognitive change is spurred by the emotion of frustration but not caused by it.

Reasoning alone is sufficient to bring cognitive change and thereby alleviate the concerns of some clients. However, this is not objective reasoning like that used when working on a logical problem, and only rarely is it contentious reasoning (argument). It is the slow, indirect dealing with cognitions as when, for example, counselors, in helping with social problems, lead clients to examine their relationship histories, to explore alternative ways to think about their concerns, and to hypothesize what others' perceptions may be. Slowly, clients become able to deal with pro and con arguments, to acquire greater understanding of themselves, and eventually to achieve new ways of thinking about other people. Other changes can be primarily cognitive, such as in religious conversions among intellectuals or in a number of career-decision matters.

## Helping Clients with Cognitive Concerns

Counseling starts cognitively even if clients' descriptions of their concerns eventually warrant their being classified as being in the affective or behavioral domain. The early minutes are cognitive because clients employ thoughts to tell why they are seeking assistance. Clients' concerns may be primarily in the cognitive domain, as illustrated when clients make derogatory comments about themselves, causing the counselor to judge that such thinking is at the root of their dissatisfactions. Although these thoughts may diminish if counseling is otherwise effective, there is no need to just hope for that outcome, because there are proven techniques for deliberately eradicating such thoughts, procedures labeled thought-stopping.

## Thought-Stopping

Thought-stopping is a valid procedure to halt compulsive, automatic, or self-negating thoughts, but as with any technical method, it is not to be used impulsively by reaching into the grab bag of tricks. It and all other cognitive change procedures are fitted into the wider perspective of clients' needs. It can be as simple a technique as a gentle admonition not to think a particular thought or an abruptly delivered negative consequence for stating a thought.* It may call for a mix of a number of procedures, including "homework" that clients are to carry out to eliminate negative cognitions and to replace them with enhancing (but correct) self-statements. One homework technique calls for putting a rubber band around a wrist and snapping it when a thought to be extinguished arises or seems imminent, thereby providing a punishing consequence which helps in stopping those thoughts. At the same time, clients direct themselves not to think those thoughts.

A negative consequence (aversive stimulus) to be used during an interview can be provided by a sudden noise presented immediately during or after the stating of an undesirable thought, along with a directive not to think that thought. For example, a high school student, Carl, had moved into the community during the summer and was concerned about his social inadequacies with girls. A "college selection" group meeting brought him into favorable contact with a counselor, which enabled Carl to take the big step of casually asking at the end of a group session if he could talk privately with the counselor.

The counselor does not know that Carl's concern relates to social relationships with girls. Only a few youths can admit to themselves that they are beset with that kind of problem, can acknowledge that they do not have the coping resources, and thus can be led to seek a professional counselor's assistance. Most, however, particularly boys, will not ask for a professional's help despite the psychological pain they may be experiencing. Other than talking out their concerns with peers, a few might look for help from a traditional counselor. They may hope in quiet desperation that the topic will be raised by some trusted adult, permitting them to talk about it without having to raise the topic themselves and thereby preventing loss of face. Some may employ a cover: "A friend of mine has a problem, and you may have some suggestions I can give." Counselors react to this statement as if it is valid, no matter if they are confident that the "friend" is the person speaking. Skillful counseling may eventually permit clients to identify themselves as the ones needing suggestions.

Carl has not yet bonded adequately with male peers with whom to talk about his concern, and he knows no trusted adults (except the counselor) to engage in

---

*Because this text provides an overview treatment of counseling, technical procedures are treated in an introductory manner. It is assumed that advanced study will bring a detailed examination of techniques, as well as the opportunity to practice them. A number of texts offer a detailed treatment of techniques—notably, one by Cormier and Cormier (1991), which also cites the research support for each procedure.

conversation about it. In any case, the heart of his concern is one that he would have trouble talking about. The counselor he has come to know is his only resource.

Although the counselor did not know Carl's concern before the initial interview, he would not have hypothesized that it centered on social concerns with girls. Carl's appearance and manner, and his effectiveness in the group activity, gave no hint of his concern. The client has some difficulty in articulating his problem, but through bits and pieces he eventually reveals what the difficulty is. It turns out that a few years ago he was told by his psychologically disheveled mother that he was illegitimate and that the person he had thought of as his father, whose surname he bore and who had since abandoned the family, was actually his stepfather. She indoctrinated him to believe that he was of less worth than others not so born. She did not know where his real father was. This awareness worked against him in his former community, and he had hoped that moving to this new area would let him start afresh. That seemed not to be happening. His increased interest in female companionship was more and more hindered by his awareness of his birth status, because he feared that if it were known, he would be rejected. He stopped reaching out to girls and did not respond to their friendliness.

The counselor does not show the surprise that this recital causes. At least Carl's behaviors show that he has unusual psychological strengths, and thus the outlook is hopeful.

The counselor acknowledges the client's concern empathically, leads Carl to review his social assets, and pledges that together they will work on removing this destructive, disparaging thought. He proposes a simple reaching-out technique to start building confidence.

The second interview provides an occasion to employ a dramatic thought-stopping technique, as shown in this exchange about a third of the way in the interview:

> **CL** (dejectedly): Yeah, I tried that a couple of times [the socially useful technique proposed and practiced in the first interview], and I kind of think it can help. But I can't stop thinking [when he is with girls] about being illegitimate and what they'll . . .
>
> **CO** (loudly slaps hand on table and almost shouts): Stop! [Client pulls back, startled.] Don't think that way about yourself, Carl. [calmly] We're going to have to keep working so you won't have those negative thoughts about your birth status.

With use of the rubber band technique, activation of further social skills, and facing up to and some acceptance of his mother's difficulties, Carl's confidence returns, mostly when he finds that he is accepted for himself when an opportunity permits him to appear to casually inform one girl in particular with whom he has started to date that his father is unknown. If future thought-stopping procedures are required, the abrupt, aversive noise procedure can be faded into a simple signal, such as a raising of the hand, palm to the client, to serve the same purpose.

Stopping negative thoughts about self is the lesser of two steps. The major one is to lead clients to acknowledge their good qualities, to reinforce positive statements they make about themselves, and to teach them schemes to use in daily situations to reinforce their positive thoughts or statements, procedures that proved effective in Carl's case. If positive thoughts do not fully displace negative ones, at least they provide the balancing corrective to them.

Thought-stopping is a professional refinement of actions that have long been a part of folk procedures. We find it in a parent's loudly and sharply delivered directive to a child who has just used a vulgar expression: "Don't you ever say that again! I don't care if your friends can talk that way, we don't use that kind of language in this family."

## *Cognitive Restructuring*

Counselors may find that clients' difficulties include specific misapprehensions about themselves, erroneous cognitions that impede their reasoning and acting. These errors must be addressed at some point, either when first identified or later, as the counselor judges appropriate. Cognitive restructuring is a broad objective attained by several techniques, one of which is thought-stopping.

The structure of cognitions is made up of beliefs about one's self, how "the world" works, and of self related to the world. The grasp of reality by mentally healthful people is more factual than not, and their self-views are generally accurate and unexaggerated. When people with distorted views of self-in-the world turn up, the counselor creates conditions that replace those distortions with accurate assessments of self and world.

For over 30 years Ellis (1962) has pointed out the commonness and potency of irrational thoughts as a cause of client dysfunction. Those thoughts may be of the objective world or of oneself, but mostly they are of self in relation to other persons. By what criteria can counselors conclude that a client's cognition is irrational—is a distortion? This sureness rests partly on commonly accepted mental-health criteria. Additionally, however, that judgment is based on counselors' values. Some ideas judged irrational by one counselor may be seen as rational and mentally healthful when judged by another. Public disputes about homosexuality and abortion clearly demonstrate life-view differences that counselors might hold, ones they would apply as criteria by which to judge clients' thoughts and behaviors. As another example, some people value demureness, a quiet self-effacement, a refraining from pushing oneself forward. Others may see that trait as a coping inadequacy that needs to be countered by assertiveness training.

There are certain extreme positions a client might hold upon which all counselors may agree. If a client were convinced that "I must make no mistakes—I must be perfect," it is highly probable that counselors would concur that the client's rule was not realistic or attainable and was a clear example of a distorted cognition. It is distortions like these that produce emotional and behavioral imbalances.

If counselors classify clients' thoughts and behavior patterns as irrational—mentally unhealthful—they explain what makes them so and how replacement of those thoughts will be a major step in helping the client. Cognitive restructuring is the objective that counselors and clients will work on together.

If a client generalizes a specific incompetency into a generality like "I just can't do anything right," the restructuring is not carried out by an immediate frontal attack. One way to eliminate overgeneralization is to lead clients to identify their competencies, past as well as present. Clients with normal mental abilities will be able to see the irrationality of their generalizations. But what if a client says, "Because everyone looks up to me, I just can't let myself make any mistakes"? The counselor is faced with an unrealistic self-view, but because it is a value statement, it will not be accessible to quick change, nor can evidence be offered to counter it rationally. A calm, extended examination of this view of self will have to include exploration of its respondently conditioned attachment to an emotion. Change in the self-view will require elimination of its conditioned linkage with that emotion.

## *Reframing*

The aphorism has it that the pessimistic sees the glass as half-empty, the optimist as half-full. Whether one or the other view is correct does not matter, because that difference in perception has no practical significance. In other matters, however, how one views (frames) a situation has significance. "My husband is always making mistakes; he's *so* incompetent" and "My husband makes mistakes, but he does the best he can" may both be factual, but the cognitive and emotional attitudes of each statement represent differences that have counseling importance because they have relationship importance.

How people describe, or cognitively frame, other people or situations is a major variable in their reaction to those people or situations. In your experience you may have come across an individual who feels compelled to identify another person with some negative label, such as stupid or uncouth, and then looks for and reports only the thoughts and behaviors of that other person that justify the negative generality. Contradictory (positive) behaviors are ignored, or if they cannot be, are grudgingly acknowledged as rare exceptions. The stereotyping of ethnic, religious, national, and racial groups is similarly tainted by generalities. Although those stereotypes are resistant to change and counselors are only rarely called upon to bring about change in them, counselors are frequently involved in changing the frame, or label, in clients' interpersonal problems, which may be in the form of helping a client stop thinking of another in undiscriminating terms. Change in thinking about another person, in contrast to changing the stereotyping of groups, can come about relatively easily because the accompanying emotional charge is less than it is in group stereotyping. People can intensely dislike other people but are inhibited by cultural mores from doing any harm to them. On the other hand, a culture can foster hate for those of another culture to the point of feeling justified in killing them or even obligated to do so.

When an unjustifiable negative label given to another person has become fixed in a client's life, a change of perception of the other can be fostered by having the client briefly take the role of the other person in a mock situation in which the counselor plays the role of the client. This step toward empathy—toward standing in the shoes of the other person and seeing the world through that person's eyes—can result in the sought-for reframing. "He's a no-good drunk" can be transformed into "He's a depressed, scared person since his wife died." This change of perception—of the perceptual frame—leads to the outcome that is the purpose of the exercise: changed relationships.

Changes of labels and statements about oneself are equally significant. An adolescent's statement "I am lazy" has no accurate reference points because there is no psychological trait of laziness. The youth's assessment is probably a selfdenouncement learned from adults. If a person can do something but does not do it, absence of motivation is shown, a lack of stimulation for action and of rewarding consequences for that action—a psychological condition. A confident, competent person may say, "I have no motivation to do that," which reflects an accurate self-perception. That person's statement "I am lazy" can be viewed as a report by one who places low worth on self because others do.

Rossi (1986) tells of the use of reframing by the Simontons (research physicians working with cancer patients). Most people who fear cancer see it as a powerful, destructive disease, a frame that may affect cures negatively. The Simontons help patients reframe that perception into the view that cancer cells are weak and confused, whereas the white cells in the body's immune system are strong and powerful, "like sharks attacking meat" (p. 163). The power of cognitions in maintaining health, but particularly in curing illness, has been reported time and again. Some instances are reported by Rossi, Cousins (1983), and Siegel (1986).

Maximum skill in reframing is shown when it enables clients to deal easily and comfortably with complex situations with which they have not been able to cope. Reframing in such instances means not just acquiring a different label for a person or situation. If it is a situation that is of concern, the counselor helps a client recall its details, identify what meaning each detail had, and determine how that detail might be construed differently but with equal accuracy, so as to be favorable, not hurtful, to the client. It is the sum of these numerous steps that makes up the changing (reframing) of the full situation.

In sum: at times, clients' developmental difficulties are rooted in inaccurate or inappropriate cognitions about self, others, or self-in-situation. Successful change cannot be predicted by countering those cognitions with disputatious reasoning only—by telling clients that their thoughts are in error, even if you know them to be so. That argumentive approach can be expected from untrained traditional counselors. To facilitate cognitive changes in clients, newly trained counselors employ techniques of proven effectiveness and then build on those techniques to generate new devices when needed.

# Helping Clients with Emotional Concerns*

Both emotion and mood, the two parts of affect, were taken up when theoretical issues were addressed. Although psychological counselors need to comprehend the nature of moods and how they color emotions, cognitions, and behaviors, they will rarely be called on to be involved in mood change. There will always be a mood in which every behavior is couched, a low-arousal-level, pervasive, relatively enduring state. This state may be either the upbeat of elation or the downbeat of depression, but more probably it will be within the midrange between those extremes and therefore not be noticeable to either client or counselor. Emotions, on the other hand, are usually noticeable, active elements in

---

*A summary of principles is not given for emotions because, unlike cognitions and behavior, they do not lend themselves readily to that treatment. This examination of techniques incorporates an examination of germane principles.

clients' concerns that must be considered when thinking about procedures to assist clients. This chapter, therefore, focuses on emotions only, and mostly negative ones.

We recall Greenberg and Safran's (1987) conclusion, from studying the literature about emotion augmented by their own experience, that emotions fall into three classes, primary, secondary, and instrumental. Primary emotions are those that most people probably think of when the word *emotion* is used. They are the spontaneous responses of change in physical homeostasis that produce exaggerated feelings caused by particular environmental conditions. For example, if a person wearing a repulsive costume jumps from a hiding place in front of another person, the departure from physical homeostasis in the latter—the sudden secretion of adrenalin, for example—is sensed as a feeling of fright. Primary emotions have commonly been given one of two labels, negative when threat is sensed or positive when desirable outcomes are anticipated or experienced. Primary emotions can be mixed, as when a person's fear is aroused (negative) by deliberately engaging in a fear-producing event that also exhilarates (positive), such as riding a roller coaster, bungee jumping, or taking a white-water trip in a kayak.

Secondary emotions, it has to be surmised, are not common: the experiencing of a primary emotion that is a response to another primary emotion, as when one becomes angry because he or she has experienced fear.

Instrumental emotions are responses that have been operantly learned, Greenberg and Safran posit, because they permit a person to influence (manipulate) other persons into providing a benefit or into behaving as the manipulator wishes. If a person's emotion in an interpersonal event results in a change favoring that person, the person subsequently may enact appearance of the emotion without the emotion being truly felt. The person may learn to show emotional behaviors without experiencing the emotion. The first time a toddler falls and scuffs a knee or otherwise experiences pain, for example, the natural response to this abrupt departure from physical homeostasis occurs: crying. This behavior elicits nurturing, doting behaviors from a bonded adult, usually the mother, and maybe even a savory treat, a response that customarily occurs. At some later point the child falls a short distance from home and easily responds with the habituated crying response despite experiencing no pain. If the mother does not hear and therefore respond, the crying is not reinforced and thus stops. The child starts for home, anticipating the usual positive response, and, let us say, en route is pleasantly distracted by a neighbor's cat for a brief time. The child then recalls the mission on which he or she embarked and continues homeward. When judging that cries can now be heard, the child is able to produce a feeling of self-pity of sufficient strength to bring forth sobs. This common anecdote may contain another lesson about learning. The mother, having come to know about this common childhood behavior (having done it herself), seeing no evidence of hurt this time, laughingly rejects the child's emotion. "You're not hurt," she may jovially exclaim. "Go back out and play." Now the child experiences and demonstrates a new and genuine emotion— anger that this ploy has been uncovered—which may bring not only a verbal but also a physical attack on the mother. How the mother handles these natural, childish behaviors has significance for the child's later behaviors.

Among older people genuine negative emotions in addition to pretended emotions (such as pouting) may be elicited not as a response to threat but because they have been reinforced as a means of manipulating another. Two persons can have the same experience, as shown in a report by a married couple who through counseling came to see that their frequent angry arguments led to sexual experiences, as part of "making up," that were far more intense than otherwise experienced.

In this section attention is given mostly to primary negative emotions, not just because they are unpleasant to experience but because they can represent inadequate responses to interpersonal situations and, thus, developmental inadequacies in clients.

Master's-level counselors can expect to bring about some changes in cognitions, negative emotions, and behavior, but because they assist normal people, their degree of involvement in those changes differs from that of clinical practitioners. Clinical practitioners (and some counseling psychologists) may see a need for and have the competence to bring about major personality restructuring. Because no attempt has been made here to provide a sharp distinction between normal and abnormal patterns of thinking, feeling, and behaving, the implication is that counselors will participate in change efforts according to the ethical limits they see on their competence to do so.

Negative emotions are a frequent variable in clients' concerns. A negative emotion experienced one time is not typically brought to a counselor but, instead, ones that have persisted, sometimes for years. Debbie, a 28-year-old client, shows the durability of negative emotion during her first interview:

> **CO:** Debbie, when you talk about your mother I notice your eyes misting a bit, and your voice seems different. Because of what you said about your past anger toward her, I'm wondering what you're feeling now when you talk about her.
>
> **CL:** I don't . . . I have so many feelings. There's hate. Yet, I guess hate's the word . . . Well, maybe that's too strong. But then I miss having a mother. Everyone's entitled to have a mother who cares about her, doesn't she? Mine just doesn't care [starts to cry].

The counselor's manner let Debbie know that the counselor understands that she is hurting and confused but also makes comments that increase the emotion felt. Debbie is urged to recall specific events in her past related to her mother, ones that caused distress, and to explore the feelings she has now when thinking about her mother. The probability is low that she will be able to bring about change in her mother's behaviors, so all that can be done is to encourage her to further express her feelings so she can accept them without putting herself down and to objectify them by acquiring a new cognitive system for handling them.

Although the counselor does not deliberately arouse Debbie's emotion, it is important to encourage its full expression so she can be brought to confront and work through these disruptive repressed feelings. Incidentally, one difference between the professional practitioner and the well-intentioned but untrained counselor can show up in traditional counseling in response to client expression of emotion. It can be expected that the untrained counselor would respond to

Debbie's crying with sympathy and consoling cooing: "Don't cry, Debbie; everything's going to be all right."

## Relaxation Procedures

That state known as tension, or stress, is a variable in many of the concerns clients have. It contributes to negative emotions, faulty cognitions, and harmful behaviors, and it works against the productivity of counseling procedures. It is often important for counselors to counter tension, and the most reliable antidote is relaxation—stress and relaxation are competing responses. If relaxation is made more potent than stress, the relaxed state will remove stress, or at least diminish it.

Three relaxation procedures are introduced here, each having a different use. They are breathing, progressive relaxation, and imagery.

**Breathing exercise.**   This is a quick, easy, all-purpose activity.* The person wishing to relax, usually while seated, takes a few deeper-than-usual breaths by filling the lungs through extending the abdomen (important!) and then takes a really deep breath. The relaxer holds the breath for a count of ten, lets it out slowly (to prevent hyperventilation), and while doing so directs himself or herself to be relaxed or says, "I am relaxed." The full process is repeated a few times. As with any skill, practice makes perfect; the quality and speed of relaxation increase with trials. It is an exercise that can be performed while waiting for a traffic light to change, for example, or in any kind of group setting, because it can be done without calling attention to oneself. It is an easy one to ask the client to do in an interview, and it produces little or no self-consciousness because counselor and client do it together.

**Progressive relaxation.**   The progressive-relaxation procedure assures deep relaxation and provides clients with an awareness of their bodies they often do not have or get from the breathing exercise. Although there is an advantage to clients if they learn this exercise first, the time it requires along with its somewhat complicated steps may cause counselors to postpone it, if they use it at all. Some relaxation is often called for in the initial interview, and the breathing one can be quickly learned.

If it is decided to use this technique, counselors must determine, based on the progress of counseling, whether the exercise will be carried out initially during a session or by the client somewhere else, for which a loaned audio tape will provide instructions. It is an exercise to use when a client can stretch out supine and has 30 or 40 minutes available.

The client, lying comfortably in bed or on the floor in a semidark, quiet room with clothing loosened and shoes off, focuses sequentially on each of the body's muscle groups, starting with the toes. For a few seconds the client increasingly tightens the muscles of each group, to which the counselor or the tape calls attention, doing so to the point of pain, and is asked to attend to how they feel when

---

*This technique, along with other stress-managing techniques, is presented more fully in a text written by a former student, George Everly (1989).

stressed. Those muscles are then quickly relaxed while the subject cognitively directs them to do so, and the client is again asked to notice how they now feel when relaxed.

The exercise proceeds up the body, ending with stressing and relaxing the head muscles: forehead, cheeks and jaw, and scalp.

This procedure will later provide clients a structure for monitoring muscles during the day from time to time, particularly facial and abdominal muscles, which noticeably tighten under stress. After a few uses of the progressive-relaxation procedure, and with self-monitoring behaviors established, the briefer breathing exercise will be adequate for use in interviews. The borrowed tape gives moment-by-moment directions to follow, so this procedure can be learned at home without a prior trial in a counseling session.

***Imagery.***   Imagery makes use of clients' abilities to imagine. Even if a screening test of those abilities shows some clients to be weak candidates for success, counselors may nonetheless decide to employ the technique along with other relaxation activities for whatever value it may have.

For this procedure, clients are asked to recall in imagery the details of a scene that in a time past was, and may still be, the scene of the best of all experiences—a scene that produced relaxation and contentment. For some this could be a major, continuing romantic activity; for others, a recalled place associated with prior "best days of my life"; for still others, an image not from memory but created because it is so pleasant—so much so that they have been using it as an aid in falling asleep.

In a comfortable chair, with eyes closed, clients begin to imagine their scene. While that is happening, the counselor instructs them to be as relaxed as possible, an outcome requiring from three to five minutes.

A common use of this procedure is to desensitize a stimulus so that it no longer elicits an anxiety-producing response. When relaxed, clients are asked to bring forward in imagery the activity (or person) that causes fear or anxiety, but to do so slowly. If the anxiety starts to overpower the imagined scene, clients are asked to remove the anxiety-producing stimulus from the imagery and to focus solely on the relaxing one. With practice the relaxation induced by the imagined scene will hold firm more and more even as the anxiety-producing stimulus becomes more vivid. It is doubtful that one trial will have the sought-after effect, and thus clients will be expected to practice this procedure numerous times. Its use, of course, can be shown to apply to any similar anxiety- or fear-causing event at any future time in clients' lives.

## *Help with Specific Emotions: Phobias*

Fear is an evolved, useful emotion because it serves a species-maintenance function in the presence of real threat. A phobia is a fear, usually intense, without there being an actual threat. Phobias are irrational in that afflicted persons can acknowledge that there is no actual threat in the experiences or things that produce fear. Nonetheless, they fear those events or things, not only when actually in their presence but also just by thinking about them. The fear of some experience can be so severe as to be described as terror, preventing the afflicted individual from carrying out essential activities. For example, some degree of fear of open spaces, empty or with crowds—agoraphobia—is common. Those experiencing its severe manifestations may be imprisoned in their houses, so great is their terror of being out of doors.

Phobia reduction calls for the usual procedures for reducing stress and removing anxiety symptoms, but modified for the conditions of this kind of concern. Phobia is not an either/or state; there are degrees of phobic responses, and for any one person with any one phobia, there may be different degrees at different times. Counselors usually learn principles and techniques sufficient to warrant their dealing with minor phobias. If clients presents phobic states beyond the knowledge and skill level of the counselor, however, referral is ethically required. The important variable for that decision is the amount and quality of supervised experience of the practitioner. A master's-level practitioner who seeks a specialty in phobia reduction may have had sufficient supervised training to help with the more severe phobias.

A common phobia of no importance in the daily lives of most people is that of snakes, called herptophobia. Steps for its removal are given here only because they demonstrate principles fundamental to one theoretical approach to the removal of phobias. (Flooding, another procedure, is not covered here.)

Herptophobia is probably an evolutionary residue from the days when poisonous reptiles were a common danger. Herptophobics dread all snakes, a condition that cannot be changed by cognitive procedures even if clients rationally know that certain snakes are harmless. Their phobia prevents them from discriminating the harmless from the dangerous or even from wanting to think about it. For herptophobics whose fear is sufficiently mild to permit them to engage in a stimulus-desensitization exercise, the removal of the phobia may be reached in less than an hour.

Desensitization eliminates the ability of a stimulus to have the effect it once did. This comes about by presenting the fear-arousing stimulus and at the same time presenting stress-reducing conditions, as in the imagery relaxation exercise. Because the two responses are incompatible, presenting them together can cause the phobic stimulus to lose its power to arouse the emotion.

Desensitization for any stimulus can occur naturally from experience, but that is a chance matter. To make certain that it happens, controlled processes can be used, as we saw with imagery or, as we now examine, by employing a different procedure based on the same principles.

The process begins with the breathing relaxation activity and the introduction of the topic for desensitization, in this case, fear of snakes. The imagery exercise is not appropriate because the fear-eliciting stimulus will be directly presented. After some relaxation occurs and is maintained by the counselor's communication skills, the counselor starts talking more specifically about reptiles' characteristics, tells how to discriminate between poisonous and nonpoisonous reptiles, answers questions, and objectively describes snakes (they are not slimy; without them, rodents would proliferate). Pictures of reptiles can be introduced and held at a distance from the client, who is invited to look more closely at them when he or she is comfortable in doing so. When the counselor judges that there is an adequate state of readiness, the client's attention is drawn to a covered box at a far part of the room. The client is told that it contains a small, nonpoisonous snake.

While relaxation is maintained and calm comments about reptiles continue, the cover is removed from the box. The counselor continues to speak relaxedly (from time to time reminding the client also to be relaxed) and then invites the client to move the chair toward the box by such steps as the client's present level of comfort permits. (The box is not brought to the client, whose phobia reduction includes acquiring approach behaviors.) At a time when the client agrees that a degree of desensitization has been reached to permit the next action, the counselor reaches in the box and says that he or she has picked up the snake. Throughout these steps, the counselor is chatting quietly about matters related to the fear-reduction objective, such as inviting the client to visualize how the counselor went about picking up the snake. When the client expresses a readiness, the snake is lifted up out of the box, while the client edges closer. If the client moves so close that he or she reports a strong fear returning (the client has been asked to monitor and report degree of fear), the client backs away—slowly—for a brief period.

The counselor asks the client to attend to certain features of the reptile, including its motion, speaking of them positively. The counselor's handling of the reptile provides modeling, and the calm speaking, slow movement, and continued reminders about relaxation will bring the client eventually to the point of looking closely at the snake, later touching it, and eventually taking hold of it. At that point, desensitization has been completed. If some phobia returns later, the process can be repeated, with quicker and more lasting fear reduction likely because of the earlier experience.

This lengthy recital was provided not because you are likely to be desensitizing a herptophobic (you may be one yourself!) but to demonstrate a process that can open up more experiences to clients who may have other fears that do interfere with living, as herptophobia does not for most. It illustrates again that relaxation, so important for mental health, is a state that clients learn during counseling and can readily produce not just to handle stress during counseling but as a valuable way to control the stress of daily life. Relaxation not only reduces stress, it prevents stress. Its use as a preventive technique is spoken of by some as stress inoculation.

Some phobias are acquired through respondent conditioning, often the aftermath of a frightening accident. Folk wisdom has long acknowledged that. For example, when a beginning horse rider is thrown off, the experienced teacher hurries the trainee right back into the saddle to prevent a phobia from building. Phobias can grow in intensity when they are continually reinforced and can thereby become more difficult to remove. If an individual experiences a sudden and very traumatic event while inside a certain building, for example, a phobic response to that building may develop. If the individual repeatedly tells himself or herself how frightening the building is, panic may be prevented initially just by not going into the building, but it may later require the advanced step of avoiding even the sight of it. Such measures prevent the pain of a phobic response, but at the same time those avoidance behaviors and phobic feelings are negatively reinforced (strengthened) because they prevent that psychological pain.

Counselors reinforce positive emotions and employ them to facilitate clients' removal of their concerns. They deal differently with different negative emotions but, in any case, seek their reduction or elimination. Phobias are an example of those negative emotions.

Other illustrations of dealing with negative emotions are given later.

## Principles of Behavior

Before attending to technical approaches that counselors apply to clients' concerns that are primarily in the behavioral domain, we will recall the principles relating to behavior covered in Chapter 7.

1. Whatever the behavior pattern, it occurs because it results in outcomes that are more desirable than undesirable. The behavior has been strengthened, or reinforced. If the punishing consequences outweigh the desirable, the probability is increased that the behavior will not be repeated.
2. Individuals can differ over which consequences of a behavior they find pleasant or painful. The folk adage states it correctly: "One person's meat is another's poison." These differences are learned. Some may be of genetic origin, but these will be modified by learning.
3. Reinforcing consequences are positive and negative. In positive reinforcement a desirable outcome follows a behavior. In negative reinforcement, a behavior is strengthened if it results in the avoidance of or escape from an unpleasant experience.
4. There are also two kinds of punishing consequences, positive and negative. Positive punishers are those in which physical hurt is the consequence. Negative punishers result in the loss of desirable conditions, such as confinement causing loss of a pleasure like watching television.
5. When possible, a desirable behavior should be created and reinforced to compete with and thus replace an undesired one rather than punishment used to eliminate the undesired behavior.
6. Behaviors typically have a cognitive component. Few changes in behaviors can be achieved fully and quickly without attending to their cognitive element.
7. To change a behavior pattern requires identifying its antecedents, those small units of which the pattern is composed, and their consequences (their reinforcers and any punishers).

The development of an athletic skill, for example, is controlled by these principles. A person tries different stances in shooting baskets or driving golf balls, modifying behaviors as a result of the consequences. If moving in a certain way produces desired outcomes, that behavior is strengthened. A coach can speed that process by being a model, instructing, and providing social reinforcers.

Countless behavior patterns are similarly established, maintained, or extinguished. Some adolescent boys acquire a "line," standard ways of behaving toward girls because those patterns "worked" in past trials. These ritual approaches to girls become part of the exchange of information (gossip) among male friends, just as girls exchange details about their verbal and behavioral rituals for either turning off a boy or showing encouragement.

Some consequences are solely environmental, whereas many are both reactions from the environment and subjective. Some are subjective only; that is, the consequences of a behavior may be solely in the person's cognitions, emotions, or both. This is so, for example, in the case of a person who does a good deed for others but without their knowing. The reinforcing consequences are in the emotion of pleasure and the cognition that an anonymous good deed has been done. These consequences illustrate the adage "Virtue is its own regard."

As early as infancy children learn how to manipulate parents and thereby demonstrate that the word *learn* is broader than the folk meaning of learning: acquiring an aware cognition about something, the meaning meant by learning in school. Some married people learn how to manipulate their spouse's behaviors to bring about pleasant consequences for themselves or prevent unpleasant behaviors. Without there also being some pleasant consequences for the other's benefit from such manipulation, it scarcely contributes to a lasting marriage.

## Helping Clients with Behavioral Concerns

Our interest is in specific procedures that counselors use to modify behaviors that are impeding clients' development. We begin by looking again at Paul's problem in order to see in detail how the school counselor used successive approximations to change one of his behavior patterns from being a punishing pattern into being a rewarding one.

### *Shaping by Successive Approximations*

Do you remember Paul from Chapter 7? He is a high school junior who asked a counselor to help him improve his grade-point average. This outcome was achieved through the steps of successive approximation.

Some might have seen his difficulty as an issue of character. "His problem," Paul's Aunt Margaret told his mother, "is just that he won't study. If he wants higher marks, all he needs to do is study more. He must be pretty weak if he can't do that." Paul's father has long wished to stop smoking, says he has tried, but just "can't" do it. Margaret thinks that he, too, has a character deficiency, one that Paul may have inherited.

Counselors do not see these as character matters (whatever character is) or solely as ones of willpower. There is no deficiency of will (eagerness, motivation) in either case, but there is a deficiency of control over behaviors. This is a really difficult matter for Paul's father, because his problem is compounded by the variable of addiction. In Paul's case, however, the issue is almost completely behavioral. There is no emotion to deal with, and the role of cognitions in maintaining the behaviors that compete with studying has changed in the previous few months. The behavior-shaping technique explained in Chapter 7 is the procedure that brought attainment of Paul's objective.

Some of the seven points given in the last section show why shaping had the desired result. The first reminds us that people seek out experiences that provide pleasing outcomes while minimizing harmful ones. At first Paul's behaviors that competed with studying were more satisfying than hurtful. Both emotional satisfaction and compatible cognitions were reinforcement for his hanging out with his buddies. Those consequences maintained behaviors that overpowered any inclination to engage in any but bare minimum studying behaviors. Maturity produces changes in what satisfies and what does not, and for Paul a change started a few months ago. He became increasingly future-oriented, a change no doubt abetted by a surge of feeling for his classmate, Renee. These changes brought him to seek different satisfactions from those of his recent past, but his friends' motivations and reinforcers did not change (as yet), a fact recorded in the second point. Paul now had strong motivation for academic success but had an inadequate behavioral repertoire to act on that motivation. He tried but was discouraged by the difficulty of breaking out of his old behavior patterns. He then turned to a counselor for help.

The contract fabricated by the counselor and agreed to by Paul, his parents, and certain teachers was based on the technical facts stated in the remaining points. The seventh emphasizes the need to attend to the molecules of a behavior pattern, as given in the terse admonition "Think small." Aunt Margaret, who would have given traditional counseling had she become involved, thought in global terms instead. "All he needs to do is study." Period. Character, in her view, cannot be broken down into small components, and because for her this is only an issue of character, the molar conceptualization of Paul's problem satisfied her.

Were Paul's father to seek help in recovering from nicotine addiction, chemical intervention would probably be provided to complement behavioral approaches. He would keep detailed records of his smoking behavior for a typical week, recording for each smoking event the time of day, the surrounding circumstances (persons, food and drink, degree of stress), and any other data deemed germane. Stimuli for smoking would be identified so that he could eventually acquire stimulus control. The chain of the smoking response would also be identified, and he would be taught how to further modify smoking behavior by breaking that chain. For both his needs and Paul's, appropriate self-instruction and self-evaluation cognitions would be learned, as would self-reinforcing techniques.

Some antismoking devices reduce smoking by mechanical means, but for Paul's father they would be ineffective because such steps do not change the behavior but merely reduce availability. One device is a box with a timed opening that permits receipt of a cigarette at lengthy intervals, such as no more than once an hour. The former Soviet leader Leonid Brezhnev employed one to control his smoking. His response to an inquiry about its effect on him was that it posed no difficulties. "See," he said with a chuckle, "I keep a regular pack in my other pocket." Motivation for and behaviors of smoking were more powerful than the motivation and behaviors for not smoking.

### *Rehearsal*

Rehearsal is usually part of a broad change strategy in which several techniques are employed. It enables clients to move from only thinking (guessing) how to act in a specific situation to acquiring a confident ability to act. A description of the desired action is followed or accompanied by demonstration and supervised practice. An earlier illustration noted how pointless it would be to expect people to become assertive just by telling them to be more assertive. Assertiveness is a behavior pattern, with emotional correlates, and must be learned. This lesson requires knowing the specific cognitions and behaviors of assertiveness and rehearsing them. The outcome of rehearsal is not just to master words and actions but also to contribute to the reduction of anxiety. The best setting for learning assertiveness is a group, a major reason being that each member's successful practice, or rehearsal, can receive the approval of other members. Desired behaviors are thereby reinforced.

Ted had a difficulty related to a lack of assertiveness, yet somewhat different. Rehearsal played a role in easing his concern.

Ted, age 29, was to have an interview for a much higher paying position in a different company. The increased brain activity gave him a sense of pleasurable excitement for a while, but as the time of the interview crept closer, he became more and more anxious. He had no employment interviewing experience. He had started work in his uncle's business upon high school graduation, and he was contented and economically secure and so had never entertained the possibility of working for another employer. He learned of the opening through a cousin, but he gave no thought to applying because in addition to his satisfaction with his present circumstances he had no perception of himself as able to undertake more responsible duties in a similar occupation.

Others, including his fiancée, pressed him to apply, and the more he thought about the additional income and prestige the other position would provide, the more he became avid for it. He experienced a mix of excitement and anxiety when completing an application form, but he was really delighted a few days later when he was invited to come for an interview in two weeks. Now not only was he faced with an event he had never experienced, by itself enough to generate anxiety, but his anxiety was compounded by prospects of a major change in his life. Stress built, accompanied by approach and avoidance urges, leading to his dominating cousin's insistence that Ted go for counseling.

Three objectives seem clear enough to the counselor: teach Ted how to relax, serve as a model, and rehearse him in the likely course of the interview. Beyond the client's objective, the counselor sees a need to provide some cognitive activities that will increase Ted's sense of self-worth.

An untrained counselor would tell Ted to do this, do that, and say this and that. Those directions would probably be fully valid, but they would be insufficient. To know cognitively what to do is one thing; to be able to act on those ideas is another. Action requires learning the process in small bites, with sufficient repetition to result in mastery of the entire process. The counselor and client play the parts of both interviewee and interviewer numerous times, with the counselor showing Ted how to think and act just prior to the interview, upon entering the room, when greeted, as the interview begins, during the body of the interview, and when the interview ends. These rehearsals shape his physical and oral responses until they are part of his way of being, and they result in his gaining confidence. They also bring about subtle personality changes.

In addition to rehearsal during interviews, Ted is shown the advantage of covert rehearsal, practicing away from the interview. To increase his confidence and further reduce his anxieties, the training includes teaching him how to give himself instructions to use in the time before the interview and during it. These include self-confidence statements to be made as well as thought-stopping procedures to eliminate the lack of confidence and deprecating evaluations he has been making. The counselor makes it clear that these are not guarantees that he will get the position, but he assures the client that they will enable him to make the best case. Furthermore, what he has learned will be of permanent value, particularly if he acquires insights, increased ambition, and confidence about future career growth.

Because a large portion of clients' concerns involves experiences with others and because those relationships are oral, rehearsals will be woven into the interviews of many clients. A counselor may say, "Let's try other ways of saying that to her" or "Let me play the part of your father to give you a chance to try out what you'd like to say to him."

### *Modeling*

Throughout everyone's life, modeling is a source of learning, although the learner is usually unaware that it is happening. Counselors deliberately foster client learning through modeling.

To help with Ted's needs, the counselor models appropriate employment-interview behaviors. Additionally, he invites the client to recall the actions of other persons who behaved effectively in interviews, to imagine how a person he admires might act when being interviewed, and, after he has sufficient skills, to use himself as a model. (The counselor's video library does not include a tape showing effective interview behaviors.)

The counselor models not just how to act but how Ted is to give himself directions for relaxation and to make self-instruction, self-enhancing, and self-reinforcing comments to himself at appropriate points. For modeling purposes, the counselor states these aloud instead of just thinking them when he plays the role of Ted. A videotape could be made of Ted performing effectively, and with several playings of the tape, or by his recalling his performance on it, the client would have had another model—himself.

In Ted's case, modeling and rehearsal are interwoven, as they often are. At other times modeling can be employed without the need for rehearsal. It is useful to know that these two processes can be relatively independent or can be intertwined along with relaxation and other procedures as counselors' professional artistry indicates.

## Helping Clients Function as Integrated Entities

At all times people function as integrated wholes: thought processes, emotions, behaviors, and physical processes are one. At the same time, these integrated people can often be helped by focusing on just one or two of those four seemingly discrete aspects. Occasionally a client will report a concern that is apparent in all four facets: cognitive, emotional, behavioral, and physical. The counselor, with client assistance, sorts out the best starting point among the first three of them. The fourth, physiological, is outside a counselor's domain, and when symptomatic of stress, it will clear up when the cognitive and behavioral aspects of a client's concerns are satisfactorily dealt with. The worries of a high-ranking army sergeant, Jerry Gilcrist, illustrate this process.

### Sergeant Gilcrist's Case

The army is Jerry's career, one in which he had felt most secure, as he also had in his marriage. Suddenly he saw challenges to this secure, predictable world, with both his career and his marriage judged by him to be in jeopardy. Most recently, his 14-year-old son, Bud, was reported by the school to have been persistently asking a female classmate, in a manner she deemed threatening, to perform a sexual act. In civilian life the matter would be dealt with between school and parents. In the military social system that event might be treated more seriously, being reported also to a person's military superior. Military personnel are responsible for the behavior of their dependents, and continuing misbehavior or a serious infraction by one of them can have a negative impact on a career. Jerry perceived the event as a career threat, especially since it occurred just after a change of commanders had left him feeling exposed and threatened. The new commander said he wanted Jerry to carry out his office-management duties in a different manner, and the client saw that order as faulting him for his past ways of working.

In the last half-year, his son, Bud, has been showing increasing resentment of Jerry's authority after years of apparently meek submission. At first this change was noticed in sullenness and surreptitious disobedience, but it has grown into more open rebellion. Bud's acting out probably reflects the flush of puberty, magnified by association with some peers who are also experiencing eagerness to test their new, puzzling selves by challenging their primary systems: family, school, and the military.

Jerry's once contentedly subordinate wife, Lois, for whom he expresses great love and with whom he has had a "great" marriage, has increasingly spoken up for their son. This has caused him to feel a growing loss of control in his family and to experience distress about the changed relations with his wife. Over the months that his conflict with his son has increased, his angry reactions have correspondingly increased, accompanied by gastric distress. For ten years he had not experienced anger toward persons in his two important social systems, the army and his family, because there had been no events that could have been perceived as a threat. To the contrary, consequences in those two systems reinforced his behavior patterns in them. He had been able to control his environments, or at least his authority in them had not been challenged.

As a child, the sergeant experienced physical punishment from his father, and he modeled that practice when dealing with his son's infractions. As career and family stress increased, he experienced increasing anger, the only device he had for coping with his growing sense of loss of control. The school complaint produced a strong surge of anger, resulting in his striking Bud with his hands rather than the customary more impersonal belt. Lois tried to restrain her husband, something she had never done before, and in the melee was shoved and fell. How much by design or accident, the client could not say. If this event were also reported, he could anticipate an additional threat to his career. There was reason for a greatly uncomprehending and distraught Sergeant Gilcrist to see his life crumbling around him.

As one who perceived himself as always able to manage his own affairs, Jerry was not a likely candidate to seek help from a professional. His coming for counseling followed a roundabout route that need not be detailed here, but its happening was enhanced because a civilian counselor was available. Otherwise he probably would have had to be driven further to the wall before he volunteered to seek help from an army psychologist, but eventually he might have been ordered to do so. There were eight interviews with the client, and two with him and his wife. The following summary does not state specific interviews in which the several procedures occurred or were introduced, although some attention is given to their sequence.

### *Counseling Features in Brief*

Listening as the client describes his concerns shows that he is experiencing seemingly separate cognitive, emotional, behavioral, and physical concerns. These elements are, in fact, separately sensed ways in which the total person is reacting to perceived threats. It becomes clear that his anger is a response to these recent specific threats, and therefore it is a state, not trait, characteristic. Because he rarely experiences digestive problems, his current distress is similarly taken to be a response to the stressful events in the two main social systems that give him existential meaning. This leads the counselor to conclude that neither the emotional nor the physical concern requires a direct approach. They will disappear with reduction in the perceived threats and changes in related behaviors.

Although Jerry's feeling of threat and resultant anger are pronounced, they are seen as those of a normal person experiencing normal developmental disruptions. There are deficits, however. A lack of challenges in recent years has led to a dearth of coping skills and has given rise to the client's perception that he is a wronged man, helpless against undeserved attacks. His rigid cognitive structure is a handicap in his present challenges, and his lack of insight, of awareness of self, and of self-in-situation are added deficiencies. These are seen as signs of a psychic fragility that make the counselor be wary that he not be seen as yet another threat. Counseling leads, therefore, will need to be noticeably empathic and nonchallenging for a longer time than usual. The normal balance between self-centeredness and attention to others is, for this client, imbalanced toward self-protection.

Following an empathic listening to his history, the counselor suggests doing the brief breathing technique for relaxation, an exercise that Jerry finds difficult to get into. After relaxation appears to be attained, the client's anger is broached as a discussion unit at his suggestion. Because he appears to have little skill in reading his own emotions, attention is given to understanding the antecedent events that caused his anger and to cognitions that preceded, accompanied, or followed those episodes.

Reframing steps are cautiously undertaken by wondering with Jerry what may be motivating his son's and wife's behaviors and how he might appear to them. This can be the most challenging part of counseling and therefore requires cautious treading by the counselor. It is easier for the client to reframe his response to his wife—from, roughly, "She's not supporting me as she should, and she's disrespecting me in front of my children" to a hypothetical view of "As a mother she has strong instincts to defend her children against any and all harm"—than it is to alter his perception of Bud. The frame from which the client views his son can be summarized as "I am the father, and in this house what I say goes. No son of mine is going to dispute my authority." The client's reactions to his son, and the success of his hopes for change, will be helped if he is able to change that view to something like "Bud is going through a confusing transition in his development. I can remember what it was like for me, how *my* father didn't understand, how he beat me, and how glad I was to get away from home. I'll have to see how I can help Bud." The client does not ever use words as empathic as that, but in the unthreatening atmosphere of counseling, given his motivation to have his life change, sufficient reframing comes about to permit a prediction that his relationship with his son can start to change.

Systematic desensitization is tried. The client's deficiency in imagining a relaxing scene requires employment of the breathing exercise to induce relaxation. While he is relaxed, an effort is made to introduce in imagery several past anger-producing episodes. These are vivid enough to be brought up in imagery so that relaxation can be competitively coupled with them. There is no experimentation in these sessions, in the sense of a controlled test of procedures. All techniques hypothesized to be useful are tried. It cannot be said, therefore, whether any one technique, such as systematic desensitization, has contributed more than others to the successful outcome of counseling.

Reducing anger through procedures such as systematic desensitization is useful, but dealing with a negative emotion cognitively must not be overlooked; that is why in this client's case anger is a discussion topic. Jerry comes to see that the only way he was able to cope with the recent perceived threats and helplessness was through the natural response of anger. Reframing is sought to alter his perception of threat in the family, along with working on more productive ways to handle anger, again using imagery.

Jerry is invited to think of an admired man of about the same age, one he sees frequently. He nominates his chaplain. The client is then asked to describe how the chaplain might handle a situation that could cause anger, such as an action of a rebellious teenage son. The client imagines him as speaking calmly, even lovingly, in face of that threat, and sees why that could be so. The counselor is causing Jerry to find a model and to imagine in detail what the model's behaviors would be, behaviors that he would think were better than impulsive anger. He then imagines himself as one named by the chaplain as having behaved in a model way in managing anger. He is asked to recall an event that recently produced anger, to imagine others who had been sent by the chaplain to watch how well he handled anger, and then to describe his actions and words. This technique moves the beneficial outcomes of modeling from other-as-model to self-as-model. It provides cognitions to be recalled and behaviors to be activated the next time the client faces a potential anger-arousing event.

In the self-as-model exercise, strong focus is placed on self-direction phrases to be used, such as "Stay cool and just listen" during a family conflict or, in contentious events with other military colleagues or nonfamily civilians, "He's [she's] not going to get your goat; keep control, Jerry; show 'em who's better." To provide the client with a wide array of coping skills, the merit of the folk practice of counting to ten to permit a surge of anger to subside is pointed out, as well as the choice of even walking away if such action will not be misunderstood.

Although Jerry's behaviors do not exist separately from his feelings, physical responses, and mentation, he can be better helped if behaviors are attended to directly. This results in the useful outcome of making him aware that positive consequences of a behavior pattern help establish and maintain a behavior. The primary targets of this topic are his actions toward family members and how children's behaviors are affected by consequences. The client can also understand that no quick or drastic changes in Bud's behaviors can be expected, no matter how diligently and craftily Jerry might apply behavioral principles. At least the consequences of his son's behaviors can now be thoughtful ones instead of just reflecting Jerry's history or resulting from impulse. The client observes that it is better to take those newer approaches with Bud, even if late, than not to do so at all. Given his son's history with his father—one of establishing rules and physical punishment for transgressions—the client becomes aware that some years may have to pass before Bud will be sufficiently mature to accept his father as a considerably different person.

Joint counseling with his wife provides the neutral and accepting climate for her to examine how she has recently changed and her desire to have a greater say in how the children are to be treated. She says emphatically that she is becoming a new person and wants acceptance of those changes. Plans are considered whereby husband and wife will work together to reinforce desirable changes in Jerry. A deeper understanding between the two is achieved, emphasizing an emerging acknowledgment and acceptance by Jerry of Lois's changed perspectives.

Counseling ends by mutual agreement. As Jerry's sense of stress was reduced in the early counseling sessions and as a result of experience, he has come to believe that he misread the new commander's evaluation of his work, therefore easing another concern about his career. His original perception, he can see, may have been an unwarranted generalization of the distress and lack of control he had recently faced in his family. Although there still are problems with Bud, the client is confident that he can cope with them in a positive manner, particularly now that he and his wife are more in agreement. He is also confident that he can constructively handle surges of anger—that all in all, he will be a more adequate husband and father.

## Concluding Reflections

The art of counseling is shown in two ways. One way involves counselors' continuing judgments about which procedures to employ from the array of established ones in their armamentarium. The other demonstration of artful practice occurs when counselors generate new techniques or modify established ones. This creativity cannot be "out of the blue," however. To be professional, the devising of new techniques must be based on principles that arise from a study of how humans come to think, feel, and act as they do. Part II provided an introduction to those topics, and it behooves you to continue with advanced study of them. This study will lead to acquiring a wider array of principles on which your professional practices can be based and will also provide you with an even more defensible basis for creating techniques.

This chapter has introduced you to some of the established techniques for helping clients remove obstacles not only to their present development but also to their continuing development. Clients will learn to apply to future situations their new insights, changed perceptions of self and environmental systems, altered cognitive structures, and improved control over their behaviors and emotions.

# ■ Points to Remember ■

1. Although humans operate as psychobiological entities that cannot be fully grasped, an effort to do so requires appraisal of and working with three facets of this totality: cognitions, affect, and behavior.
2. To meet some clients' concerns, it may be sufficient to work with just one or two of these facets. Counselors use as many facets with as much depth as is required to assist clients.
3. Cognitions not only are powerful variables in the control of emotion and behavior but also affect the quality of people's physical functioning.
4. Among the technical procedures for altering cognitions are thought-stopping and cognitive restructuring through reframing. Clients' directions to themselves and use of self-reinforcement statements are applicable no matter the facet through which clients' concerns are approached.
5. Procedures for helping clients cope with affect include relaxation exercises of three kinds: controlled breathing, progressive relaxation, and imagery. Desensitization activities can remove negative emotions.
6. Behavioral approaches not only can alter how people act but also are useful in reducing negative affect when used as supplements to the procedures named in point 5. Some behavioral techniques are shaping through successive approximations; inducing clients' control over behavior stimuli and consequences by manipulation of reinforcing and punishing activities; rehearsal; and modeling of others' coping thoughts and behaviors. Later, after having acquired appropriate cognitions and behaviors, clients can serve as their own models.
7. The needs of some clients require moving back and forth among established cognitive, affective, and behavioral techniques and creating new techniques based on established principles.

# ■ Complementary Reading ■

A scholarly grasp of counseling is useless without the technical skill to apply those ideas. Although this chapter has introduced you to some counseling techniques, their number is greater and more complex than covered here. Each class of techniques requires coverage to a degree beyond the scope of this book. Before the prepracticum or practicum course in your program, you will need not only familiarity with the uses of a number of techniques but also the ability to state when each would be appropriate and some budding skill in employing them.

To complement your knowledge, I recommend Cormier and Cormier (1991), all chapters beginning with "Selecting Helping Strategies." For another wide-ranging coverage of techniques organized around 11 intervention methods, I recommend:

KANFER, F. H., & GOLDSTEIN, A. P. (1980). *Helping People Change*: 4th ed. New York: Pergamon Press.

Helping clients manage their emotions may call for a rather straightforward technique such as counterconditioning (Cormier & Cormier, 1991) or the more subtle, advanced therapeutic techniques found in:

GREENBERG, L. R., RICE, L. N., & ELLIOTT, R. (1993). *Facilitating Emotional Change*. New York: Guilford Press.

Chapters 8–13 explicate the procedures, but if time permits I also urge study of at least Chapters 1–5.

Because cognitions and behaviors are usually intertwined, it is appropriate for techniques to change them to be presented together, as they are in the volumes above. If you plan to specialize in a child and youth clientele, I suggest you complement your knowledge of cognitive and behavioral techniques with:

FINCH, A. J., NELSON, W. M., & OTT, E. S. (1983). *Cognitive-Behavioral Procedures with Children and Adolescents*. Needham Heights, MA: Allyn & Bacon.

Helping clients change does not need to be limited to procedures that emanate from interview rooms. There are aesthetic, literary, musical, game, movement, and physical-challenge activities that have proven records in client change. Even if you will never be employing procedures such as these, knowing about them will broaden your understanding of how humans change. To this end, I recommend:

NICKERSON, E. T., & O'LAUGHLIN, K. (1982). *Helping through Action: Action-Oriented Therapies*. Amherst, MA: Human Resources Development and Press.

## CHAPTER

# 13

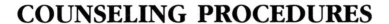

# COUNSELING PROCEDURES

## Overview

Counseling is carried out by numerous agencies, public and independent, and deals with a multiplicity of clients' psychological concerns. Some agencies also attend to clients' physical or spiritual needs. This chapter is about psychological counseling in a variety of professional settings; specialized agencies may require training beyond that common to all settings.

Occupation is the most common developmental subject, the core topic in school and university counseling centers, public and private employment agencies, rehabilitation centers, and correctional institutions. Thus, occupational counseling is discussed first.

Many changes have occurred in all aspects of formal vocational counseling since its inception almost a century ago, and so have career assessment devices. Because these instruments are among the most common measures employed in counseling, a few are examined, along with a sample of instruments in other counseling topics.

The detailed examination of careers includes procedures for acquiring skills to address career concerns, especially in schools. A counselor's professional skills are most evident when he or she is helping a client plan a life that centers around the occupational variable, be it the first serious career investigation of an adolescent or the job change of a mature adult. We examine the relationships of five clients and their counselors, and look at the role of career counseling among the elderly, adolescents and young adults, and clients in a rehabilitation center in three distinct environments.

The chapter closes by considering clients from varying cultural minorities and procedures that supplement interviews in meeting clients' developmental needs.

## Counseling and Occupational Careers

Of the ways in which adults are maximized as humans, three are common for most people: (1) by bonding, particularly with one person in a way that permits confident expression of sexual and other positive emotions; (2) by regularly engaging in satisfying activities that, in most cases, provide income for the person and any dependents; and (3) by holding to a comforting spirituality. The second of these, called the occupational career (an occupation and other systematic activities, such as hobbies, make up the person's total career), is one with which counselors commonly become involved.

Individuals differ greatly in the strength of the drive they experience toward a specific occupation. Each of us knows people who were sure from childhood that they just "had to" do things found in a certain occupation. We may know a pilot whose childhood fascination with aircraft was continuous and pronounced. Some may recall another child whose fascination with fine art matured into one aesthetic creativity. Then there are people who from their earliest years have engaged in entrepreneurial activities, have earned a bachelor's degree in business, and have persistently engaged in those activities. We assume that the drive to engage in these activities is as inherent as a person's gender. All of those individuals might have been less fulfilled had they not pursued the desired occupation. The psychological counselor, as a developmentalist, is interested in helping clients maximize themselves; therefore, a central topic for counselors is the individual's occupational life.

The agencies in which counselors work determine the nature of the interventions in career development that counselors provide. The programmatic activities of counselors employed with groups in elementary and secondary schools and in universities are amply detailed in other literature. Some adolescents will begin to experience an urgency to commit to a career or to plan and act on the specifics of career entrance. For them counselor assistance must be fully individualized. Counseling individuals in career matters will be a frequent activity and one through which the counselor will make a major contribution to the individual's development. To do so requires comprehension of the subtle psychological forces at work and an awareness that thinking about a career with an individual is, in effect, thinking about the maximization, about the psychological completeness, of that individual.

In nonliterate, nontechnological, hunting/gathering tribes, work was a necessity because the tribes' members had to be nourished and sheltered. Men, except one or a few who were designated to deal with the tribe's religious rituals, did the same kind of work—they had identical occupations. In addition to child-rearing activities, women also engaged in similar occupations: processing food and preparing clothing.

Millennia later there appears to be no similarity between Western cultures and those of early tribes. Yet there is a major similarity: the need to work to provide maintenance for oneself and dependents. That there have been great changes in the characteristics of occupations since then is obvious, and to three of these our thoughts are directed.

## Changes in Job Quantity, Occupational Concepts, and Counseling Procedures

The great array of occupations that came to be, and the changes in political and psychological concepts about humans, stimulated the start and growth of counseling.

## *The Proliferation of Occupations*

By the Middle Ages in Western civilization, occupations had slowly evolved from those that required no preparation through crafts, for which training was needed, and on to work that required literacy. That proliferation did not mean that anyone could enter any occupation or training. Gender, class, and, later on, guild memberships were channels into which the course of one's occupational life ran.

By the end of the 19th century the number of occupations had multiplied geometrically as a result of the technological revolution begun a few centuries earlier. In European countries at that time cultural restrictions on which occupations individuals could enter remained. In contrast, the principles of equality, individual freedom, and initiative planted at the time of North America's colonization had developed into a belief that "you can be anything you want to be—this is the land of opportunity; the sky's the limit; write your own ticket." Except for men from somewhat affluent families of European origin, however, those ideals could not be readily translated into reality. Still, there was a plethora of occupations that poorer Euro-American men could enter. At the start of the 20th century a few socially oriented intellectuals saw the problems faced by children of immigrants, who knew only of parents' occupations or the ones they saw in their neighborhood. They commonly had no vision of how to reach beyond their present condition to use the freedoms inherent in their families' new country. The result was the emergence of a new movement.

## *Changes in Occupational Concepts and the Start of Counseling*

The new movement, called vocational guidance, resulted in another new occupation, that of vocational counseling. It provided assistance to youths in selecting and entering occupations with deliberation instead of through the old route of chance based on ignorance. The children addressed were mostly boys, because the mores consigned most girls to a domestic lot, although they might work for a time before marriage. The social forces and demographics of that time also precluded Native Americans, Asiatics, or the descendants of former slaves from the benefits of vocational guidance. The occupation of vocational counseling mutated during succeeding decades into the profession addressed here, psychological counseling.

**Definitions.**   Four terms with differing connotations will be employed in this chapter:

1. *Career* is often used elsewhere as a synonym for occupation. It is used here to refer to the full array of major activities in which a person engages with some consistency. For some very few persons, indeed, the word *occupation* is synonymous with career. For most adults, the occupation is probably the major activity, but there are other activities consistently—perhaps even urgently—pursued. A hobby may be one, a marriage another.
2. *Occupation* distinguishes one set of work behaviors from another. Well-known craft occupations are mechanic, plumber, and carpenter. There are trade occupations, artistic ones, and professional occupations, for example.

3. *Job* denotes an occupation found in one business establishment or enterprise. A city's transit authority will employ bus drivers, a large corporation will employ tax attorneys and accountants, for example; these are jobs within those enterprises.
4. *Position* denotes the physical element implied in the word. A person whose occupation is that of lathe operator is employed in a lathe-operator job in Noahasark Shipbuilding Company, where he or she is assigned to lathe No. 7, a position. Sylvia is a counselor (occupation) holding a position as one of the 11 counselors in the job of counselor in Trivium University's Counseling Center.

The career emphasis in this section is on occupations, and indeed at times the two words may be used as if synonymous. It is the total text that attends to careers as broadly defined.

To the historical perspective that a job was something that had to be done for sustenance there came to be wedded the broader idea that each person had the right to seek maximization as a unique individual. A century ago chance permitted few people to achieve a broad image of self or gave them any opportunity to implement that image. Human existence then was viewed as separate expressions of self, as if one's occupation, sexuality, spirituality, and culture were only slightly overlapping but generally independent manifestations of being. Today the being of a person is seen as totality, a truly broad and realizable image of self. People may have an occupational persona—that is, the behaviors presented to others in the workplace—and that may differ from their persona in the family, yet personae are relatively surface adaptations to different social systems. The defensible view is of persons-as-entities, as integrated wholes.

We have seen that counselors address either a client behavior or a cognition. At the same time, counselors know that although these two may appear to be independent functions, they are, in fact, facets of a unified entity. Similarly, when clients approach counselors for help in laying out an occupational career, counselors intellectually frame this concern as a life-development matter, because people's occupational career is not separable from their entire career as a complete human. In accepting this totality of people, counselors are acting existentially and humanistically as well as psychologically.

To reverse the argument: when providing assistance to clients as they face broadly envisioned life-development tasks, counselors bring them to examine the occupational facet of their being. Incidentally, in light of the acknowledgment in the counseling literature that people's occupation is coextensive with their total being, it is particularly perplexing that one can hear reports that counselors, and particularly doctoral-level ones, show so little interest in the occupational career of their clients. Developmental matters, with careers as a feature, are at the heart of the counseling profession—they are the historical commitment of counseling, in contrast to the restorative focus of therapy.

To whatever degree this playing-down of career concerns has occurred, it may reflect confusion of the primitive concepts of what was called vocational guidance or counseling with the advanced and complex concepts that are germane today. We look again at the history.

***Selecting an occupation from among the many: vocational guidance.***  Systematic, intentional vocational counseling started in the first years of the 20th century as an expression of the vocational guidance movement. It was described by a major contributor, Frank Parsons (1909), as a process for (1) identifying the characteristics of the person ready to enter an occupation, (2) causing that person to learn about the world of work, and then (3) applying "true reasoning" to these two sets of data. Assessment of counselees' characteristics ("clients" seems too overblown a word for this primitive encounter) was made by vocational counselors using homemade devices. Assessment included counselors' evaluation of counselees' characteristics and required counselees also to carefully examine their own characteristics, facing up to any negative traits they might uncover.

Knowledge of the working world, the second step, was provided by counselors using such information as they could acquire. The vocational counselors were expected to do the true reasoning in the third step, although the counselees would be involved as far as their reasoning capacities permitted.

***Further concept changes.***  In Parsons's day, a person's occupation was acknowledged as essential for physical maintenance, as it still is, but it was considered unrelated to the way humans functioned in other seemingly distinct areas. As other apparently independent areas of human concerns were identified, each in turn was seen as requiring its own unique guidance approaches. This led to an expanded classification of guidance into the three areas reported extensively in the literature of the 1950s and 1960s—vocational, educational, and personal.

Educational guidance called for help to high school students in making selections from among the proliferating curricula and subjects and from among the puzzlingly different institutions available to the small minority going on to higher education. Later the third area emerged, helping students with concerns that were neither occupational nor educational and therefore were "personal." This breakdown is unacceptable by today's conceptual standards, a point conveyed by the observation that there is nothing more personal than an individual's occupation. Education is strongly oriented to occupations, so counseling relative to education cannot be justified outside general development, which always includes career matters. All counseling is developmental; all counseling is personal counseling.

The professional literature shows that this conceptual shift is now nearing consensus. It maintains that a person's career is only one (albeit central) expression of the interrelated wholeness that marks human existence measured over the life span. In ideally functioning people, all characteristics and stages of development, including occupational commitments and activities, are integrated into a reasonably smooth-running unity with each part complementing all others. This ideal is not commonly reached, and sometimes the parts are in conflict, a condition producing the need for counseling. Psychological counselors, through group activities and individual counseling, help individuals move toward the ideal. That is why counseling about careers is, in fact, counseling about a client's current stage of development. It provides a contextual framework, Blustein (1992) observes, that "allows for an understanding of the complex relationships between vocational behavior and collateral lines of development and functioning" (p. 720).

This changed concept is found in dropping the modifier *vocational* from the word *rehabilitation* in the federally funded programs under that title. If, a number of decades ago, a worker lost a right arm in some industrial accident, for example, the view was that the worker had to be retrained to enter a different occupation. The loss of an arm is now viewed as something more than an event requiring occupational adjustment. It requires the readjustment of the person as an entirety, because that is the way people function. The rehabilitation needed is not vocational (better that than nothing, however), but personal. And rehabilitation counseling is offered to those facing readjustment needs from a much wider array of circumstances than occupational accidents.

Another conceptual shift is the viewing of occupations not just as patterns of activities to do but as activities to be. An occupational career, particularly in the professions, gives an opportunity to individuals to express being, to maximize themselves. An occupation provides a major opportunity to fulfill the psychological need to be all that one can be. The word *dedication* is commonly used to describe those who find maximum meaning in life by giving themselves over completely to occupations such as physician, educator, or law enforcer, to name a few. The role of occupations in giving maximum meaning to life is suggested by the question "Why do millionaires work?" Without a consistent, organized, creative regimen, there is diminished being.

A different question can be asked: "Why do some lottery winners quit work and then, after a period, long to return to their former occupation?" Hunter/gatherers had to work to live, as do the vast majority of people today. There is no support for the thought that if most people had no need to work for sustenance and luxuries, they would not work. The evidence is on the other side. Moreover, there is substantial anecdotal evidence that wealthy people not regularly employed in a creative occupation experience anomie—existential anxiety—manifested in mentally unhealthy behaviors. It is no surprise that some people suddenly made wealthy by a lottery are reported to have become existentially disoriented, a state relieved by their return to the work force.

This recent view of an occupation as a prime source of a sense of completeness has contributed to a major social change. If it is a right in this culture to have this sense of fulfillment, it is a right for all people. With that commitment attained, no longer would occupations that required professional preparation, risk, and dedication be limited to men, and predominantly those of European origin. Women would now decide for themselves whether their full-time occupation was in the home, in the working world, or in both at different times. The psychological and legal commitments now are that the workplace is open without reference to gender, race, religion, or ethnic identification. That commitment is short of full realization, but the path is marked, and even if social obstacles are still in the path, the motion toward the ideal is eroding those obstacles.

Although the first two parts of Parsons's formula, knowledge of self and of occupations, are still valid in rough form, they are now couched in these broader conceptualizations about the meaning of occupations in human lives and the wholeness of human functioning. These newer visions of the role of careers in life, plus new methods of appraisal, make up the great change found today in counseling about careers. Parsons's middle step, learning about occupations, is still essential, but again there has been a great change in the amount and accessibility of accurate information. The third of Parsons's steps, true reasoning, was applied to the first two steps. Based on today's knowledge, this third step is no longer sufficient as he expressed it. It is, in fact, made up of the three counseling focuses: clients' cognitions, affect, and behaviors. Reasoning occurs, of course, but it is not the primitive activity that Parsons once envisioned.

### *The Third Change: Assessment Devices*

Changes in concepts and counseling competencies in the career area are reflected in the psychological instruments developed for this area. Their changing content both reflected and abetted change in concepts about the role of occupations in life. In Parsons's time there were no instruments to assist in counseling; today there is an assessment device for each facet, or variable, of career-decision activity that can be thought of, and multiple instruments each for a number of these.

It may be claimed, with partial accuracy, that the data provided by the variety of inventories and other assessment devices could be acquired through the verbal exchange of counseling. Even if it were possible and desirable to acquire the same data from interviews only, the following superiorities of published instruments would justify their use:

1. They ensure getting all useful information instead of depending upon counselors' memories.
2. Valuable counseling time is not required to assemble data that can be acquired outside of interviews.
3. The procedure of responding to a printed instrument is, for most clients, more interesting than responding to a series of detailed oral questions.
4. Counselors could not acquire by interview procedures alone the kind of data yielded by the subtle measures that some instruments employ. For instance, answers to the items in the instruments that bear the surname of their author, Kuder, are all forced choices.
5. Published instruments provide more than data about any one client; they permit comparing a client's responses with those of others. They also provide information from the developer about how best to employ the data produced by the instrument.

## Assessment Instruments

For some people with minimal education reared in a restricting culture, entry into the world of work, either the first time or at any subsequent times, can mean just finding any kind of employment. For them choice does not mean assessment of self, looking to how self can be implemented in the occupational world, and then developing and working on a plan to achieve that goal. For others not so limited, questions about the future are addressed cognitively, not in some vague, global way but by employing specific but somewhat overlapping cognitions. These include concepts of self, values, interests, and assumptions, along with aspirations and life objectives. There are also cognitive abilities, such as aptitudes for dealing with verbal and numerical data or physical aptitudes. The assessment of occupational interests has a long history, with change occurring as concepts about the psychological meaning of occupations changed.

## Interest Inventories

By the middle decades of this century, scholarly interest in the similarities and differences among people had provided both a rationale for understanding clients and the standardized instruments needed to collect occupationally related data. An early major instrument came from the research of Edward K. Strong, Jr. He had studied the characteristics of successful workers in a number of occupations, notably the higher level ones appropriate for university graduates. Those findings provided the basis for a vocational-interest inventory, published first in 1927 and still widely used today in revised form. Clients' interests are surveyed, and the results are organized into patterns. A match with similar patterns is sought from among the occupational families on the inventory.

Another major development had remote origins in the proposition that people in the Western world, far from being alike, were distributed among six modes of thinking and acting, labeled values. Allport, Vernon, and Lindsey later developed a scale based on those six values. This scale provided a general understanding of clients but had only hypothetical significance for career choice. Research and theorizing about the construct called "personality" similarly had identified different kinds of personalities, again with only conjectural use in occupational matters. Types of values and types of personalities were spoken of as if these were two discrete categories of human functioning, but they are only partially so. Each is an effort to analyze the totality of human thought and action into large, distinctive patterns.

A major advancement accompanied the publication of the results of John Holland's research (1966, 1985). He offered six vocational personalities and corresponding work environments, findings that were solidly substantiated. Unlike earlier, only loosely empirically supported classifications of values and personality, Holland's rigorous, empirically supported conclusions were aimed solely at the occupational facet of human existence, and thus they have had continuously increasing significance for counseling.

Holland's study of the psychological aspects of careers showed that Western workers, using measures Holland developed, fell into one of six career-significant types, realistic, investigative, artistic, social, enterprising, and conventional. Individuals were found to have a main orientation to one of these but also to have two minor orientations. A three-letter code is created for each subject, comprising the initials of three of the six types that receive the highest scores. The first letter shows the primary type, and the other two letters report the next two ranked types. From the three-letter code, a person can find the occupations that match that code, ranging from lower level ones (in terms of complexity of functions and education required) to professions and similar occupations.

An important finding is that the relationships among the six types run from compatible to incompatible. These degrees of affinity are shown by arraying the

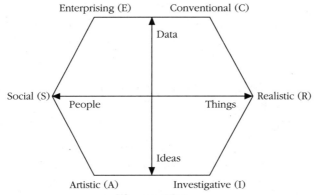

**Figure 13-1**

Holland's hexagon of career types, with four dimensions added later. Reprinted from Prediger, Swaney, and Mau, 1993, Vol. 71, p. 423. Copyright © ACA. Reprinted with permission. No further reproduction authorized without written permission of the American Counseling Association. Originally adapted by permission of American College Testing from Lamb and Prediger, 1981, p. 2.

types on a hexagonal figure (see Figure 13-1). Compatible types are found at adjacent angles, while incompatible ones are found on opposite angles. An unconflicted person's three-letter score, therefore, will contain three adjacent letters.

The importance of Holland's studies for counseling with a career emphasis is demonstrated by the widespread adaptation and extension of the hexagon concept by other occupational psychologists and test developers. One that adds a useful new dimension to the hexagon and overcomes some counseling inadequacies of the original figure has been developed by Prediger, Swaney, and Mau (1993). The U.S. Department of Labor has been studying and classifying occupations for many years. It has identified every occupation as being characterized by some degree of involvement of data, people, and things (DPT). The numerical code for each of the over 20,000 occupations given in the *Dictionary of Occupational Titles* (1977) includes three numerals showing the occupational involvement of each occupation in the DPT domains. Prediger and his colleagues find that occupations have an additional dimension, ideas. They employ these four, not in the coding procedure of the Department of Labor's occupational classification scheme but to extend Holland's hexagon by adding all four classifications to it, as shown in Figure 13-1.

Whereas Holland's hexagon was not designed to have a counseling function, being offered only to illustrate his theory, the addition of these four characteristics permits plotting occupational families at precise points on the hexagon, thereby eliminating some inadequacies and providing a counseling function by allowing clients to visualize more precisely the relationships among occupations.

The variety of inventories beyond the two mentioned above reflects different concepts about occupational interests. To be justified in the use of any, counselors need hands-on familiarity with a variety of interest inventories and other instruments and need to study experts' evaluations, such as those found in the Mental Measurement Yearbooks (Mitchell, 1985); Hood and Johnson's (1991) book, which reviews instruments used in a number of counseling areas; and Kapes and Mastie's (1988) review and analysis attending specifically to career-assessment instruments.

## *Values Inventories*

The physical scientist's work has the advantage of dealing with precisely defined elements. In the less exact, probabilistic science of psychology, researchers and practitioners deal with cognitive entities labeled interests and values and wonder about their differences. In some ways, interests are values, and vice versa. Nonetheless, there is enough that is distinctive in an inventory of values that if a full assessment of a client's cognitions is deemed appropriate, values inventories are available. Hood and Johnson (1991) evaluate the *Minnesota Importance Question-naire* and the two values inventories developed by Donald Super, with observations about their usefulness.

## *Assessing Assumptions*

The way an individual confronts any domain of life is partly determined by the person's assumptions and beliefs about that domain. No matter what clients' concerns are, therefore, it behooves counselors to know an individual's assumptions and beliefs about the domain of those concerns. As with other cognitive areas that have counseling significance, a counselor can acquire this knowledge just by asking clients to report their beliefs. The alternative to this haphazard and time-consuming approach is to provide them with a researched array of beliefs and assumptions to which they can respond. John Krumboltz makes this possible with the *Career Beliefs Inventory* (1993) which provides clients with 96 statements to which they respond on a 5-point scale running from strong disagreement to strong agreement.

It is essential, not just a useful starting point, to know clients' assumptions and beliefs about the occupational world, particularly to know those of adults concerned about occupational matters.

# Group and Individual Career Needs

Counselors' functions in certain agencies—notably, schools—include proposing and often directing group activities to enhance the development of the agency's members, particularly in career matters. For schools, as an example, there are activities to impart decision-making skills, teach information-seeking behaviors, and create opportunities to clarify values. If training in seeking information is offered, the counselor is not obligated to give information about occupations and higher education, because students will acquire the motivation and skills needed to acquire that kind of information, a lesson of lifelong value.*

Institutions of higher education similarly offer group experiences related to careers. For example, the University of Maryland (College Park) offers one-credit

---

*A middle school program for building information-seeking behaviors is described in Chapter 12 of Byrne (1977). Catalogs of career and other school-oriented developmental materials are given at the end of the chapter.

courses in a number of personal development areas, including these career-related topics: career planning and decision making, job-search strategies, and academic and career advancement.

## *Individual Counseling*

The first fact to remember is that counseling about the career aspect of life differs greatly with clients' developmental levels and among individuals at any level. Counselors in secondary schools, for example, help students whose career-exploration history is in its infancy, who are facing concurrent needs to adapt in such complex areas as families and sexuality, and whose life goals are undefined or only weakly defined. There are considerable differences in the counseling required by that population and that required by more mature clients who are contemplating career changes at the middle of the developmental scale.

Counselors need to be informed about development over the life span, with emphasis on the specific population each plans to serve, because counseling that emphasizes career concerns is counseling about life-span development. In working with youths, counselors convey that the counseling sessions are built on the client's past and present and are directed as much as possible to a tenable future. Clients are not given reason to assume that if one or more interviews result in the choice of an occupational family to enter, career concerns are over for life. What is conveyed is that career shifts and adjustments are lifelong because developmental concerns are lifelong. (To understand careers from this perspective, see Zunker, 1990, and Herr and Cramer, 1992.) Counselors in agencies that serve mature clients will be called upon to help adults in transition, and for that population particular developmental knowledge is needed (Lea & Leibowitz, 1992; Schlossberg, 1984).

By attending to clients' developmental histories, counselors can close a gap of which Parsons had little cause to be aware when he identified the first two of the three elements that constitute vocational counseling, a gap between knowing oneself and the working world. To identify those two elements was adequate for that time and that place (New England), but it is not today, anywhere in the country. Before clients' self-knowledge can be translated into the working world, it has to be passed through the filters of their gender, race, and ethnicity. Such a process is necessary in order to assess how those characteristics may inhibit or facilitate acceptance in a work environment. Based solely on clients' interests and abilities, any choice could have been viewed as tenable (Sherman, 1992).

Most white men of European descent can move directly from self-knowledge (Parsons's first need) to a chosen occupation (result of meeting his two other stated needs). Matters are different when race is a variable. This fact requires counselors to be knowledgeable about developmental and counseling issues relative to each racial subpopulation before assuming that they have sufficient information to deal with career specifics.

Developmental level and race as counseling variables are further affected by the variable of gender. The male psyche has been examined for years; the female psyche has only recently been the focus of scholarly studies. Material about women in general has become abundant, and publications are now available that are specifically related to counseling with women, including career concerns unique to them (Cook, 1993).

Although counselors may have completed their training programs before age 25, the average age is higher. It can be assumed, therefore, that counselors have sufficient maturity, enhanced by a study of development, to be effective with clients regardless of their age. However, ample anecdotal evidence does point to counselors' gender and ethnicity as variables in their effectiveness when dealing with concerns that involve value and other issues of affect.

Given the fact that client variables are countless, there can still be general prescriptions for counseling individuals, some of which can be identified by thinking about these diverse individuals in the age range 30–50:

1. June, age 32, recently divorced, must support a daughter, 10, and son, 13. High school education, waitress before and occasionally during marriage. Needs help with son.
2. Roger, age 42, African descent, married, four children: daughter a senior in HS, son 15, son 13, daughter 8. Was in charge of shipping for medium-sized manufacturing concern when it suddenly closed. Has looked for over six months for regular employment; has taken occasional part-time work, which he finds demeaning. Thinks he must change occupation but has no idea to what, and claims he cannot afford training.
3. Charles, age 34, seeking to determine an occupation after six years served of a ten-year sentence for drug dealing. Had been licensed in a health field and had practiced for three years. The license will not be reissued. Single.

Someone observing the counseling of these three clients would note the similarity with which it began. The communication skills described in Chapter 10 would be easy to identify in each instance: simple reinforcers, invitations, reflection of feeling, paraphrasing, and clarification would dominate, at least in the first part of the initial interview, and be apparent at times in all interviews. What could not be observed is the way the counselor frames each client's problems as a long-term developmental matter, involving not only immediate occupational concerns but also the other areas in which each client's wholeness as a person is manifested, such as in marital and family relationships.

The topic of developmental levels, or stages, is not an academic one; it bears importantly on the readiness of each client to deal effectively with his or her career concern. Study by counselors of developmental stages, such as those proposed by Super (1957) or Erickson (1968), permits the counselor to make such assessments mentally. The laid-off shipping manager, Roger, would probably be found to have an occupational maturity that could be built upon, but the recently divorced June is likely to have the occupational maturity of a teenager. The released convict, Charles, likewise would be found to be of arrested developmental maturity, higher than June but lower than Roger. Counseling would have to take those levels into account, particularly in interpreting appraisal devices, such as that all-important one, the interest inventory.

Assessments of values and assumptions, supplemented by some measure of competence in verbal and mathematical reasoning (information that would be available to counselors in educational institutions), will help construct a matrix for understanding each client. Another aspect of cognitions is important—the quality of the cognitive process that each client can apply to the task. This issue is addressed by Knefelkamp and Slepitza (1976) in a model that adapts Perry's (1970) intellectual and ethical model to the assessment of clients' stages of cognitive development as they apply to careers.

The premise is that people have relatively independent cognitive systems for each distinct area in which they must apply reasoning, one such being a career. Each system has four cognitive stages, each of which has substages. Those stages, as applied to careers, start with dualism. ("There is a correct occupation for me, and the rest are incorrect. An authority [test, counselor] will tell me which is the correct one.") In the next stage, multiplicity, the person is beginning to see that more than one career choice is likely to be tenable and becomes interested in the process through which a desirable career can be identified. The counselor remains dominant, however—the determiner of the process. In stage three, relativism, people have advanced cognitively from looking for help from elsewhere or other persons to taking charge of the reflective process by which decisions are made. The final stage, commitment within relativism, is the level of maximum cognitive maturity. It comprises three substages. When clients have reached the highest substage, they:

> have a firm knowledge of who they are and how that affects all aspects of one's life . . . They are aware of the effects they have on others and the effects others have on them.
>
> They . . . seek new ways to express what they are about [and] are characterized by an active seeking out and processing of information. [They take] on more risks to their self esteem in an effort to fully attain their potential. They are about new things, new challenges, new ways to interact, but tempered by an insightful realization of the potential positive and negative effects on their actions on self and others [Knefelkamp & Slepitza, 1976, p. 56].

Like Piaget's findings in child development, this scheme is also a developmental epistemology; that is, it is correlated with age and experience. Counseling can accelerate upward movement through the stages, but it is important to know at what stage a client starts so that counseling will not presume capacities that are not there. Given their past histories, it is tenable to expect June to be at the dualism stage, Roger to be in an early stage of relativism, and Charles to be at the multiplicity stage.

## *The Case of June*

These three clients are functioning as entireties in the several systems in which they live and in the psychological processes of cognitions, affect, and actions. The concern that June brought to the counselor, for example, was management of her son's behaviors. She lives her life as an entirety, so consideration for her total existence requires paying attention to other aspects of her life. Because an occupation can be a major way of expressing one's being, that topic has to be raised. She was a waitress from time to time during her marriage and is now employed as one full time, thus having two occupations, the other being homemaker. When she is faced with the question "Does the occupation of waitress express to the world who you are—does it accurately define you?"—her hesitations, her arguments with herself, indicate a level of thinking that had never occurred to her.

Interest and aptitude assessment reveals potentials for higher order occupations that quite surprised June. She was counting on the counselor to tell her what occupation would be best for her. Her cognitive development, along with other facets of maturity, had been stunted by events following her early marriage and past life, both causing and resulting from her low opinion of herself.

Just as the several facets of her life are expressions of her whole being, so are her cognitions, emotions, and behaviors. June as an entity has to be understood and helped by approaching that entirety through delving into each of those. Low self-worth and regret about her early marriage and interrupted education, all negative cognitions about self, are colored by negative emotions. Her behaviors express insufficient assertiveness, as would be expected when there is a cognition of low self-worth. This lack of assertiveness contributed to her sense of loss of control over her son.

Cognitive restructuring, assertiveness training, and help in finding a support group for recently divorced women with children lead June to new views of herself and to a conviction that she is not to be defined for life by her current occupation. She now sees herself with excitement as a new person, with opportunities she never could have imagined open to her. She has become almost grateful that the divorce happened. She enrolls in a community college, where she can receive such further counseling as she feels she needs.

## *The Case of Roger*

Roger also experienced negative emotion, but it was aroused by circumstances different from those of June. He and his wife expected to send their soon-to-be-graduated daughter to college, but after his job loss they see no way. If she were able to get financial aid, it might be possible. He has not found a job as a shipping manager, he is embarrassed about taking unemployment checks, and even that income will end in a few months.

Counseling requires looking at life as a whole, how his job loss has affected other aspects of life, and how to insulate those other aspects from the ill effects of unemployment. His identity was tied up with his occupation, which he had done well and which had brought him praise and an income that satisfied family needs. The effect of the job loss was almost as devastating as an accidental loss of a limb. Frustration and despair followed anger—emotions that spilled over into his family life. His development appeared appropriate for his age and experience.

The counseling need is to induce flexibility into Roger's view of an appropriate occupation. An interest inventory makes him aware of his managerial competencies, which could be applied to other occupations. He has counted primarily on the state employment office as the source of openings for a shipping manager, although he went to the personnel offices of two nearby industries to inquire if they needed help in their shipping departments. To counter these inadequate approaches, he learned from a handbook how to write a résumé and how to pursue employment.

Roger's negative emotions recede as he gains confidence about how to seek employment and as he becomes flexibile about the kinds and locations of jobs he could fill. He comes to see that retraining is not the radical and expensive matter he thought, depending upon what sort of training he undertakes. He operated on the common fallacy: education or training is acquired early in life, and then you go to work. He comes to accept the desirability of education and training continuing throughout life. His daughter is granted a scholarship at a state institution and locates employment in the university library to supplement her scholarship funds.

Roger had only minor career development difficulties; his problems were unemployment, with greatly reduced income, and keeping the rest of his life stabilized until he found satisfactory employment. When he was employed, he had an excellent image of himself as worker, husband, and father. Reemployment would cause those self-views to return. At no time was race seen as a variable in his career concerns.

## *The Case of Charles*

Charles is now "clean" and knows he is so for life. During imprisonment he underwent a major cognitive restructuring, from which emerged a radically new self. He is most eager to implement his new views of himself. Clinical and standardized assessment show him to be alert, of above average intellectual abilities, and strongly motivated to cut out a new life that will restore the prestige he lost when he became addicted and then a minor drug dealer.

Counseling with Charles is counseling about his future life and the role an occupational career can play in maximizing the person he sees himself becoming. His needs are for insights that will be important in achieving this new self, and for knowledge of procedures for reentering the occupational world, outcomes both relatively easily brought about. His cognitive maturity lets him take initiatives and responsibilities for his future. No affect or behavioral liabilities are identified.

## *Nancy's Career Concerns*

Nancy's needs and counseling about them differ noticeably from the concerns of June, Roger, and Charles. She is the daughter, and only child, of a homemaker mother and lawyer father. The father's practice is solely as corporate attorney for a large manufacturing company in a small city. The parents are conservative elitists, keeping a watchful eye on their daughter. It is reasonable to expect that if an independent girls' high school had been at hand, Nancy would have been enrolled in that. A boarding school was rejected because of the parents' preference to have her at hand. Some fellow students in the public high school she attended recall her as intellectual and genteel to the point of stuffiness. Some thought of her as shy, and some as "stuck-up."

It was assumed from Nancy's earliest days that she would attend college, but at no point was she pushed by her family to commit to a career. She entered a large university after graduating from high school, enrolling in a variety of liberal arts courses. During most of her first semester she maintained the cognitive structures and behaviors with which she had entered. By December, however, she could see changes in her perspectives and assessments of self. Of considerable influence were the female friends she admired, all of whom were career oriented and some of whom had made career decisions.

Nancy was ignorant of the occupational world, except for a vague knowledge of what it meant to be a lawyer and an even vaguer knowledge of the occupations of some relatives and of some friends' parents. She was aware that some of her friends' mothers were employed but knew little of the nature of their occupations.

What started off as a mild but growing curiosity about occupations during the latter part of the first semester had, by the middle of the second semester, become a strong interest in a career. With encouragement from friends to do so, she turned up at the university counseling center.

Perhaps because there have been no disruptions in her life to require cognitive growth, the radius of her personality is short. She is a naive youth, both occupationally and socially. With so little in her occupational history to build on, the counselor moves to a battery of assessment instruments, the central one being an interest inventory. (The counseling center routinely uses the Strong-Campbell Interest Inventory.) The results are, unsurprisingly, a rather flat profile, but with some prominence of a pattern of results that, to Nancy's surprise, point to science. She did well in high school science courses, as she did in all other studies, but did not feel a noticeable interest in that field over others. They were required courses, so you just took them and did your best, a "B" student earning "A"s because of conscientious study.

Although in her sophomore year Nancy enrolls in physics along with psychology and sociology, by her junior year her major is sociology, with a minor in psychology. She decides upon a career in anthropology, a decision validated in another series of counseling interviews. Nancy's occupational maturing is uncomplicated, growing with her general maturing. Counseling shortens the decision process and reduces chance factors.

The counselor viewed assisting Nancy as being concerned with her as a totality, but it was only the cognitive aspect of her life, specifically focused on occupations, that the counselor had to work with. Other cognitive components and affective and behavioral aspects of her being were insignificant variables in resolving her concern.

## *The Case of Sandra*

Matters are somewhat different for Sandra, a high school senior of African heritage. Although younger than Nancy, she is more mature generally as well as occupationally. Her call upon a counselor is for help not only in making a occupational decision but also help in finding scholarship assistance for the college studies she hopes for. Her father recently lost his job and is existing on unemployment insurance, soon to run out. For a time she was dejected about this turn of events and assumed that she would look for a job after graduation. However, her parents are adamant that she continue with college plans if she can get financial help.

Sandra has always found some kind of work, and as a result of employment in a gift shop during the previous summer developed an interest in having her own business sometime. This is an idea she wants to check out with the counselor. An interest inventory confirms that she has an appropriate entrepreneurial interest. (It cannot, of course, be so specific as to name the particular business she would do well to enter.) There is discussion of the difficulty of that kind of career in general and the specific obstacles in capitalizing that kind of venture, which might apply not only to a woman but particularly an African-American woman. These are not issues to be resolved now, however; for now it is sufficient to courageously and persistently push on, continuing her scholarly achievements and school activities.

By the end of the interview series, Sandra has increased enthusiasm about her career aim and has sent for scholarship and college-entrance materials.

### *Counseling Commonalities*

Under the definitions employed here, there was no need for therapy in any of these five instances—no need for personality reconstruction. All of the clients were normal persons with normal concerns. Passing the five cases through a mental-health filter, we find that June had the most aggravated problems and Charles, Nancy, and Sandra the least. In any case, psychological counselors are sensitive to the mental health of their clients, knowing causes of normal disturbances and how they can be eased. A person labeled a mental-health counselor would have engaged in no different practices with June and Roger (but could have better served other, more complex mental-health needs than this counselor because of his or her supplemental specialized preparation).

Successful counseling outcomes required conceptualizing each client as a totally functioning individual while exploring cognitive, affective, and behavioral components. It meant getting a grasp of the client's social system, including the bondings and affiliations that were significant variables. It attended to development as it had occurred over time and might proceed in the future. Particular thought was given to the facilitation of June's development.

Counseling in the cases of June, Roger, and Charles included occupational specifics but was not centered on them. Those particulars were brought into the discussion when life goals were considered to understand their part in achieving maximum fulfillment. Had counseling been held to whatever narrow limits the clients expressed, June's counseling would have focused on the concern she presented—that of child management. That topic was addressed, but it became subsidiary to opening up her development so she would be enabled to introduce new satisfactions into her life. This led, of course, to consideration of occupations that would support that outcome.

Interest, aptitude, and cognitive standardized instruments supplemented clinical information in June's and Charles's instances. The limits on June's cognitive maturity required delaying the use of an interest inventory until she was beyond the dualism stage. With Roger there was no need for any instrumentation other than an inventory that pointed to clusters of occupations that were tenable for him. These provided a basis for helping him achieve more cognitive flexibility.

## Career Counseling with Three Types of Clients

### *The Elderly*

Imagine a counselor employed in a community of retired people. Does that counselor have to deal with occupational concerns? By older conceptualization, no. But the answer is yes if the issue is reframed so that the focus is not on a consistent pattern of activities that is carried out for remuneration. (Homemakers are in an unremunerated occupation.) If the counselor is concerned instead with helping ensure each individual's sense of worth and with maximizing each individual's potential for that particular developmental stage, occupations are defined not solely as remunerated activities but as those that enhance and fulfill. In that sense, a counselor would be involved with occupational matters in this ever-increasing subpopulation.

Those concepts define the significance of the term *occupation* at all adult ages, not just the elderly, a stance that emphasizes mentally healthy, continuing development. It is the stance with which June, Roger, and Charles were approached. It permits placing occupational matters in perspective by giving rise to the question of how people can experience the most fulfilling lives through the work they do. A person may give his or her life to an occupation; the occupation should also give life to the person.

## Adolescents and Young Adults

By now the principles on which counseling about occupations is based have been delineated to the point where you can speak to this next population with little tutelage. It is the population of the most avid seekers of the "right" occupation, as well as the "right" mate. It is also the population with many members whose developmental levels are not sufficiently mature to make those "right" decisions, if by that is meant permanent commitments that will yield lifelong satisfactions.

The principles offered here propose that a high school career-guidance program is, in effect, a life-guidance program in which students become aware of issues of fulfillment and of the role of occupations as a major route to that end. They also become aware that development is lifelong and that therefore they can expect changes in how that fulfillment is provided. On this point, it is essential that adolescents become aware of and see the occupational significance of the fact that interests are likely to change during the following ten years as physical and psychological maturation continues. Some will make commitments in their teens that provide lifetime satisfaction. Others, however, are likely to experience at least one major change of occupational interest by their mid-20s. Witness the academically competent person reported earlier who had been a space scientist, had left that occupation to prepare for and become the Wall Street financial wizard he was, and at the time of the report about him was preparing for a lifetime occupation as a clown.

One goal is to build flexibility into clients' assumptions and beliefs about the future and to provide skills to process developmental changes. With this orientation, students can see the results of an occupational-interest inventory for what it is, a report of the present level of development. That is a good starting point and can fruitfully occur even in middle schools. The message to those early adolescents is that just because their current occupational interests were obtained by responses to printed instruments, the sum of those responses may have no more lifetime validity than their "fire fighter," "law enforcer," "nurse," or "astronaut" responses when they were 6 or 7 to Aunt Mary's "What do you want to be when you grow up?"

A wealth of specialized, empirically tested information is available to counselors in secondary schools and universities about career-development practices for use in group and individual approaches. Coverage of that material is beyond the purview of this text. Some sources for that information are given at the end of the chapter.

### *Rehabilitation Counseling*

The central emphasis of rehabilitation counseling since the 1920s has been on occupations (Rubin & Roessler, 1987). In recent years there have been major changes in emphases, particularly in the effort to draw those who are the natural clients of rehabilitation counselors into life's mainstream. Legislation requires that society is no longer to be structured for the majority "we" who have no physical disabilities, with a "Too bad for them, but that's the way it is" stance for the disabled. Society is to be restructured as necessary to accommodate all people, regardless of their physical competence, a parallel to the recasting of society into one that accords accommodation in all matters to all people without reference to gender or race. Little change in social attitudes toward the physically disadvantaged was required to alter their status from "them" to "us." The change relative to gender and race is a much more complex one, with incomplete achievements.

Counselors in a rehabilitation setting function professionally like those in any other setting, but they are required to have additional knowledge about physical and other restrictions on occupational functioning. Because rehabilitation counselors serve clients from start to finish, including job placement, they need coordinating skills in addition to counseling competencies as part of their supplemental training.

Psychological counselors attend to the normal development of psychologically normal persons. The relationship between careers and desirable normal development has been explored, along with counselor assistance when occupational questions are a developmental focus. In the next section we examine the functions of counselors when the developmental emphasis is a topic different from careers. After that examination, we will briefly consider counseling procedures by which occasional clients can be assisted.

## Other Common Client Concerns

We are reminded that only career concerns were emphasized in the prior three clientele groups for reasons explained earlier. Within each of the three, of course, there will be found a variety of client concerns in addition to or different from the career topic. At the same time, some of these other concerns are common among many clients. Three of these will be briefly examined, each served by a counseling speciality.

### *Marriage*

Marriage is the one of the three arenas for which counselors are rarely asked for assistance in the entering or starting-anew stages. In this culture marriage partner selection is commonly held to be primarily a matter of emotion, one syruped over with romance. Family, friends (particularly friends), and the clergy will be the primary consultants in mate-selection. Adjustment concerns (marriage difficulties) may also bring consultation with those familiar persons, but there has been an increase in the view that amelioration of marriage difficulties is best served by an objective, professionally trained person, hence the surge in professional marriage counseling.

The principles applied in this activity are those on which counseling about any facet of living is based. A number of the concepts relative to occupations are applicable generally, and therefore apply to distinct topics such as marriage. One difficulty in counseling discordant married couples lies in the need to deal simultaneously with two or more persons, some of whom can be assumed to be incompatible on some significant matters. In that kind of situation, counseling is like helping to arbitrate differences between parents and a rebellious child. Indeed marriage difficulties can stem from different views in just such matters as child rearing. In any case, because counseling even one person about marriage requires consideration of all persons locked in a social system, it is common to label counseling with this focus not just as marriage, but as marriage and family. Counselors who engage in marriage and family counseling also serve individuals, and therefore need preparation for that function. When functioning as marriage counselors, the goal is restoration to health of a system that has become "ill." This focus requires supplemental specialized preparation to be certified or licensed in this topic.

## Sex

Sexual problems can appear in any post-puberty developmental period, well into seniority. In years past, if counseling was sought about those concerns in high probability it was from a person in the clergy, given the view that sexuality was a moral issue, or from a physician on the premise that the sexual difficulty was a medical one. If help was sought from trained counselors, the counselors likely had only little specialized knowledge to inform their functions. The complexity of this essential aspect of existence and the specialized nature of counseling around sexual matters earned increasing professional attention some decades ago which led to the emergence of specialized training, certification, and licensing for those wishing to enter this specialized counseling pursuit. Those in marriage and family counseling typically have acquired this specialized training, or at least a specialist is available if marriage and family counseling is provided by an agency.

## Mental Health

All professional counselors are mental-health counselors. Whatever concerns clients have are reflections of their mental health, and whatever professional actions counselors take with clients bear on their mental health. Nonetheless some normal people can experience aberrations in cognitions, emotions, or behaviors of a severity that is better served by those with the specialized training received as mental-health counselors. No sharp line delineates the practice of psychological counselors functioning under the title of mental-health counselors from psychological counselors who function with other titles. The difference between the two groups is found in the greater amount of study in aberrant behavior acquired by mental-health counselors.

A secondary school counseling center is ideally staffed with a variety of practitioners. Typical psychological counselors assist students in groups and individually to master developmental concerns, a major one being occupational careers, as we saw. Students with persistent cognitive, emotional, or behavioral imbalances can profit greatly if one or a few mental-health counselors are included on the guidance team to deal with the youths' time-consuming specialized concerns—if necessary to serve as links in helping those clients receive assistance from clinical psychologists.

## Clients from Varying Subcultures

Few countries come near the United States in the matter of cultural diversity. Some are at the other extreme of cultural uniformity, Japan for one. This diversity is compounded by being the product of two variables, ethnic and racial differences. A variable in counselor competence, therefore, is knowledge of and sensitivity to culturally determined thinking, feeling, and behavior. This complex and important topic cannot be considered here at any other than introductory length; therefore, you are urged to examine the documents on multicultural issues cited in the Complementary Reading section.

The complexity of the topic can be grasped by awareness of essential differences among three major groups that cut across race and ethnic origin: the population before European immigration began, voluntary immigrants, and involuntary immigrants.

Decade by decade after the American Revolution, common cultural characteristics emerged, based on a common language, which characterized the new country. An "American" culture had taken root. The European immigrants retained as much of their culture as necessary to ease the transition to the new one. Immigrants would speak their native language, but also expected their children to speak English. The grandchildren might know only a little of their grandparents' native tongue and in most ways acted "American." To be Polish Americans means being Americans who retain elements of a former culture, just as it does for numerous other willing immigrant groups.

By plan, some citizens of this new American culture brought about the destruction of another culture almost completely—that of the original inhabitants, the so-called Indians. The cultures of the millions of African natives who were here involuntarily were also deliberately destroyed by the citizens who controlled that outcome. There is no African culture remaining among their descendants, even though the term *African American* is becoming common. Since the abolition of slavery, the social climate dominated by whites has made it difficult for blacks to develop a culture in which there could be a sense of pride to replace the lost African one and the rejected slave culture. The culture that did emerge following the end of slavery was for years marked by basic survival needs, both physical and psychological. New black cultures have since emerged, the need for physical survival is a reduced concern in contrast to a half-century ago, and conditions for desirable psychological outcomes have improved somewhat for some black subcultures. The existence of several black subcultures points to the dangers of stereotyping, found in the remarks of people who speak of African Americans as if their individual and small-group commonalities exceeded their differences. However, the original deculturation of black Americans continues to have harmful effects on many who have been unable to break the cycle of imposed poverty and ignorance. Even the natives of this continent, for all the damage done to their cultures, did not experience so complete a loss.

When counselors of any cultural origin are called on to serve clients from any other culture, as happens in schools, they must know about and be sensitive to culture variables that may be significant for those clients. This also means avoiding stereotyping.

Everyone has stereotypes; they are part of one's life view. They can be inaccurate, which is undesirable enough, but when inaccurate perceptions of others are tied to strong emotions, considerable individual and community harm may result. Objective study about other cultures counters those harmful stereotypes, replacing them with accurate generalizations. Because counselors work with individuals, they must be wary of stereotypes of whatever quality. A counselor of North European heritage may hold inaccurate stereotypes of recent Spanish-speaking immigrants. Objective study may replace some of those inaccuracies but still leave the insufficiently accurate label "Hispanic." Chilean, Puerto Rican, and Mexican immigrants speak Spanish, but that fact does not justify assumption of other major cultural similarities among them. At a microcosmic level, stereotyping of families buries the uniqueness of its members: "Well, what can you expect from a Casbel; they're all alike."

Although the thoughts, feelings, and behaviors of all people are genetic dispositions modified by cultures, there are variables such as their socioeconomic class and gender that affect what individuals will acquire from a culture. On the one hand, to be a counselor in the United States imposes an ethical as well as a civic obligation to be steeped in the cultures of clients each counselor seeks to help and to know how those varying cultures may affect approaches for attaining counseling objectives. On the other hand, because counselors serve individuals, what is more important is the need for them to guard against approaching any client as if gross cultural characteristics that apply to the many also apply to this person.

# Other Counseling Procedures

## *Counseling with Groups*

The effectiveness of such groups as Alcoholics Anonymous in facilitating change is well recognized. Counselor-led groups are equally effective, although known to only a portion of the general population. A counselor in a school may gather small groups of students who are facing similar developmental difficulties and who have agreed to meet. Often the purpose is not to provide support but to promote change, such as in the case of racial disharmony or chronic tardiness. The primary objective is cognitive and affective change, which can be brought about by the interplay of group members led by the skilled counselor.

Psychodrama requires some dramatic sense as well as special training on the part of the counselor. Members of a group of, say, eight individuals are assigned roles through which they can address interpersonal problems in a session that may go on for an hour or more, with the roles that individuals play switched from time to time. The drama's intensity and realism can result in cognitive restructuring, emotional release and modification, and behavior change. For example, if the group has eight members, four might start the drama, with others called on to replace an "actor" when the counselor judges that that would further individual change.

## *Other Procedures*

Some procedures and techniques are used with all clients, some, with many clients, and a few, far less commonly or even rarely. The frequency of use appears to depend on the training that counselors receive and their experience with these supplemental activities. The supplemental procedures and techniques are numerous. Bibliotherapy is an example.

Bibliotherapy refers to the benefit to clients that comes from prescribed or suggested reading to be done outside the counseling interview. As an illustration, if the difficulties experienced by a counseling psychologist's client show the high likelihood of mood disorder, a book that describes a person's success in combating the malady may be a useful recommendation. Even a technical treatment of the topic can be informative to a client who shows academic interest in the disorder. This kind of reading, if suggested at all, is intended only as a supplement to the normal interview approaches that counselors employ with any particular concern. Of course, only counselors trained to counsel about biogenic or other complex disorders would suggest readings for clients in such topics.

Biographies, particularly autobiographies, can present models for clients, thereby extending the benefits of counseling beyond interviews. Clients can also be referred to some of the many how-to books that address their problems or interests. Some catalogs of materials are listed in the Complementary Reading section.

## Concluding Reflections

With this chapter we have come to the end of the academic and technical portion of a journey that began with seeking to understand the characteristics of the profession of psychological counselor. Upon reaching the conclusion of this scholarly venture we see counselors artfully, skillfully, and professionally employing a variety of knowledge-based procedures that will bring about the variety of psychological changes sought by clients. With scholarly matters now beyond us, all that remains for our inquiry are the professional issues examined in Chapter 14.

Our study confirms what new students will have anticipated: clients can be expected to differ in significant ways, even if it appears justifiable to use the same label to describe the concerns of some. I am comfortable with the hypothesis that a surgeon will find more similarity among patients needing an appendectomy than a counselor will among clients, no matter the similarity suggested by the counseling topic. It is for this reason that counselors cannot be instructed in "what to dos" that apply to all client concerns falling under common labels, such as careers, getting along with some other person(s), or poor self-concepts. The directions to new surgeons for the removal of an appendix have little variability. Conversely, psychological counselors cannot be told that when clients come with a labeled concern, "Follow these procedures with each client." The brief presentations in this chapter of five clients who told a counselor that their concerns were occupational ones let us see that there could be only minor similarities in procedures followed and techniques employed.

Counselors need not be concerned primarily about "how to"; that is the role of a technician. The professional knows "why" and, based on that knowledge, can artfully develop the procedures and appropriate techniques to suit each client's unique being. The "why" requires study of factors that bear on development. It is equally imperative for counselors to continue to advance their knowledge of development and counseling skills to match the constant evolution of such material. Changes in psychology are less rapid than the dramatic changes in the healing arts, but our professional ethics require, and our clients expect, that we give clients help based on the best evidence available. Continuing education is the lot of all who wish to claim with pride that they are competent, professional counselors.

■                        **Points to Remember**                        ■

1. Occupations are not just one of an equal number of ways for individuals to fill in time. They are a major source of individuals' fulfillment. Occupational matters, therefore, are central concerns of counselors.
2. Counselors in settings such as schools, universities, and rehabilitation agencies address this central counseling topic partly through group programs that meet common needs and teach personal skills related to making occupational decisions.
3. Group activities serve useful functions in providing common knowledge and skills, but they must be supplemented by individual counseling. Just as men's suits bought "off the rack" must be adjusted to each person's unique physical characteristics, counselors adjust the knowledge and skills they acquire to the unique psychological needs of individuals.
4. Almost a century ago, Parsons reported two client needs for making an occupational selection, knowledge of self and knowledge of the occupational world. These two needs are still valid, but great changes in them have come about, particularly in the past 30 years. (Parsons's third need is "right thinking.")
5. A major change in knowing oneself results from the development of valid career assessment devices. These measures provide clients with systematic knowledge about such cognitive variables as interests, aptitudes, and assumptions. Other cognitions must be explored but are completely unique to the individual. Counselors' skills facilitate bringing these into consideration.
6. Knowledge for knowledge's sake is not the sole intent of counseling about career matters. The intent is also to help clients create, sharpen, recast, or increase a sense of personal meaning, autonomy, purposefulness, and competency to cope in the occupational world. Counselors' sensitivity to general mental-health criteria and the part an occupation has in the total existence of each client are always present, although these topics may not need to be specifically addressed.
7. Career topics are tenable ones for all kinds of counseling agencies. However, some agencies, such as those providing marriage and family counseling, may

need to attend to careers only a little or not at all. An agency that specializes in career counseling may have more need to consider clients' marriage status than a marriage and family agency needs to deal with careers.

8. Counselors in marriage and family agencies need special preparation to attend to a system created by the interaction of individuals. Even though the system itself is the focus, counselors must be sensitive to the role of occupations in clients' lives and understand how the occupation of each individual affects the family as a system.

9. Of the several life circumstances that are variables in occupational matters, such as age and gender, a major one is client race or ethnicity. It is incumbent upon counselors to examine their values regarding this matter to see which may be negatively emotionally driven and to scrutinize the negative stereotypes that they may hold about differing ethnic or racial subpopulations, with the intention of altering those values and stereotypes.

# ■  Counselor Formation Activities  ■

Study of this text probably denotes your interest in becoming a counselor. Although your counselor-preparation curriculum may require you to discuss your motivation to be a counselor with a faculty member or an advanced student, you can benefit by examining this topic on your own. This requires searching out the origins of your interest in this occupation by reaching back at least to adolescence. You will profit from the experience by focusing on specific topics such as:

1. What part did role models play?
2. Have you experienced counseling? If the quality was inadequate, why did that not affect you negatively?
3. Did you know what knowledge and skills were required for counseling before you decided to enter the profession?
4. What evidence was available to you that supports your decision? Was any of this evidence supplied by an occupational-interest inventory?
5. What support for or objections to this decision have you received from other persons?
6. In what ways will the profession of counselor complement other activities in your life to provide maximum fulfillment. What part did the lure of money, power, and status play in your decision to be a counselor?
7. If you have selected a specialized group to serve as a counselor, what variables determined that selection?

# ■  Complementary Reading  ■

The assumption of this text is that all counselors, except those dealing with children, will at some time or another have to be concerned with clients' occupations, because they have to be concerned with life careers. Some counselors, of course, specialize in the psychology of occupational careers—in any case, it is a topic calling for supplemental reading. Certain groups of clients have common concerns in addition to career ones, and this chapter gives a few examples of some diverse client populations. Some are found in agencies, such as rehabilitation agencies, but other clientele are those with even more uniform concerns. These are illustrated in the list of *The Counseling Psychologist* issues below.

Although there may not be time now to peruse a full-length text, you should take time shortly to scan a text that examines psychological issues related to occupations. One is proposed here, although most any will be helpful. For those interested in either the rehabilitation or mental-health settings, two texts worth scanning are also proposed. You will also need familiarity with multicultural issues in counseling, so literature to begin that complementary study is found below.

### Counseling about Occupational Careers

ISAACSON, L., & BROWN, D. (1993). *Career Information, Career Counseling, and Career Development.* Needham Heights, MA: Allyn & Bacon.

### Rehabilitation Counseling

PARKER, R. M., & SZYMANSKI, E. M. (1992). *Rehabilitation Counseling: Basics and Beyond* (2nd ed.). Austin, TX: Pro-Ed.

### Mental-Health Counseling

HERSHENSON, D., & POWER, P. (1987). *Mental Health Counseling: Theory and Practice.* Needham Heights, MA: Allyn & Bacon.

### Multicultural Counseling

A useful start for your complementary readings in this topic is:

"Multiculturalism as a Fourth Force in Counseling." (1991). *Journal of Counseling and Development, 70*(1).

Give particular attention to the articles in Part I, "A Conceptual Framework."

For a unified treatment of topics, I recommend:

AXELSON, J. A. (1993). *Counseling and Development in a Multicultural Society*, 2nd ed. Pacific Grove, CA: Brooks/Cole.

Two texts that focus on counseling are:

SUE, D. W., & SUE, D. (1991). *Counseling the Culturally Different*, 2nd ed. New York: Wiley.

PEDERSON, P. B., DRAGUNS, J. G., LONNER, W. J., & TRIMBLE, J. E. (Eds.). (1989). *Counseling across Cultures*, 3rd ed. Honolulu: University of Hawaii Press.

Although the special considerations appropriate in counseling Native Americans are considered in the two books above, an informative introduction to the topic is provided in:

THOMASON, T. C. (1991). Counseling Native Americans. *Journal of Counseling and Development,* 69(4), 321–327.

## *The Counseling Psychologist Series*

The Division of Counseling Psychology issues a quarterly publication, *The Counseling Psychologist* (Sage Publications), addressing specific counseling topics. Some in that series deal with counseling of particular subpopulations. Recent ones are given here; one may be appropriate complementary reading for the counseling specialty you plan to pursue.

"Religious Faith across the Life Span." (1989). Volume *17*(4).
"Counseling Lesbian Women and Gay Men." (1991). Volume *19*(2).
"Counseling Psychology and Health Applications." (1991). Volume *19*(3).
"Counseling the HIV-Infected Client." (1991). Volume *19*(4).
"Major Social Theories of Aging and Implications." (1992). Volume *20*(2).
"Feminist Counseling and Therapy." (1993). Volume *21*(1). This volume is
    not about counseling women but about counseling from a feminist per-
    spective.

## 14

CHAPTER

# Our Profession

## Overview

A profession is defined by concepts and the procedures and techniques through which the concepts are made operative. New students are eager to learn counseling's procedures and techniques (hands-on behaviors are always attractive), and they accept studying theory because they want to be professional practitioners. But concepts and techniques alone do not a profession make—they are two legs of the stool. The third leg requires attention to the profession's culture, which comprises like practitioners whose interactions with other practitioners and with the general society are structured partly by the practitioners themselves and partly by society. However the structure may come about, it has to be there, or there is no profession. This chapter examines the issues that can make or break a profession, issues that require the studied attention of all who look forward to bearing the title of counselor.

This examination takes us first to consideration of the word *profession*. In exploring the characteristic of professions, we lean upon the conclusions of sociologists who have studied the histories and roles of occupations. Five generally accepted characteristics are examined. That requires the consideration of how professions ensure the quality of preparation of their practitioners through the process of accrediting training programs. Professions must also attest to the quality of the practitioners themselves, and we explore the topics of certification and licensure. Additionally, societies expect professions to police the professional activities of their members. This is done by first issuing a code of ethics and then erecting a structure for ensuring adherence to that code. The chapter closes with an introductory consideration of counselor liability.

# But *Is* Counseling a Profession?

Is counseling a profession? Does it matter? It depends on who is asking and answering. It will be informative to examine the issues that determine the answers that different people will give.

The first issue is approached by asking who is authorized to designate certain occupations as professions. One answer: social custom. The word *profession* is loosely used, particularly in our egalitarian society where high-status titles are often given to occupations for which little education or skill is required. In common parlance, one use of the word distinguishes an occupation carried out full time from an activity engaged in as a sideline, not a major source of income. A person called a professional plumber, for example, is one who is trained and licensed and works at plumbing full time. In contrast, the neighborhood handyperson, who knows enough to counsel about typical plumbing problems and to carry out common repairs, may be spoken of as a plumber but not as a professional one.

In the matter of psychological concerns, a young person may report that Uncle Gus or Aunt Emma counseled him or her about a problem, just as either of those adults may say that he or she counseled a niece or nephew. Whether or not the words *counselor* or *counseling* are employed in those situations, in this text the label "professional counselor" is reserved for trained, perhaps certified or licensed, usually full-time practitioners.

Two groups have a need for defined classifications of occupations: government agencies and those scholars who study the occupational facet of life. Two federal agencies, the U.S. Bureau of the Census and the Department of Labor, are required by law to classify occupations. For the Labor Department, occupations are differentiated by the level of functions performed in relation to things, data, and people and the level of preparation required to carry out those functions. In the classification schemes of those two government agencies, the term *profession* is limited to the highest level, one that does not include the oldest profession or plumbing or, as yet, the occupation of psychological counselor.

# Characteristics of a Profession

Scholars who study social forces and the history of occupations have recorded the characteristics of groups of occupations. Greenwood (1962)*, summarizing sociological findings, identifies six characteristics of a profession. These provide one basis for judging whether psychological counseling is fully a profession.

## 1. *The Occupation Is Based on a Systematic Theory*

There are theoretical variations in every acknowledged profession; the issue is whether variations are merely minor differences about major tenets or major differences about entire theories. When the major precepts of astronomy are considered, it can be said that its theoretical base is uniform. But theoretical bases

*From *Man, Work and Society* by Sigmund Nosow and William H. Form (Eds.). Copyright © 1962 by Basic Books, Inc. Copyright Renewed. Reprinted by permission of Basic Books, a division of HarperCollins Publishers, Inc.

can change. Consider geology. Over recent decades the hypothesis of plate tectonics, a newer accounting for major geological phenomena, has been increasingly supported and consequently accepted by geologists. For the transition period it could not be said that there was a single theory on which geology was based. The steady influx of new geologists has brought common commitment to plate tectonic theory, so again it can be said that geology is based on a uniformly accepted theory. There have been similar theoretical shifts in astronomy, with periods of transition sandwiched between times of widely accepted theory. Overall, however, the theoretical differences among astronomers and geologists can be described as minor.

Psychologists can carry out laboratory experiments, whereas astronomers and geologists cannot. But there is more agreement among theorists in those two professions than there is in psychology. Why? Astronomy and geology involve relatively fixed relationships among objective things that are relatively unchanged over time, a circumstance that imposes limits on the possible range of theories. The subjects for observation in psychology, humans, are diverse, complicated, and in flux—circumstances that permit broad differences in the way theorists account for thinking, feeling, and acting. Additionally, there has always been a fundamental philosophical disagreement over whether psychology must be limited to objective study (thus corresponding in rigor with other sciences), must engage only in the study of subjective phenomena, or should conduct research on both objective and subjective human phenomena. A social phenomenon probably contributes to this difference between the relative uniformity of theory in astronomy and geology and the diversity in psychological theorizing: few laypersons are concerned with theories in astronomy or geology. When it comes to explanations of why people think and act as they do, everyone, both lay and professional, has an interest—and a theory. Each different theory proposed by individuals in this area acquires adherents, and so theoretical diversity is increased. Some theories take on theological or ethical qualities, a position that may be justifiable when humans are the topic but is not germane to the material sciences. With the removal of the domination of theology from astronomy and geology, those qualities are no longer issues among the professional practitioners of those two sciences. Some theorists about human action and thought subscribe inflexibly to a positivist view of science. Others, reflected in this text, accept a middle ground that holds to the reality of both the objective and subjective worlds of individuals. Still others propose that "truth" lies only in people's subjective world.

Is there a systematic theory subscribed to by the majority of counselors? No. Does each counselor subscribe to some theory? Probably yes. All counseling practice is theoretically based, but theories differ. Counseling is not the only human-service occupation afflicted with theoretical confusion: social work experiences the tugs between its historic commitment to psychoanalytic positions and more scientific stances; some clinical-psychology and psychiatric training programs are also in the process of replacing analytic roots with empirically supported theoretical commitments.

## 2. Society Views Members of the Occupation as Authorities

When a society subscribes uniformly to a theology, the religious leaders of that society are seen as persons of great authority—in some societies, even over life itself. Physicians in the United States are commonly viewed with the awe that attaches to authority, a response encouraged until recently by the way physicians dealt with patients. Up to recent times it was common for physicians to order patients to take certain medicines with no explanation of the content or effect. Many people do not seek medical help from physicians, but a number of those who do so appear to take the stance of "I'll put myself in your hands and do as you tell me." Medically, most patients appear to be cognitive dualists.

Are counselors viewed similarly? The proportion of the population needing medical help that seeks it from physicians is probably larger than the proportion of people needing assistance with developmental matters that seeks it from counselors. With only anecdotal data available to examine this question, it is tenable to say that an increasing proportion of citizens views counselors as authorities in their field. Whereas physicians are taught to encourage their role as authorities for their patients' own good, and for that reason maintain a social separation between themselves and patients, the nature of counseling requires counselors to be personally close to clients. However, this does not appear to diminish their authority among those who seek assistance.

### 3. The Society Grants Powers to the Occupation

To provide a basis for comparison, we can look at the ways society grants powers to physicians. The stance of our society is that certain drugs may not be legally given or used unless a physician so directs. Physicians are accorded the sole right to declare someone dead, and if they are psychiatrists, they have the authority to commit patients without their consent. Physicians are given the legal right to keep patients' medical records confidential. Lawyers are given similar control over clients' records. Counselors do not have this right. The authority and powers ascribed by society to professions is shown most clearly in the legal right of the profession to control who is permitted to practice in it. States acknowledge that right by licensing physicians and lawyers only after they have met the training criteria set by the professions. Counselors have recently begun to come into this status. A decade ago only a few states provided some form of legal acknowledgment of counselors: certification, registration, or licensing. Now more than 30 states do, an outcome of efforts of the American Counseling Association (ACA) and its state branches. On this criterion there is an advance toward professionalism, but at this time, in general, counselors have weak legal status and no community powers. By this criterion we are not yet a profession.

### 4. The Profession Has Created a Code of Ethics

In exchange for the privileges society accords a profession, setting it off from the rest of society as a self-governing body, it expects that the profession will police its members. Some psychological counselors are counseling psychologists and are members of the American Psychological Association (APA). This professional body has an ethical code and a structure to police its members. At intervals the APA issues a list of disbarred members and identifies the ethical standard that was violated. Most psychological counselors are not qualified for membership in the APA, but a substantial portion are members of the ACA, which also has a code of ethics but lacks adequate enforcement machinery.

In 1982 the National Board for Certified Counselors (NBCC), an agency to be reported on in detail shortly, established a code of ethics for counselors it certifies. Counselors who are members of the ACA and are certified by the NBCC seemingly have two codes of ethics by which their professional conduct is to be guided. This should create no problem, because the essential points of each code are similar. The ACA code of ethics and germane portions of the APA code are found in Appendixes A and B.

## 5. There Is an Occupational Culture

Again we can be informed by two professions with long histories, law and medicine. Both occupations clearly have a robust culture. The building of an occupational culture starts with the selectiveness of its practitioners and then must have a sufficient span of time to become established and gain a reputation in the general society. With time there will emerge notable saints and sinners and even figures of national importance. Most of all, there will be a sense of "we-ness" among its practitioners, separating "us" from "them" and thereby providing a sense of identity. Entry is formal and in most cases is for life. The way each profession is practiced is similar for most practitioners: office and hospital for physicians, office and courtroom for lawyers. Society accords them status as a subsociety.

Counselors are found in a diverse array of settings, attending to an equally diverse clientele. Thirty years ago, relative to counseling in schools, I could write:

> There is no guarded door leading into the inner sanctum of [school] counsel-
> ing. It is a wide-open door, with no initiation rites, and with only the threshold
> of state certification to step over. There are ways to enter without even crossing
> that threshold. Because it is not a culture difficult to enter or leave, there is
> constant coming and going. The culture is so sparse that it exerts little gravity
> pull on those who do become school counselors [Byrne, 1977, p. 281].

The counseling culture in schools has improved steadily since then, but there is still no substantial culture encompassing counselors in general. There are distinctive cultures of the specialized divisions to which ACA members belong, such as rehabilitation, mental health, college, and employment agencies, but an ACA culture is only slowly building, reflected in the association's need to change its name two times. Through national, regional, and state conventions, increasing membership requirements, increasing training substance, and common publications, however, a counseling culture has been thickening to a point where it is defensible now to say that it does meet this one of the sociologists' criteria. Counselors now have an occupational identity given to them partly by their professional culture.

## 6. A Profession's Practitioners Have Occupational Autonomy

The autonomy of professionals is usually identified by their independence to make professional judgments that significantly affect people's lives. Counselors have much more independence now than they did 30 years ago. At that time most counselors were employed in educational institutions, with those in public secondary schools generally having no more autonomy than any teacher, although the autonomy of counselors in institutions of higher education has always been high. The evidence points to the ever-increasing right of counselors in secondary schools to engage in practices they deem professionally appropriate, with school principals consulting them more often for their developmental expertise. These changes have probably been accelerated by the notable improvement in counselors' preparation. Marriage, rehabilitation, and mental-health counselors, among others, are professionally autonomous, exercising independence of judgment.

Another measure of autonomy is the prevalence of independent practice. Thirty years ago, counselors practicing independently were a rarity; today it is an option selected by a noticeable minority.

Psychological counseling began as vocational counseling in public institutions, and the majority of counselors are still employed by them. This does not detract from their autonomy per se. Many physicians and lawyers are also employed in agencies. Autonomy is not to be judged on where a professional practitioner is employed but on the presence or absence of limits on practicing as one determines to be professionally required.

It is true that counseling may not be classified as a profession on some governmental list, and it may not fully meet sociological criteria. On the other hand, there is ample justification for trained, full-time counselors, with some association or state authentication, to call themselves members of a profession.

## Accreditation and Licensing: Steps in Professionalization

Major forces in professionalization are quality professional preparation and the identification of individuals who meet training and other requirements stipulated by the profession. At the doctoral level, practitioners are counseling psychologists if they are members of Division 17 (Counseling Psychology) of the APA. Preparation programs in counseling psychology were established decades ago, with the quality of the 60 currently accredited institutions ascertained by regular review by an APA board. Upon completion of training, graduates apply to the appropriate board of their state to be evaluated for licensing as a psychologist. As in the case of other professions, this permits them to offer services to the public under the title of psychologist. Without being certified by a state to do so, no one is permitted to advertise to the public as a psychologist.

Most counselors have not earned doctorates and therefore are not counseling psychologists. They too can be graduates of accredited programs and can earn certification by a national agency. (Such agencies typically certify professionals, while state boards license them.) These actions, taken in recent decades after years of little change, represent great steps toward professionalization. In the 1950s, for example, completion of six graduate courses was the common requirement in most of the states that certified school counselors (not all did). Additionally, each applicant for certification was required to have had a year's employment outside the field of education. The six required courses were typically offered by colleges of education, but not in departments organized for counselor preparation. Because preparation of school counselors was financially supported by the U.S. Office of Education (USOE) and focused on vocational guidance, the six courses had to be offered in order for a college to receive the USOE subsidy for faculty to teach those courses. Without that subsidy, many institutions would not have prepared counselors. The USOE grants also supported employment of state supervisors of counselors and, in some states, even of counselors in schools.

Today, counselors for schools can be prepared in departments whose programs for counselors in general and for a specialty in school counseling meet the requirements of a national accreditation agency. After completing training, the counselor can apply for certification by a national certifying board and, depending on the state, for certification, registration, or licensing by a state board of examiners. The movement toward professionalization from the six-course preparation programs and the absence of licensure of 40 years ago to present standards has been marked by gains and some setbacks, with the greatest gains made in the past 10 years.

## *Accreditation of Counselor Education Programs*

The history of the march toward a national accreditation program is offered elsewhere (Sweeney, 1992). From early efforts by states' counselor associations, and particularly through the efforts of the ACA (at that time called the American Association for Counseling and Development), there has evolved a national accreditation body, the Council for Accreditation of Counseling and Related Educational Programs (CACREP). Does CACREP have suitable status? Who accredits the accreditors? Accreditation of undergraduate educational institutions and programs has a long history. The agencies that accredit graduate programs established the Council on Postsecondary Accreditation (COPA) and set standards by which applicants for membership in COPA could be evaluated. COPA recently disbanded, but CACREP earned COPA recognition before it did so. Evaluation has now reverted to the separate agencies that at one time composed COPA.

The drive toward professionalism by state and national groups is evidence of and contributes further to the occupational culture, the fifth of Greenwood's criteria of professional status. As of mid-1992, the counselor-education programs of 62 institutions had earned CACREP accreditation.

To qualify for CACREP accreditation there must be a training of a minimum of 48 semester-hours of stipulated graduate courses or 60 hours for program specialties in mental health and in marriage and family counseling/therapy. Students must complete 100 hours of supervised practicum in their counselor-education institution and 600 hours of a supervised internship or externship.

These accreditation requirements illustrate a chicken-or-egg dilemma common to movement toward professionalism by any occupation. For example, if a current licensing or certification requirement calls for completion of 30 prescribed semester-hours of preparation but experienced practitioner/scholars deem that to be an insufficient amount, how can the substance of programs be increased? For one thing, state professional associations can push state licensing or certification boards to raise their training requirements.

Then, too, national professional associations may set higher standards for accreditation of training programs, and that action can stimulate universities to extend the length of their training. For a period, however, the training programs of accredited institutions may exceed state certification or licensing requirements, an anomaly that creates problems for students who are eager to complete training and be employed. They are ready, naturally, to accept existing requirements and resist having to now complete much higher ones—which they deem to be inflated only so a university's program can be accredited—because their employment will be delayed. Some institutions that have struggled over the years to offer a 30-semester-hour program now may need to find scarce resources to increase to a 48-hour program if they wish to attain CACREP accreditation. Without it they must expect to lose prospective students to programs that are CACREP accredited.

State boards and institutions are not the only forces affecting this issue. National professional associations set standards for membership that bear on employment. For example, an agency may stipulate that applicants for an opening must meet the requirements for certification of the National Academy of Certified Clinical Mental Health Counselors. If a professional association's certification carries employment clout, that group may be impelled to require 60 hours of preparation, a move that would in turn require training institutions to judge whether they should follow that lead. With such push and pull, the training aspect of occupations makes its slow way toward increased professionality.

Training programs in larger institutions prepare for a number of specialized counseling settings or clientele. Some departments qualify to offer federally supported programs in rehabilitation counseling. The first national independent accreditation of a counselor-preparation program was carried out by the Council on Rehabilitation Education (CORE), which was established in 1971 and recognized by COPA. CORE became a model for the development of CACREP.

## *Documenting Counselors' Professional Status*

Documenting the status of counselors must be the next step toward professionalization. It will require acknowledgment by state legislatures that a national professional association supervises the training of counselors and will undertake responsibility for their licensing by guaranteeing that they will demonstrate competence. At present each state that has enacted some form of credentialing legislation (about 70% of all states) stipulates how counselors are to be "papered" (credential, registration, license), what training and experience are required, whether titles are mandated or restricted, and to what kind of service the credentialing applies. In 1986 coordination of the activities of boards in the states which have them fell to American Association of State Counseling Boards. If the inconsistency among states appears to be chaotic, keep in mind that any form of state legal acknowledgment of counselors is comparatively recent. The oldest form has been the certification accorded to counselors in schools by state education boards.

A step toward national certification followed the setting up of the board (CORE) in 1971 to accredit rehabilitation counseling programs. Almost 80 have earned this recognition. In 1972 the Commission on Rehabilitation Counselor Certification (CRCC) was established to certify rehabilitation counselors, permitting those certified to place "CRC" after their names ("C-CRC" in Canada), a qualification earned by more than 12,000 people. This step was followed in 1979 by the establishment of a certificate for the clinical mental-health counselor by the National Academy of Certified Mental Health Counselors. That certificate, also available in Canada, has been earned by around 2000 people.

A major step toward a national certification program for all counselors was taken in 1982 with the establishment of the NBCC. The board originated in actions by the ACA but now functions as an independent body. The generic certification by the board is made upon successful completion of a written examination of knowledge of counseling information and skills. Specialists in career counseling, gerontology, and school counseling may take additional examinations through the NBCC.

The examination is in eight areas: (1) human growth and development, (2) social and cultural foundations, (3) the helping relationship, including counseling theories, (4) group dynamics, processes, and counseling, (5) lifestyle and career development, (6) appraisal of individuals, (7) research and evaluation, and (8) professional orientation.*

## Professional Associations

The persistent advance toward professionalization on different fronts, with the consequently increased status of counselors, is a result of counselors' united efforts to bring about such change. The establishment of government agencies to support counseling and the obtaining of governmental financial support for agencies and their programs have similarly come about because of professional associations' legislative efforts. This is as it should be. Those efforts characterize a profession, and a characteristic of professionals is their support of, if not participation in, those actions. Such support can be given only by membership in the appropriate professional body, at whatever level it exists—local, state, and national.

Frequent note has been made of two national associations through which efforts are carried out on behalf of psychological counseling. For counselors with a doctorate, participation in the continuing professionalization of counseling is through the APA, specifically in the Division of Counseling Psychology. Chapter 1 provided ample testimony about the great contribution to the professionalization of counseling that has been made by that division over four decades. The ACA has also been cited numerous times as a source of the professional growth of psychological counseling (but without use of the modifier "psychological"). The three names under which this association has functioned represent the professional growth that has occurred as a consequence of the efforts of its members. For years it was called the American Personnel and Guidance Association, a name that reflected the effort to blend separately existing groups whose occupational interests overlapped to varying degrees. Later the name was changed to the American Association for Counseling and Development, a title that appropriately recognized the developmental focus of its members. Professional change is reflected also by the words dropped in that change. One was the vague "Personnel," a label that originally included a variety of helping associations, but ones related to counseling

---

*Some of the material above is adapted from Glosoff (1992).

only because they were also helping occupations. The deletion of "Guidance" did not signal a diminution of interest in the developmental activities of counselors in schools but simply discontinuance in the association's title of a specialized counseling activity. In 1992 the present name was adopted, one that identifies its members as professional psychological counselors in a wide array of settings and topics, as shown by the 16 division titles:*

> Association for Assessment in Counseling
> Association for Adult Development and Aging
> American College Counseling Association
> Association for Counselor Education and Supervision
> Association for Humanistic Education and Development
> Association for Multicultural Counseling and Development
> American Mental Health Counselors Association
> American Rehabilitation Counseling Association
> Association for Spiritual, Ethical, Religious, and Values Issues in Counseling
> American School Counselor Association
> Association for Specialists in Group Work
> International Association of Addictions and Offender Counselors
> International Association of Marriage and Family Counselors
> Military Educators and Counselors Association
> National Career Development Association
> National Employment Counseling Association

### Codes of Ethics

Society's expectancy is that in return for acknowledging an occupation's existence as a separate subsociety called a profession, the occupation's practitioners will be joined into an association that will monitor the occupational behavior of its members. The association does this by adopting rules by which professional behaviors of its members can be guided and measured. These rules are called codes of ethics. Both the APA and the ACA have created ethical codes as has the NBCC. Fortunately for an NBCC counselor who is a member of the APA and the ACA, these codes do not conflict. A sizable proportion of psychological counselors who are counseling psychologists and therefore APA members are also ACA members. They will be familiar with the codes of each association.

Entrants to a profession likely (and fortunately) hold to high ideals and the expectancy of adherence to the standards of the profession by members of its association. Nevertheless, because all professional practitioners are of a lesser order than angels, each profession accumulates its roster of sinners. Transgressions

---

*Although it is correct to identify the ACA as an association for professional counselors, through some divisions people may join it who are not prepared as counselors. They are supportive of the association's objectives and offer that support through their membership. By some standards, this policy classifies the ACA as an interest association, rather than a professional one. The eligibility requirements of a professional association stipulate that applicants shall have completed professional preparation. It seems appropriate, however, to identify the ACA as both a professional and interest association because it is the association "home" of the majority of professional counselors in the United States.

against ethical codes are held by society to be more egregious in some professions than others. It is apparently more newsworthy when a member of the clergy or a psychiatrist is charged with stealing or sexual abuse than when a counselor is guilty of similar acts. The ministry and psychiatry are long-established professions around which the public has cast an aura of incorruptability.

A recent APA survey of psychologists reports their ethical dilemmas (Pope & Vetter, 1992). The authors note that the greatest number of ethical conflicts involves confidentiality (18%), with equally troubling dilemmas found in blurred, dual, or conflicting relationships. Because of the intensity of the unique relationship that can develop between a distraught client and an empathic person helping to remove distress, it is not unnatural for that relationship to acquire sexual overtones. Although the ethical burden is on the counselor to keep the relationship professional, it is in this difficult-to-control emotional area that occasional ethical violations are reported.

In each profession there are occasional egregious violations of the code of ethics. Many psychologists were dismayed some years back when it was found after the death of an internationally renowned psychologist that he had deliberately falsified data in his research on racial differences. For every one of these violators there are thousands of ethically dedicated professionals outside the scan of the public press.

Leaders of professional associations and groups within them at times nudge the membership toward ethical stances that have not welled up from all the members. In recent years the attention of society has been placed on subpopulations that may not have received social benefits accorded to the majority. This awareness has been carried into professional associations to find reflection not just in ethical codes but in both literature and convention activities that increase their members' awareness of the significance for both clients and counselors of minority status.

Both the ACA and the APA publish ethical-standards workbooks through which individuals and groups during training can be helped to translate specific standards in the codes into counseling experiences.

## *Liability*

Ethical violations are concerns of the professional society. Those violations become the concern of the general society when harm is done to a client, such as by sexual abuse. At times, however, despite a counselor's best efforts, a client may claim that harm was done and hence sue the counselor, a contingency against which counselors protect themselves by malpractice insurance.

At times an unexpected suit may be brought against a counselor, as has occasionally happened when parents of a child who has committed suicide charged the counselor with culpability for not having reported the possibility of suicide to the parents. New counselors can become informed about this issue by reference to a report covering a number of cases (Pate, 1992).

Counselors need to be aware of the legal rights and prohibitions provided them by state laws. Confidentiality laws differ, but generally the knowledge that counselors have about clients may be subject to subpoena, unlike the status of records in medicine and law. At the same time, counselors will be made aware by their ethical codes that they are required to disclose some information they learn from clients, such as suicide threats or admission of felonies. Ethical casebooks clarify these matters.

## Concluding Reflections

The present stage of professionalization of counseling has been reached by the efforts of committed, thoughtful, practitioner/scholars joined together in professional associations. Continuance toward improvement of quality calls for maintaining those efforts. The right of any counselor to claim to be a professional imposes an obligation to join with fellow professionals to bring about continuous improvements in the quality of service offered our clients, and that goal requires maintenance of the health of professional associations that only we as individuals can provide.

## ■        Counselor Formation Activities        ■

1. Ask one or more counselors for a few comments about their professional history:
    a. What factors led to their first employment as a counselor?
    b. To what national, state, and local professional associations do they belong? Why not to others?
    c. What certifications or licenses do they hold or are they working toward? What role does such licensure or certification play in their professional life?
2. Ask those counselors to describe ethical dilemmas with which they were faced and how they resolved those issues. Inquire whether they consulted ethical codes and casebooks to help them in that resolution.
3. Ethical concerns are one matter, legal ones another. Have these counselors ever been faced with or been threatened with legal action? Have they maintained insurance to cover legal actions?
4. In your small group, each student presents a dilemma taken from an ethical standards casebook. The group seeks to reach a satisfying adjudication before consulting the judgment offered in the casebook.

## ■        Complementary Reading        ■

The American Counseling Association in Alexandria, Virginia, offers a number of publications on legal concerns. Of particular note is the *ACA Legal Series* of seven publications, each of 75 pages. The series is edited by T. P. Remley, Jr. Two titles illustrate the topics addressed by the series:

GIBBS, L. A., & SWANSON, C. D. (1993). *Confidentiality and Privileged Communication.*

WEIKEL, W. J., & HUGHES, P.R. (1993). *The Counselor as Expert Witness.*

A general treatment of legal matters is provided in these two publications:

MCCARTHY, M. M., & SORENSON, G. P. (1993). "School Counselors and Consultants: Legal Duties and Liabilities." *Journal of Counseling and Development,* 72(2), 159–167.

HOPKINS, B. R., & ANDERSON, B. (1990). *The Counselor and the Law*, 3rd ed. Alexandria, VA: American Counseling Association.

The nature of an association's ethical standards is that they are phrased in general terms. On the other hand, events that may arouse ethical challenges may not be open to clear evaluation by broad ethical standards. ACA has prepared a casebook to help solve ethical dilemmas of this sort:

HERLIHEY, B., & GOLDEN, L. B. (1988). *Ethical Standards Casebook*, 4th ed. Alexandria, VA: American Counseling Association.

An evaluation of the advantages of a National Board for Certified Counselors presents some thought-arousing arguments. They can be examined in:

WEINRICH, S. G., & THOMAS, K. R. (1993). "The National Board for Certified Counselors: The Good, the Bad, and the Ugly." *Journal of Counseling and Development,* 72(1).

Some counseling students are planning to complete a doctor's degree and seek licensure as a counseling psychologist. Issues of entry into occupations employing counseling psychologists are examined in:

"New and Early Professionals." (1992, January). *The Counseling Psychologist, 20.*

# Ethical Standards of the American Counseling Association

## Preamble

*The Association is an educational, scientific, and professional organization whose members are dedicated to the enhancement of the worth, dignity, potential, and uniqueness of each individual and thus to the service of society.*

*The Association recognizes that the role definitions and work settings of its members include a wide variety of academic disciplines, levels of academic preparation, and agency services. This diversity reflects the breadth of the Association's interest and influence. It also poses challenging complexities in efforts to set standards for the performance of members, desired requisite preparation or practice, and supporting social, legal, and ethical controls.*

*The specification of ethical standards enables the Association to clarify to present and future members and to those served by members the nature of ethical responsibilities held in common by its members.*

*The existence of such standards serves to stimulate greater concern by members for their own professional functioning and for the conduct of fellow professionals such as counselors, guidance and student personnel workers, and others in the helping professions. As the ethical code of the Association, this document establishes principles that define the ethical behavior of Association members. Additional ethical guidelines developed by the Association's Divisions for their specialty areas may further define a member's ethical behavior.*

## Section A
### General

1. The member influences the development of the profession by continuous efforts to improve professional practices, teaching, services, and research. Professional growth is continuous throughout the member's career and is exemplified by the development of a philosophy that explains why and how a member functions in the helping relationship. Members must gather data on their effectiveness

and be guided by the findings. Members recognize the need for continuing education to ensure competent service.

2. The member has a responsibility both to the individual who is served and to the institution within which the service is performed to maintain high standards of professional conduct. The member strives to maintain the highest levels of professional services offered to the individuals to be served. The member also strives to assist the agency, organization, or institution in providing the highest caliber of professional services. The acceptance of employment in an institution implies that the member is in agreement with the general policies and principles of the institution. Therefore the professional activities of the member are also in accord with the objectives of the institution. If, despite concerted efforts, the member cannot reach agreement with the employer as to acceptable standards of conduct that allow for changes in institutional policy conducive to the positive growth and development of clients, then terminating the affiliation should be seriously considered.

3. Ethical behavior among professional associates, both members and nonmembers, must be expected at all times. When information is possessed that raises doubt as to the ethical behavior of professional colleagues, whether Association members or not, the member must take action to attempt to rectify such a condition. Such action shall use the institution's channels first and then use procedures established by the Association.

4. The member neither claims nor implies professional qualifications exceeding those possessed and is responsible for correcting any misrepresentations of these qualifications by others.

5. In established fees for professional counseling services, members must consider the financial status of clients and locality. In the event that the established fee structure is inappropriate for a client, assistance must be provided in finding comparable services of acceptable cost.

6. When members provide information to the public or to subordinates, peers, or supervisors, they have a responsibility to ensure that the content is general, unidentified client information that is accurate, unbiased, and consists of objective, factual data.

7. Members recognize their boundaries of competence and provide only those services and use only those techniques for which they are qualified by training or experience. Members should only accept those positions for which they are professionally qualified.

8. In the counseling relationship, the counselor is aware of the intimacy of the relationship and maintains respect for the client and avoids engaging in activities that seek to meet the counselor's personal needs at the expense of that client.

9. Members do not condone or engage in sexual harassment which is defined as deliberate or repeated comments, gestures, or physical contacts of a sexual nature.

10. The member avoids bringing personal issues into the counseling relationship, especially if the potential for harm is present. Through awareness of the negative impact of both racial and sexual stereotyping and discrimination, the counselor guards the individual rights and personal dignity of the client in the counseling relationship.

11. Products or services provided by the member by means of classroom instruction, public lectures, demonstrations, written articles, radio or television programs, or other types of media must meet the criteria cited in these standards.

## Section B
## *Counseling Relationships*

This section refers to practice and procedures of individual and/or group counseling relationships.

The member must recognize the need for client freedom of choice. Under those circumstances where this is not possible, the member must apprise clients of restrictions that may limit their freedom of choice.

1. The member's primary obligation is to respect the integrity and promote the welfare of the client(s), whether the client(s) is (are) assisted individually or in a group relationship. In a group setting, the member is also responsible for taking reasonable precautions to protect individuals from physical and/or psychological trauma resulting from interaction within the group.

2. Members make provisions for maintaining confidentiality in the storage and disposal of records and follow an established record retention and disposition policy. The counseling relationship and information resulting therefrom must be kept confidential, consistent with the obligations of the member as a professional person. In a group counseling setting, the counselor must set a norm of confidentiality regarding all group participants' disclosures.

3. If an individual is already in a counseling relationship with another professional person, the member does not enter into a counseling relationship without first contacting and receiving the approval of that other professional. If the member discovers that the client is in another counseling relationship after the counseling relationship begins, the member must gain the consent of the other professional or terminate the relationship, unless the client elects to terminate the other relationship.

4. When the client's condition indicates that there is clear and imminent danger to the client or others, the member must take reasonable personal action or inform responsible authorities. Consultation with other professionals must be used where possible. The assumption of responsibility for the client's(s') behavior must be taken only after careful deliberation. The client must be involved in the resumption of responsibility as quickly as possible.

5. Records of the counseling relationship, including interview notes, test data, correspondence, tape recordings, electronic data storage, and other documents are to be considered professional information for use in counseling, and they should not be considered a part of the records of the institution or agency in which the counselor is employed unless specified by state statute or regulation. Revelation to others of counseling material must occur only upon the expressed consent of the client.

6. In view of the extensive data storage and processing capacities of the computer, the member must ensure that data maintained on a computer is: (a) limited to information that is appropriate and necessary for the services being provided; (b) destroyed after it is determined that the information is no longer of any value in providing services; and (c) restricted in terms of access to appropriate

staff members involved in the provision of services by using the best computer security methods available.

7. Use of data derived from a counseling relationship for purposes of counselor training or research shall be confined to content that can be disguised to ensure full protection of the identity of the subject client.

8. The member must inform the client of the purposes, goals, techniques, rules of procedure, and limitations that may affect the relationship at or before the time that the counseling relationship is entered. When working with minors or persons who are unable to give consent, the member protects these clients' best interests.

9. In view of common misconceptions related to the perceived inherent validity of computer-generated data and narrative reports, the member must ensure that the client is provided with information as part of the counseling relationship that adequately explains the limitations of computer technology.

10. The member must screen prospective group participants, especially when the emphasis is on self-understanding and growth through self-disclosure. The member must maintain an awareness of the group participants' compatibility throughout the life of the group.

11. The member may choose to consult with any other professionally competent person about a client. In choosing a consultant, the member must avoid placing the consultant in a conflict of interest situation that would preclude the consultant's being a proper party to the member's efforts to help the client.

12. If the member determines an inability to be of professional assistance to the client, the member must either avoid initiating the counseling relationship or immediately terminate that relationship. In either event, the member must suggest appropriate alternatives. (The member must be knowledgeable about referral resources so that a satisfactory referral can be initiated.) In the event the client declines the suggested referral, the member is not obligated to continue the relationship.

13. When the member has other relationships, particularly of an administrative, supervisory, and/or evaluative nature with an individual seeking counseling services, the member must not serve as the counselor but should refer the individual to another professional. Only in instances where such an alternative is unavailable and where the individual's situation warrants counseling intervention should the member enter into and/or maintain a counseling relationship. Dual relationships with clients that might impair the member's objectivity and professional judgement (e.g., as with close friends or relatives), must be avoided and/or the counseling relationship terminated through referral to another competent professional.

14. The member will avoid any type of sexual intimacies with clients. Sexual relationships with clients are unethical.

15. All experimental methods of treatment must be clearly indicated to prospective recipients, and safety precautions are to be adhered to by the member.

16. When computer applications are used as a component of counseling services, the member must ensure that: (a) the client is intellectually, emotionally, and physically capable of using the computer application; (b) the computer application is appropriate for the needs of the client; (c) the client understands the purpose and operation of the computer application; and (d) a followup of client

use of a computer application is provided to both correct possible problems (misconceptions or inappropriate use) and assess subsequent needs.

17. When the member is engaged in short-term group treatment/training programs (e.g., marathons and other encountertype or growth groups), the member ensures that there is professional assistance available during and following the group experience.

18. Should the member be engaged in a work setting that calls for any variation from the above statements, the member is obligated to consult with other professionals whenever possible to consider justifiable alternatives.

19. The member must ensure that members of various ethnic, racial, religious, disability, and socioeconomic groups have equal access to computer applications used to support counseling services and that the content of available computer applications does not discriminate against the groups described above.

20. When computer applications are developed by the member for use by the general public as self-help/stand-alone computer software the member must ensure that: (a) self-help computer applications are designed from the beginning to function in a stand-alone manner, as opposed to modifying software that was originally designed to require support from a counselor; (b) self-help computer applications will include within the program statements regarding intended user outcomes, suggestions for using the software, a description of the conditions under which self-help computer applications might not be appropriate, and a description of when and how counseling services might be beneficial; and (c) the manual for such applications will include the qualifications of the developer, the development process, validation data, and operating procedures.

## Section C
### Measurement and Evaluation

The primary purpose of educational and psychological testing is to provide descriptive measures that are objective and interpretable in either comparative or absolute terms. The member must recognize the need to interpret the statements that follow as applying to the whole range of appraisal techniques including test and nontest data. Test results constitute only one of a variety of pertinent sources of information for personnel, guidance, and counseling decisions.

1. The member must provide specific orientation or information to the examinee(s) prior to and following the test administration so that the results of testing may be placed in proper perspective with other relevant factors. In so doing, the member must recognize the effects of socioeconomic, ethnic, and cultural factors on test scores. It is the member's professional responsibility to use additional unvalidated information carefully in modifying interpretation of the test results.

2. In selecting tests for use in a given situation or with a particular client, the member must consider carefully the specific validity, reliability, and appropriateness of the test(s). General validity, reliability, and related issues may be questioned legally as well as ethically when tests are used for vocational and educational selection, placement, or counseling.

3. When making any statements to the public about tests and testing, the member must give accurate information and avoid false claims or misconceptions.

Special efforts are often required to avoid unwarranted connotations of such terms as IQ and grade equivalent scores.

4. Different tests demand different levels of competence for administration scoring and interpretation. Members must recognize the limits of their competence and perform only those functions for which they are prepared. In particular, members using computer-based test interpretations must be trained in the construct being measured and the specific instrument being used prior to using this type of computer application.

5. In situations where a computer is used for test administration and scoring, the member is responsible for ensuring that administration and scoring programs function properly to provide clients with accurate test results.

6. Tests must be administered under the same conditions that were established in their standardization. When tests are not administered under standard conditions or when unusual behavior or irregularities occur during the testing session, those conditions must be noted and the results designated as invalid or of questionable validity. Unsupervised or inadequately supervised test-taking, such as the use of tests through the mails, is considered unethical. On the other hand, the use of instruments that are so designed or standardized to be self-administered and self-scored, such as interest inventories, is to be encouraged.

7. The meaningfulness of test results used in personnel, guidance, and counseling functions generally depends on the examinee's unfamiliarity with the specific items on the test. Any prior coaching or dissemination of the test materials can invalidate test results. Therefore, test security is one of the professional obligations of the member. Conditions that produce most favorable test results must be made known to the examinee.

8. The purpose of testing and the explicit use of the results must be made known to the examinee prior to testing. The counselor must ensure that instrument limitations are not exceeded and that periodic review and/or retesting are made to prevent client stereotyping.

9. The examinee's welfare and explicit prior understanding must be the criteria for determining the recipients of the test results. The member must see that specific interpretation accompanies any release of individual or group test data. The interpretation of test data must be related to the examinee's particular concerns.

10. Members responsible for making decisions based on test results have an understanding of educational and psychological measurement, validation criteria, and test research.

11. The member must be cautious when interpreting the results of research instruments possessing insufficient technical data. The specific purposes for the use of such instruments must be stated explicitly to examinees.

12. The member must proceed with caution when attempting to evaluate and interpret the performance of minority group members or other persons who are not represented in the norm group on which the instrument was standardized.

13. When computer-based test interpretations are developed by the member to support the assessment process, the member must ensure that the validity of such interpretations is established prior to the commerical distribution of such a computer application.

14. The member recognizes that test results may become obsolete. The member will avoid and prevent the misuse of obsolete test results.

15. The member must guard against the appropriation, reproduction, or modification of published tests or parts thereof without acknowledgment and permission from the previous publisher.

16. Regarding the preparation, publication, and distribution of tests, reference should be made to:

   a. "Standards for Educational and Psychological Testing," revised edition, 1985, published by the American Psychological Association on behalf of itself, the American Educational Research Association and the National Council of Measurement in Education.
   b. "The Responsible Use of Tests: A Position Paper of AMEG, APGA, and NCME," *Measurement and Evaluation in Guidance,* 1972, *5,* 385–388.
   c. "Responsibilities of Users of Standardized Tests," APGA, *Guidepost,* October 5, 1978, pp. 5–8.

## Section D
## Research and Publication

1. Guidelines on research with human subjects should be adhered to, such as:

   a. *Ethical Principles in the Conduct of Research with Human Participants* Washington, D.C.: American Psychological Association, Inc., 1982.
   b. Code of Federal Regulation, Title 45, Subtitle A, Pan 46, as currently issued.
   c. *Ethical Principles of Psychologists,* American Psychological Association, Principle #9: Research with Human Participants.
   d. Family Educational Rights and Privacy Act (the Buckley Amendment).
   e. Current federal regulations and various state rights privacy acts.

2. In planning any research activity dealing with human subjects, the member must be aware of and responsive to all pertinent ethical principles and ensure that the research problem, design, and execution are in full compliance with them.

3. Responsibility for ethical research practice lies with the principal researcher while others involved in the research activities share ethical obligation and full responsibility for their own actions.

4. In research with human subjects, researchers are responsible for the subjects' welfare throughout the experiment, and they must take all reasonable precautions to avoid causing injurious psychological, physical, or social effects on their subjects.

5. All research subjects must be informed of the purpose of the study except when withholding information or providing misinformation to them is essential to the investigation. In such research the member must be responsible for corrective action as soon as possible following completion of the research.

6. Participation in research must be voluntary. Involuntary participation is appropriate only when it can be demonstrated that participation will have no harmful effects on subjects and is essential to the investigation.

7. When reporting research results, explicit mention must be made of all variables and conditions known to the investigator that might affect the outcome of the investigation or the interpretation of the data.

8. The member must be responsible for conducting and reporting investigations in a manner that minimizes the possibility that results will be misleading.

9. The member has an obligation to make available sufficient original research data to qualified others who may wish to replicate the study.

10. When supplying data, aiding in the research of another person, reporting research results, or making original data available, due care must be taken to disguise the identity of the subjects in the absence of specific authorization from such subjects to do otherwise.

11. When conducting and reporting research, the member must be familiar with and give recognition to previous work on the topic, as well as to observe all copyright laws and follow the principles of giving full credit to all to whom credit is due.

12. The member must give due credit through joint authorship, acknowledgments, footnote statements, or other appropriate means to those who have contributed significantly to the research and/or publication, in accordance with such contributions.

13. The member must communicate to other members the results of any research judged to be of professional or scientific value. Results reflecting unfavorably on institutions, programs, services, or vested interests must not be withheld for such reasons.

14. If members agree to cooperate with another individual in research and/or publication, they incur an obligation to cooperate as promised in terms of punctuality of performance and with full regard to the completeness and accuracy of the information required.

15. Ethical practice requires that authors not submit the same manuscript or one essentially similar in content for simultaneous publication consideration by two or more journals. In addition, manuscripts published in whole or in substantial part in another journal or published work should not be submitted for publication without acknowledgment and permission from the previous publication.

## *Section E*
## *Consulting*

Consultation refers to a voluntary relationship between a professional helper and help-needing individual, group, or social unit in which the consultant is providing help to the client(s) in defining and solving a work-related problem or potential problem with a client or client system.

1. The member acting as consultant must have a high degree of self-awareness of his/her own values, knowledge, skills, limitations, and needs in entering a helping relationship that involves human and/or organizational change and that the focus of the relationship be on the issues to be resolved and not on the person(s) presenting the problem.

2. There must be understanding and agreement between member and client for the problem definition, change of goals, and prediction of consequences of interventions selected.

3. The member must be reasonably certain that she/he or the organization represented has the necessary competencies and resources for giving the kind of

help that is needed now or may be needed later and that appropriate referral resources are available to the consultant.

4. The consulting relationship must be one in which client adaptability and growth toward self-direction are encouraged and cultivated. The member must maintain this role consistently and not become a decision maker for the client or create a future dependency on the consultant.

5. When announcing consultant availability for services, the member conscientiously adheres to the Association's Ethical Standards.

6. The member must refuse a private fee or other remuneration for consultation with persons who are entitled to these services through the member's employing institution or agency. The policies of a particular agency may make explicit provisions for private practice with agency clients by members of its staff. In such instances, the clients must be apprised of other options open to them should they seek private counseling services.

## Section F
### Private Practice

1. The member should assist the profession by facilitating the availability of counseling services in private as well as public settings.

2. In advertising services as a private practitioner, the member must advertise the services in a manner that accurately informs the public of professional services, expertise, and techniques of counseling available. A member who assumes an executive leadership role in the organization shall not permit his/her name to be used in professional notices during periods when he/she is not actively engaged in the private practice of counseling.

3. The member may list the following: highest relevant degree, type and level of certification and/or license, address, telephone number, office hours, type and/or description of services and other relevant information. Such information must not contain false, inaccurate, misleading, partial, out-of-context, or deceptive material or statements.

4. Members do not present their affiliation with any organization in such a way that would imply inaccurate sponsorship or certification by that organization.

5. Members may join in partnership/corporation with other members and/or other professionals provided that each member of the partnership or corporation makes clear the separate specialities by name in compliance with the regulations of the locality.

6. A member has an obligation to withdraw from a counseling relationship if it is believed that employment will result in violation of the Ethical Standards. If the mental or physical condition of the member renders it difficult to carry out an effective professional relationship or if the member is discharged by the client because the counseling relationship is no longer productive for the client, then the member is obligated to terminate the counseling relationship.

7. A member must adhere to the regulations for private practice of the locality where the services are offered.

8. It is unethical to use one's institutional affiliation to recruit clients for one's private practice.

## Section G
## Personnel Administration

It is recognized that most members are employed in public or quasi-public institutions. The functioning of a member within an institution must contribute to the goals of the institution and vice versa if either is to accomplish their respective goals or objectives. It is therefore essential that the member and the institution function in ways to: (a) make the institutional goals specific and public; (b) make the member's contribution to institutional goals specific; and (c) foster mutual accountability for goal achievement.

To accomplish these objectives, it is recognized that the member and the employer must share responsibilities in the formulation and implementation of personnel policies.

1. Members must define and describe the parameters and levels of their professional competency.

2. Members must establish interpersonal relations and working agreements with supervisors and subordinates regarding counseling or clinical relationships, confidentiality, distinction between public and private material, maintenance and dissemination of recorded information, work load, and accountability. Working agreements in each instance must be specified and made known to those concerned.

3. Members must alert their employers to conditions that may be potentially disruptive or damaging.

4. Members must inform employers of conditions that may limit their effectiveness.

5. Members must submit regularly to professional review and evaluation.

6. Members must be responsible for inservice development of self and/or staff.

7. Members must inform their staff of goals and programs.

8. Members must provide personnel practices that guarantee and enhance the rights and welfare of each recipient of their service.

9. Members must select competent persons and assign responsibilities compatible with their skills and experiences.

10. The member, at the onset of a counseling relationship, will inform the client of the member's intended use of supervisors regarding the disclosure of information concerning this case. The member will clearly inform the client of the limits of confidentiality in the relationship.

11. Members, as either employers or employees, do not engage in or condone practices that are inhumane, illegal, or unjustifiable (such as considerations based on sex, handicap, age, race) in hiring, promotion, or training.

## Section H
## Preparation Standards

Members who are responsible for training others must be guided by the preparation standards of the Association and relevant Division(s). The member who functions in the capacity of trainer assumes unique ethical responsibilities that frequently go beyond that of the member who does not function in a training capacity. These ethical responsibilities are outlined as follows:

1. Members must orient students to program expectations, basic skills development, and employment prospects prior to admission to the program.

2. Members in charge of learning experiences must establish programs that integrate academic study and supervised practice.

3. Members must establish a program directed toward developing students' skills, knowledge, and self-understanding stated whenever possible in competency or performance terms.

4. Members must identify the levels of competencies of their students in compliance with relevant Division standards. These competencies must accommodate the paraprofessional as well as the professional.

5. Members, through continual student evaluation and appraisal, must be aware of the personal limitations of the learner that might impede future performance. The instructor must not only assist the learner in securing remedial assistance but also screen from the program those individuals who are unable to provide competent services.

6. Members must provide a program that includes training in research commensurate with levels of role functioning. Paraprofessional and technician-level personnel must be trained as consumers of research. In addition, personnel must learn how to evaluate their own and their program's effectiveness. Graduate training, especially at the doctoral level, would include preparation for original research by the member.

7. Members must make students aware of the ethical responsibilities and standards of the profession.

8. Preparatory programs must encourage students to value the ideals of service to individuals and to society. In this regard, direct financial remuneration or lack thereof must not be allowed to overshadow professional and humanitarian needs.

9. Members responsible for educational programs must be skilled as teachers and practitioners.

10. Members must present thoroughly varied theoretical positions so that students may make comparisons and have the opportunity to select a position.

11. Members must develop clear policies within their educational institutions regarding field placement and the roles of the student and the instructor in such placement.

12. Members must ensure that forms of learning focusing on self-understanding or growth are voluntary, or if required as part of the educational program, are made known to prospective students prior to entering the program. When the educational program offers a growth experience with an emphasis on self-disclosure or other relatively intimate or personal involvement, the member must have no administrative, supervisory, or evaluating authority regarding the participant.

13. The member will at all times provide students with clear and equally acceptable alternatives for self-understanding or growth experiences. The member will assure students that they have a right to accept these alternatives without prejudice or penalty.

14. Members must conduct an educational program in keeping with the current relevant guidelines of the Association.

# Policies and Procedures for Processing Complaints of Ethical Violations

## Section A
### General

1. The American Counseling Association, hereinafter referred to as the "Association" or "ACA," as an educational, scientific, and charitable organization, is dedicated to enhancing the worth, dignity, potential, and uniqueness of each individual and rendering service to society.

2. The Association, in furthering its objectives, administers Ethical Standards that have been developed and approved by the ACA Governing Council.

3. The purpose of this document is to facilitate the work of the ACA Ethics Committee by specifying the procedures for processing cases of alleged violations of the ACA Ethical Standards, codifying options for sanctioning members, and stating appeal procedures. The intent of the Association is to monitor the professional conduct of its members to ensure sound ethical practices.

## Section B
### Ethics Committee Members

1. The Ethics Committee is a standing committee of the Association. The Committee consists of six (6) appointed members, including the Chairperson. The editor of the *Ethical Standards Casebook* serves as an *ex officio* member of this Committee without vote. Two members are appointed annually for a three (3) year term by the President-Elect; appointments are subject to confirmation by the ACA Governing Council. Any vacancy occurring on the Committee will be filled by the President in the same manner, and the person appointed shall serve the unexpired term of the member whose place he or she took. Committee members may be reappointed to not more than one (1) additional consecutive term.

2. The Chairperson of the Committee is appointed annually by the incumbent President-Elect, subject to confirmation by the ACA Governing Council. A Chairperson may be reappointed to one additional term during any three (3) year period.

## Section C
### Role and Function

1. The role of the Ethics Committee of the Association is to assist in the arbitration and conciliation of conflicts among members of the Association, except where appropriate client concerns may be expressed. The Committee also is responsible for:

A. Educating the membership as to the Association's Ethical Standards,

B. Periodically reviewing and recommending changes in the Ethical Standards of the Association as well as the Policies and Procedures for Processing Complaints of Ethical Violations,

C. Receiving and processing complaints of alleged violations of the Ethical Standards of the Association, and

D. Receiving and processing questions.

2. In processing complaints about alleged ethical misconduct, the Committee will compile an objective, factual account of the dispute in question and make the best possible recommendation for the resolution of the case. The Committee, in taking any action, shall do so only for cause, shall only take the degree of disciplinary action that is reasonable, shall utilize these procedures with objectivity and fairness, and in general shall act only to further the interests and objectives of the Association and its membership.

3. The ACA Ethics Committee itself will not initiate any ethical violation charges against an ACA member.

4. Of the six (6) voting members of the Committee, a vote of four (4) is necessary to conduct business. In the event the Chair or any other member of the Committee has a personal interest in the case, he or she shall withdraw from reviewing the case. A unanimous vote of those members of the Committee who reviewed the case is necessary to expel a member from the Association.

5. The Chairperson of the ACA Ethics Committee and/or the ACA Executive Director (or his/her designee) may consult with ACA legal counsel at any time.

## Section D
## Responsibilities of Committee Members

1. The members of the Ethics Committee must be conscious that their position is extremely important and sensitive and that their decisions involve the rights of many individuals, the reputation of the counseling and human development community, and the careers of the members. The Committee members have an obligation to act in an unbiased manner, to work expeditiously, to safeguard the confidentiality of the Committee's activities, and to follow procedures that protect the rights of all individuals involved.

## Section E
## Responsibilities of the Chairperson

1. In addition to the above guidelines for members of the Committee, the Chairperson, in conjunction with Headquarters staff, has the responsibilities of:

A. Receiving (via ACA Headquarters) complaints that have been certified for membership status of the accused,

B. Notifying the complainant and the accused of receipt of the case,

C. Notifying the members of the Ethics Committee of the case,

D. Presiding over the meetings of the Committee,

E. Preparing and sending (by certified mail) communications to the complainant and accused member on the recommendations and decisions of the Committee, and

F. Arranging for legal advice with assistance and financial approval of the ACA Executive Director.

## Section F
## Complaints

1. All correspondence, records, and activities of the ACA Ethics Committee will remain confidential.
2. The ACA Ethics Committee will not act on anonymous complaints, nor will it act on complaints currently under civil or criminal litigation.
3. The ACA Ethics Committee will act only on those cases where the accused is a current member of ACA or was a member of ACA at the time of the alleged violation. State Division and State Branch Ethics Committees may act only on those cases where the accused is a member of the State Division or State Branch and not a member of ACA.

## Section G
## Submitting Complaints—Procedures for ACA Members

1. The procedures for submission of complaints to the Ethics Committee are as follows:
    A. If feasible, the complainant should discuss with utmost confidentiality the nature of the complaint with a colleague to see if he or she views the situation as an ethical violation.
    B. Whenever feasible, the complainant is to approach the accused directly to discuss and resolve the complaint.
    C. In cases where a resolution is not forthcoming at the personal level, the complainant shall prepare a formal written statement of the complaint and shall submit it to the ACA Ethics Committee. Action or consideration by the ACA Ethics Committee may not be initiated until this requirement is satisfied.
    D. Formal written complaints must include a statement indicating the behavior(s) that constituted the alleged violation(s), and the date(s) of the alleged violation(s). The written statement must also contain the accused member's full name and complete address. Any relevant supporting documentation may be included with the complaint.
    E. All complaints that are directed to the ACA Ethics Committee should be mailed to the Ethics Committee, c/o The Executive Director, American Counseling Association, 5999 Stevenson Avenue, Alexandria, Virginia 22304. The envelope must be marked "CONFIDENTIAL." This procedure is necessary to ensure the confidentiality of the person submitting the complaint and the person accused in the complaint.

## Section H
## Submitting Complaints—Procedures for Non-members

1. The ACA Ethics Committee recognizes the rights of non-ACA members to file grievances concerning a member. Ordinarily this non-member will be a client or student of an ACA member who believes that the ACA member has acted unethically.
2. In such cases, the complainant shall contact the ACA Executive Director (or his/her designee) and outline, in writing, those behaviors he or she feels were

unethical in nature. Headquarters staff will delineate the complaint process to the complainant.

## Section I
## Processing Complaints

1. When complaints are received at Headquarters, the ACA Executive Director (or his/her designee) shall: (a) check on the membership status of the accused, (b) acknowledge receipt of the complaint within ten (10) working days after it is received in ACA Headquarters, and (c) consult with the Chairperson of the ACA Ethics Committee within ten (10) working days after the complaint is received in ACA Headquarters to determine whether it is appropriate to proceed with the complaint. If the Director (or designee) and Chairperson determine it is in-appropriate to proceed, the complainant shall be so notified. If the Director (or designee) and Chairperson determine it is appropriate to proceed with the complaint, they will identify which Ethical Standard(s) are applicable to the alleged violation. A formal statement containing the Ethical Standard(s) that were allegedly violated will be forwarded to the complainant for his/her signa-ture. This signed formal statement will then become a part of the formal complaint.

2. Once the formal complaint has been compiled (as indicated above), the Chair-person of the ACA Ethics Committee shall do the following:
   A. Inform the complainant in writing that the accused member has been noti-fied of the charges,
   B. Direct a letter to the accused member informing the member of accusations lodged against him or her, including copies of all materials submitted by the complainant, asking for a response, and requesting that relevant information be submitted to the Chairperson within thirty (30) working days.

3. The accused is under no duty to respond to the allegations, but the Committee will not be obligated to delay or postpone its review of the case unless the accused so requests, with good cause, in advance. Failure of the accused to respond should not be viewed by the Committee as sufficient ground for taking disciplinary action.

4. Once the Chairperson has received the accused member's response or the thirty (30) days have elapsed, then the Chairperson shall forward to the members of the ACA Ethics Committee legal counsel's opinion (if applicable), staff verifica-tion of membership status, allegations, and responses, and direct the Committee to review the case and make recommendations for its disposition within two (2) weeks of receipt of the case.

5. The ACA Ethics Committee will review the case and make recommendations for its disposition and/or resolution within two hundred (200) working days follow-ing its receipt.

6. The ACA Ethics Committee Chairperson may ask the President of ACA to appoint an investigating committee at the local or state level to gather and submit relevant information concerning the case to the Committee.

## Section J
### Options Available to the Ethics Committee

1. After reviewing the information forwarded by the Chairperson, the Ethics Committee shall have the power to:

   A. Dismiss the charges, find that no violation has occurred, and dismiss the complaint, or
   B. Find that the practice(s) in which the member engages that is (are) the subject of the complaint, is (are) unethical, notify the accused of this determination, and request the member to voluntarily cease and desist in the practice(s) without impositions of further sanctions, or
   C. Find that the practice(s) in which the member engages, that is (are) the subject of the complaint, is (are) unethical, notify the accused of this determination, and impose sanctions.

## Section K
### Appropriate Sanctions

1. The Committee may consider extenuating circumstances before deciding on the penalty to be imposed. If the Committee finds the accused has violated the Ethical Standards and decides to impose sanctions, the Committee may take any of the following actions:

   A. Issue a reprimand with recommendations for corrective action, subject to review by the Committee, or
   B. Place the member on probation for a specified period of time, subject to review by the Committee, or
   C. Suspend eligibility for membership in ACA for a specified period of time, subject to review by the Committee, or
   D. Expel the member from ACA permanently.

## Section L
### Consequences of Sanctions

1. Both a reprimand and probation carry with it no loss of membership rights or privileges.

2. A suspended member forfeits the rights and privileges of membership only for the period of his or her suspension.

3. In the event a member is expelled from ACA membership, he or she shall lose all rights and privileges of membership in ACA and its divisions permanently. The expelled member shall not be entitled to a refund of dues already paid.

4. If the member is suspended or expelled, and after any right to appeal has been exhausted, the Committee will notify the appropriate state licensing board(s) of the disciplined member's status with ACA. Notice also will be given to the National Board for Certified Counselors, the ACA Divisions of which the disciplined party is a member, the State Branch of ACA in which the member resides, the members of ACA, the complainant, and other organizations as the Committee deems necessary. Such notice shall only state the sanctions imposed and the sections of the ACA Ethical Standards that were violated. Further elaboration shall not be disclosed.

5. Should a member resign from the Association after a complaint has been brought against him or her and before the Ethics Committee has completed its deliberations, that member is considered to have been expelled from the Association for failure to respond in a timely and complete manner to the Ethics Committee.

## Section M
## Hearings

1. At the discretion of the Ethics Committee, a hearing may be conducted when the results of the Ethics Committee's preliminary determination indicate that additional information is needed. The Chairperson shall schedule a formal hearing on the case and notify both the complainant and the accused of their right to attend.

2. The hearing will be held before a panel made up of the Ethics Committee and, if the accused member chooses, a representative of the accused member's primary Division. This representative will be identified by the Division President and will have voting privileges.

## Section N
## Recommended Hearing Procedures

1. Purposes of Hearings. The purposes for which hearings shall be conducted are: (a) to determine whether a breach of the Ethical Standards of ACA has occurred, and (b) if so, to determine what disciplinary action should be taken by the ACA. If a hearing is held, no disciplinary action will be taken by ACA until after the accused member has been given reasonable notice of the hearing and the specific charges raised against him or her and has had the opportunity to be heard and to present evidence in his or her behalf. The hearings will be formally conducted. The Committee will be guided in its deliberations by principles of basic fairness and professionalism, and will keep its deliberations as confidential as possible, except as provided herein.

2. Notice. At least forty-five (45) working days before the hearing, the accused member should be advised in writing of the time and place of the hearing and of the charges involved. Notice shall be given either personally or by certified or registered mail and shall be signed by the Committee Chair. The notice should be addressed to the accused member at his or her address as it appears in the membership records of the ACA. The notice should include a brief statement of the complaints lodged against him or her, and should be supported by the evidence. The accused is under no duty to respond to the notice, but the Committee will not be obligated to delay or postpone its hearing unless the accused so requests in writing, with good cause, in advance. Failure of the accused to appear at the hearing should not be viewed by the Committee as sufficient ground for taking disciplinary action.

3. Conduct of the Hearing.

    A. Accommodations. The Committee shall provide a private room to conduct the hearings, and no observers shall be permitted. The location of the hearing shall be determined at the discretion of the Committee, taking into consideration the convenience of the Committee and the parties involved.

B. Presiding Officer. The Chair of the Ethics Committee shall preside over the hearing and deliberations of the Committee. In the event the Chair or any other member of the Committee has a personal interest in the case, he or she shall withdraw from the hearing and deliberations and shall not participate therein. The Committee shall select from among its members a presiding officer for any case where the Chair has excused himself or herself. At the conclusion of the hearing and deliberation of the Committee, the Chair shall promptly notify the accused and complainant of the Committee's decision in writing.

C. Record. A record of the hearing shall be made and preserved, together with any documents presented as evidence, at the ACA Headquarters for a period of three (3) years following the hearing decision. The record may consist of a summary of testimony received, or a verbatim transcript, at the discretion of the Committee.

D. Right to Counsel. The parties shall be entitled to have counsel present to advise them throughout the hearing, but they may not participate beyond advising. Legal Counsel for ACA shall also be present at the hearing to advise the Committee and shall have the privilege of the floor.

E. Witnesses. Either party shall have the right to call witnesses to substantiate his or her version of the case. The Committee shall also have the right to call witnesses it believes may provide further insight into the matter before the Committee. Witnesses shall not be present during the hearings except when they are called upon to testify. The presiding officers shall allow questions to be asked of any witness by the opposition or members of the Committee and shall ensure that questions and testimony are relevant to the issues in the case. Should the hearing be disturbed by disparaging or irrelevant testimony or by the flareup of tempers, the presiding officer shall call a brief recess until order can be restored. Witnesses shall be excused upon completion of their testimony. All expenses associated with witnesses or counsel on behalf of the parties shall be borne by the respective parties.

F. Presentation of Evidence.

1. A member of the Committee shall be called upon first to present the charge(s) made against the accused and to briefly describe the evidence supporting the charge(s).

2. The complainant or a member of the Committee shall then be called upon to present the case against the accused. Witnesses who can substantiate the case shall be called upon to testify and answer questions of the accused and the Committee.

3. If the accused has exercised the right to be present at the hearing, he or she shall be called upon last to present any evidence which refutes the charges against him or her. This includes the presentation of witnesses as in Subsection (E) above. The accused member has the right to refuse to make a statement in his or her behalf. The accused will not be found guilty simply for refusing to testify. Once the accused chooses to testify, however, he or she may be cross-examined by members of the Committee or the complainant.

4. The Committee will endeavor to conclude the hearing within a period of approximately three (3) hours. The parties will be requested to be considerate of this time frame in planning their testimony. Testimony that is merely cumulative or repetitious may, at the discretion of the presiding officer, be excluded.

5. The accused has the right to be present at all times during the hearing and to challenge all of the evidence presented against him or her.

G. Relevancy of Evidence. The Hearing Committee is not a court of law and is not required to observe the rules of evidence that apply in the trial of lawsuits. Consequently, evidence that would be inadmissible in a court of law may be admissible in the hearing before the Committee, if it is relevant to the case. That is, if the evidence offered tends to explain, clarify, or refute any of the important facts of the case, it should generally be considered. The Committee will not receive evidence or testimony for the purpose of supporting any charge that was not set forth in the notice of the hearing or that is not relevant to the issues of the case.

4. Burden of Proof. The burden of proving a violation of the Ethical Standards is on the complainant and/or the Committee. It is not up to the accused to prove his or her innocence of any wrong-doing. Although the charge(s) need not be proved "beyond a reasonable doubt," the Committee will not find the accused guilty in the absence of substantial, objective, and believable evidence to sustain the charge(s).

5. Deliberation of the Committee. After the hearing with the parties is completed, the Committee shall meet in a closed session to review the evidence presented and reach a conclusion. The Committee shall be the sole trier of fact and shall weigh the evidence presented and judge the credibility of the witnesses. The act of a majority of the members of the Committee shall be the decision of the Committee and only those members of the Committee who were present throughout the entire hearing shall be eligible to vote.

6. Decision of the Committee. The Committee will first resolve the issue of the guilt or innocence of the accused. Applying the burden of proof in paragraph 4 above, the Committee will vote by secret ballot, unless the members of the Committee consent to an oral vote. In the event a majority of the members of the Committee do not find the accused guilty, the charges shall be dismissed and the parties notified. If the Committee finds the accused has violated the Ethical Standards, it must then determine what sanctions to impose in accord with Section K: Appropriate Sanctions.

## *Section O*
## *Appeal Procedures*

1. Appeals will be heard only in such cases wherein the appellant presents evidence that the sanction imposed by the Committee has been arbitrary or capricious or that the procedures outlined in the "Policy Document" have not been followed.

2. The complainant and accused shall be advised of the appeal procedure by the Chairperson of the ACA Ethics Committee. The following procedures shall govern appeals:

   A. A three (3) member review committee composed of the Executive Director of the ACA, the President of the ACA Division with which the accused member is most closely identified, and the immediate Past President of ACA. The ACA attorney shall serve as legal advisor and have the privilege of the floor.

   B. The appeal with supporting documentation must be made in writing within sixty (60) working days by certified mail to the ACA Executive Director and indicate the basis upon which it is made. If the member requires a time extension, he or she must request it in writing by certified mail within thirty (30) working days of receiving the decision by the ACA Ethics Committee. The extension will consist of ninety (90) working days beginning from that request.

   C. The review committee shall review all materials considered by the ACA Ethics Committee.

   D. Within thirty (30) working days of this review, the members on the review committee shall submit to the President of the ACA a written statement giving their opinion regarding the decision of the Ethics Committee. Each member shall concur with or dissent from the decision of the Ethics Committee.

   E. Within fifteen (15) working days of receiving this opinion, the President of ACA will reach a decision based on the considered opinions of the review committee from the following alternatives:

      (1) support the decision of the Ethics Committee, or
      (2) reverse the decision of the Ethics Committee.

3. The parties to the appeal shall be advised of the action in writing.

## Section P
## Records

1. Records of the ACA Ethics Committee and the review committee shall remain at the ACA Headquarters.

## Section Q
## Procedures for Submitting and Interpreting Questions of Ethical Conduct

1. The procedures for submitting questions to the Ethics Committee are as follows:

   A. Whenever possible, the questioner is first advised to consult other colleagues seeking interpretation of questions.

   B. If a national level resolution is deemed appropriate, the questioner shall prepare a written statement, which details the conduct in question. Statements should include the section or sections of the Ethical Standards to be interpreted relative to the conduct in question. All questions that are directed to the Ethics Committee should be mailed to: Ethics Committee, c/o ACA Executive Director.

C. The ACA Ethics Committee Chairperson or his/her designee:

   (1) may confer with legal counsel, and
   (2) shall direct a letter to the questioner acknowledging receipt of the question, informing the member that the questions will be interpreted by the Committee, and outlining the procedures to be involved in the interpretation.

D. The Ethics Committee will review and interpret the question and, if requested by the questioner, make recommendations for conduct.

# B

# Excerpts from Ethical Standards of the American Psychological Association That Apply to Psychological Counseling

## 2. Evaluation, Assessment, or Intervention

### 2.01 Evaluation, Diagnosis, and Interventions in Professional Context

a. Psychologists perform evaluations, diagnostic services, or interventions only within the context of a defined professional relationship. (See also Standard 1.03, Professional and Scientific Relationship.)

b. Psychologists' assessments, recommendations, reports, and psychological diagnostic or evaluative statements are based on information and techniques (including personal interviews of the individual when appropriate) sufficient to provide appropriate substantiation for their findings. (See also Standard 7.02, Forensic Assessments.)

### 2.02 Competence and Appropriate Use of Assessments and Interventions

a. Psychologists who develop, administer, score, interpret, or use psychological assessment techniques, interviews, tests, or instruments do so in a manner and for purposes that are appropriate in light of the research on or evidence of the usefulness and proper application of the techniques.

b. Psychologists refrain from misuse of assessment techniques, interventions, results, and interpretations and take reasonable steps to prevent others from misusing the information these techniques provide. This includes refraining from releasing raw test results or raw data to persons, other than to patients or clients as appropriate, who are not qualified to use such information. (See also Standards 1.02, Relationship of Ethics and Law, and 1.04, Boundaries of Competence.)

### *2.03 Test Construction*

Psychologists who develop and conduct research with tests and other assessment techniques use scientific procedures and current professional knowledge for test design, standardization, validation, reduction or elimination of bias, and recommendations for use.

### *2.04 Use of Assessment in General and with Special Populations*

a. Psychologists who perform interventions or administer, score, interpret, or use assessment techniques are familiar with the reliability, validation, and related standardization or outcome studies of, and proper applications and uses of, the techniques they use.
b. Psychologists recognize limits to the certainty with which diagnoses, judgments, or predictions can be made about individuals.
c. Psychologists attempt to identify situations in which particular interventions or assessment techniques or norms may not be applicable or may require adjustment in administration or interpretation because of factors such as individuals' gender, age, race, ethnicity, national origin, religion, sexual orientation, disability, language, or socioeconomic status.

### *2.05 Interpreting Assessment Results*

When interpreting assessment results, including automated interpretations, psychologists take into account the various test factors and characteristics of the person being assessed that might affect psychologists' judgments or reduce the accuracy of their interpretations. They indicate any significant reservations they have about the accuracy or limitations of their interpretations.

### *2.06 Unqualified Persons*

Psychologists do not promote the use of psychological assessment techniques by unqualified persons. (See also Standard 1.22, Delegation to and Supervision of Subordinates.)

### *2.07 Obsolete Tests and Outdated Test Results*

a. Psychologists do not base their assessment or intervention decisions or recommendations on data or test results that are outdated for the current purpose.
b. Similarly, psychologists do not base such decisions or recommendations on tests and measures that are obsolete and not useful for the current purpose.

### *2.08 Test Scoring and Interpretation Services*

a. Psychologists who offer assessment or scoring procedures to other professionals accurately describe the purpose, norms, validity, reliability, and applications of the procedures and any special qualifications applicable to their use.

b. Psychologists select scoring and interpretation services (including automated services) on the basis of evidence of the validity of the program and procedures as well as on other appropriate considerations.
c. Psychologists retain appropriate responsibility for the appropriate application, interpretation, and use of assessment instruments, whether they score and interpret such tests themselves or use automated or other services.

## 2.09 Explaining Assessment Results

Unless the nature of the relationship is clearly explained to the person being assessed in advance and precludes provision of an explanation of results (such as in some organizational consulting, preemployment or security screenings, and forensic evaluations), psychologists ensure that an explanation of the results is provided using language that is reasonably understandable to the person assessed or to another legally authorized person on behalf of the client. Regardless of whether the scoring and interpretation are done by the psychologist, by assistants, or by automated or other outside services, psychologists take reasonable steps to ensure that appropriate explanations of results are given.

## 2.10 Maintaining Test Security

Psychologists make reasonable efforts to maintain the integrity and security of tests and other assessment techniques consistent with law, contractual obligations, and in a manner that permits compliance with the requirements of this Ethics Code. (See also Standard 1.02, Relationship of Ethics and Law.) . . .

# 4. Therapy

## 4.01 Structuring the Relationship

a. Psychologists discuss with clients or patients as early as is feasible in the therapeutic relationship appropriate issues, such as the nature and anticipated course of therapy, fees, and confidentiality. (See also Standards 1.25, Fees and Financial Arrangements, and 5.01, Discussing the Limits of Confidentiality.)
b. When the psychologist's work with clients or patients will be supervised, the above discussion includes that fact, and the name of the supervisor, when the supervisor has legal responsibility for the case.
c. When the therapist is a student intern, the client or patient is informed of that fact.
d. Psychologists make reasonable efforts to answer patients' questions and to avoid apparent misunderstandings about therapy. Whenever possible, psychologists provide oral and/or written information, using language that is reasonably understandable to the patient or client.

## 4.02 Informed Consent to Therapy

a. Psychologists obtain appropriate informed consent to therapy or related procedures, using language that is reasonably understandable to participants. The content of informed consent will vary depending on many circumstances; however, informed consent generally implies that the person (1) has the capacity to consent, (2) has been informed of significant information concerning the procedure, (3) has freely and without undue influence expressed consent, and (4) consent has been appropriately documented.

b. When persons are legally incapable of giving informed consent, psychologists obtain informed permission from a legally authorized person, if such substitute consent is permitted by law.

c. In addition, psychologists (1) inform those persons who are legally incapable of giving informed consent about the proposed interventions in a manner commensurate with the persons' psychological capacities, (2) seek their assent to those interventions, and (3) consider such persons' preferences and best interests.

### 4.03 *Couple and Family Relationships*

a. When a psychologist agrees to provide services to several persons who have a relationship (such as husband and wife or parents and children), the psychologist attempts to clarify at the outset (1) which of the individuals are patients or clients and (2) the relationship the psychologist will have with each person. This clarification includes the role of the psychologist and the probable uses of the services provided or the information obtained. (See also Standard 5.01, Discussing the Limits of Confidentiality.)

b. As soon as it becomes apparent that the psychologist may be called on to perform potentially conflicting roles (such as marital counselor to husband and wife, and then witness for one party in a divorce proceeding), the psychologist attempts to clarify and adjust, or withdraw from, roles appropriately. (See also Standard 7.03, Clarification of Role, under Forensic Activities.)

### 4.04 *Providing Mental Health Services to Those Served by Others*

In deciding whether to offer or provide services to those already receiving mental health services elsewhere, psychologists carefully consider the treatment issues and the potential patient's or client's welfare. The psychologist discusses these issues with the patient or client, or another legally authorized person on behalf of the client, in order to minimize the risk of confusion and conflict, consults with the other service providers when appropriate, and proceeds with caution and sensitivity to the therapeutic issues.

### 4.05 *Sexual Intimacies with Current Patients or Clients*

Psychologists do not engage in sexual intimacies with current patients or clients.

### 4.06 *Therapy with Former Sexual Partners*

Psychologists do not engage as therapy patients or clients persons with whom they have engaged in sexual intimacies.

### 4.07 *Sexual Intimacies with Former Therapy Patients*

a. Psychologists do not engage in sexual intimacies with a former therapy patient or client for at least two years after cessation or termination of professional services.

b. Because sexual intimacies with a former therapy patient or client are so frequently harmful to the patient or client, and because such intimacies undermine public confidence in the psychology profession and thereby deter the public's use of needed services, psychologists do not engage in sexual intimacies with former therapy patients and clients even after a two-year interval except in the most unusual circumstances. The psychologist who engages in such activity after the two years following cessation or termination of treatment bears the burden of demonstrating that there has been no exploitation, in light of all relevant factors, including (1) the amount of time that has passed since therapy terminated, (2) the nature and duration of the therapy, (3) the circumstances of termination, (4) the patient's or client's personal history, (5) the patient's or client's current mental status, (6) the likelihood of adverse impact on the patient or client and others, and (7) any statements or actions made by the therapist during the course of therapy suggesting or inviting the possibility of a posttermination sexual or romantic relationship with the patient or client. (See also Standard 1.17, Multiple Relationships.)

## *4.08 Interruption of Services*

a. Psychologists make reasonable efforts to plan for facilitating care in the event that psychological services are interrupted by factors such as the psychologist's illness, death, unavailability, or relocation or by the client's relocation or financial limitations. (See also Standard 5.09, Preserving Records and Data.)
b. When entering into employment or contractual relationships, psychologists provide for orderly and appropriate resolution of responsibility for patient or client care in the event that the employment or contractual relationship ends, with paramount consideration given to the welfare of the patient or client.

## *4.09 Terminating the Professional Relationship*

a. Psychologists do not abandon patients or clients. (See also Standard 1.25e, under Fees and Financial Arrangements.)
b. Psychologists terminate a professional relationship when it becomes reasonably clear that the patient or client no longer needs the service, is not benefiting, or is being harmed by continued service.
c. Prior to termination for whatever reason, except where precluded by the patient's or client's conduct, the psychologist discusses the patient's or client's views and needs, provides appropriate pretermination counseling, suggests alternative service providers as appropriate, and takes other reasonable steps to facilitate transfer of responsibility to another provider if the patient or client needs one immediately.

# 5. Privacy and Confidentiality

These Standards are potentially applicable to the professional and scientific activities of all psychologists.

## 5.01 Discussing the Limits of Confidentiality

a. Psychologists discuss with persons and organizations with whom they establish a scientific or professional relationship (including, to the extent feasible, minors and their legal representatives) (1) the relevant limitations on confidentiality, including limitations where applicable in group, marital, and family therapy or in organizational consulting, and (2) the foreseeable uses of the information generated through their services.

b. Unless it is not feasible or is contraindicated, the discussion of confidentiality occurs at the outset of the relationship and thereafter as new circumstances may warrant.

c. Permission for electronic recording of interviews is secured from clients and patients.

## 5.02 Maintaining Confidentiality

Psychologists have a primary obligation and take reasonable precautions to respect the confidentiality rights of those with whom they work or consult, recognizing that confidentiality may be established by law, institutional rules, or professional or scientific relationships.

## 5.03 Minimizing Intrusions on Privacy

a. In order to minimize intrusions on privacy, psychologists include in written and oral reports, consultations, and the like, only information germane to the purpose for which the communication is made.

b. Psychologists discuss confidential information obtained in clinical or consulting relationships, or evaluative data concerning patients, individual or organizational clients, students, research participants, supervisees, and employees, only for appropriate scientific or professional purposes and only with persons clearly concerned with such matters.

## 5.04 Maintenance of Records

Psychologists maintain appropriate confidentiality in creating, storing, accessing, transferring, and disposing of records under their control, whether these are written, automated, or in any other medium. Psychologists maintain and dispose of records in accordance with law and in a manner that permits compliance with the requirements of this Ethics Code.

## 5.05 Disclosures

a. Psychologists disclose confidential information without the consent of the individual only as mandated by law, or where permitted by law for a valid purpose, such as (1) to provide needed professional services to the patient or the individual or organizational client, (2) to obtain appropriate professional consultations, (3) to protect the patient or client or others from harm, or (4) to obtain payment for services, in which instance disclosure is limited to the minimum that is necessary to achieve the purpose.

b. Psychologists also may disclose confidential information with the appropriate consent of the patient or the individual or organizational client (or of another legally authorized person on behalf of the patient or client), unless prohibited by law.

### 5.06 Consultations

When consulting with colleagues, (1) psychologists do not share confidential information that reasonably could lead to the identification of a patient, client, research participant, or other person or organization with whom they have a confidential relationship unless they have obtained the prior consent of the person or organization or the disclosure cannot be avoided, and (2) they share information only to the extent necessary to achieve the purposes of the consultation. (See also Standard 5.02, Maintaining Confidentiality.)

### 5.07 Confidential Information in Databases

a. If confidential information concerning recipients of psychological services is to be entered into databases or systems of records available to persons whose access has not been consented to by the recipient, then psychologists use coding or other techniques to avoid the inclusion of personal identifiers.
b. If a research protocol approved by an institutional review board or similar body requires the inclusion of personal identifiers, such identifiers are deleted before the information is made accessible to persons other than those of whom the subject was advised.
c. If such deletion is not feasible, then before psychologists transfer such data to others or review such data collected by others, they take reasonable steps to determine that appropriate consent of personally identifiable individuals has been obtained.

### 5.08 Use of Confidential Information for Didactic or Other Purposes

a. Psychologists do not disclose in their writings, lectures, or other public media, confidential, personally identifiable information concerning their patients, individual or organizational clients, students, research participants, or other recipients of their services that they obtained during the course of their work, unless the person or organization has consented in writing or unless there is other ethical or legal authorization for doing so.
b. Ordinarily, in such scientific and professional presentations, psychologists disguise confidential information concerning such persons or organizations so that they are not individually identifiable to others and so that discussions do not cause harm to subjects who might identify themselves.

### 5.09 Preserving Records and Data

A psychologist makes plans in advance so that confidentiality of records and data is protected in the event of the psychologist's death, incapacity, or withdrawal from the position or practice.

## *5.10  Ownership of Records and Data*

Recognizing that ownership of records and data is governed by legal principles, psychologists take reasonable and lawful steps so that records and data remain available to the extent needed to serve the best interests of patients, individual or organizational clients, research participants, or appropriate others.

## *5.11  Withholding Records for Nonpayment*

Psychologists may not withhold records under their control that are requested and imminently needed for a patient's or client's treatment solely because payment has not been received, except as otherwise provided by law.

# References

AINSWORTH, M. D. (1989). Attachments beyond infancy. *American Psychologist, 44,* 709–716.

ALSCHULER, S. S., IVEY, A. E., & HATCHER, C. (1977). Psychological education. In C. Hatcher et al. (Eds.), *Innovations in Counseling Psychology*. San Francisco: Jossey-Bass.

AMERICAN PSYCHIATRIC ASSOCIATION (1987). *Diagnostic and statistical manual of mental disorders, 3rd ed., revised.* Washington, DC.

ASIMOV, I. (1981). *New guide to science.* New York: Basic Books.

AXELSON, J. A. (1993). *Counseling and development in a multicultural society* (2nd ed.). Pacific Grove, CA: Brooks/Cole.

BAKER, L., & CLARK, R. (1990). Genetic origins of behavior: Implications for counselors. *Journal of Counseling and Development, 68*(6), 597–600.

BANDURA, A. (1977). *Social learning theory.* Englewood Cliffs, NJ: Prentice-Hall.

BANDURA, A. (1986). *Social foundations of thought and action.* Englewood Cliffs, NJ: Prentice-Hall.

BANDURA, A. (1989). Human agency in social cognitive theory. *American Psychologist, 44,* 1175–1184.

BECK, A. T. (1964). Thinking and depression: II. Theory and therapy. *Archives of General Psychiatry, 10,* 561–571.

BECK, A., FREEMAN, A., et al. (1990). *Cognitive therapy of personality disorders.* New York: Guilford Press.

BECK, A. T., RUSH, A. J., SHAW, B. F., & EMERY, G. (1979). *Cognitive therapy of depression.* New York: Guilford.

BENJAMIN, H. (1949). *The cultivation of idiosyncrasy.* The 1949 Inglis Lecture. Cambridge, MA: Harvard University Press.

BERNE, E. (1961). *Transactional analysis in psychotherapy.* New York: Grove Press.

BISHOP, J. B. (1990). The university counseling center: An agenda for the 1990's. *Journal of Counseling and Development, 68,* 408–413.

BLUSTEIN, D. L. (1992). Applying current theory and research in career exploration and practice. *Career Development Quarterly, 40*(4), 313–323.

BLY, R. (1990). *Iron John.* Reading, MA: Addison-Wesley.

BRABECK, M. M., & WERFEL, E. R. (1985). Counseling theory: Understanding the trend toward eclecticism from a developmental perspective. *Journal of Counseling and Development, 63,* 343–348.

BUCK, R. (1985). Prime theory: An integrated view of motivation and emotion. *Psychological Review, 92,* 389–413.

BYRNE, R. H. (1977). *Guidance: A behavioral approach.* Englewood Cliffs, NJ: Prentice-Hall.

CANTOR, N. (1990). From thought to behavior: "Having" and "doing" in the study of personality and cognition. *American Psychologist, 45,* 735–750.

CAPLE, R. B. (1985). Counseling and the self-organization paradigm. *Journal of Counseling and Development, 64,* 173–178.

CATTELL, R. B., & KLINE, P. (1977). *The scientific analysis of personality and motivation.* New York: Academic Press.

CLAIBORN, C. D., & LICHTENBERG, J. W. (1989). Interactional counseling. *The Counseling Psychologist, 17*(3), 355–453.

COMMITTEE ON DEFINITION, DIVISION OF COUNSELING PSYCHOLOGY. (1980). Counseling psychology as a specialty. In J. M. Whiteley (Ed.), *The history of counseling psychology.* Pacific Grove, CA: Brooks/Cole.

COOK, E. P. (1993). *Women, relationships, and power: Implications for counseling.* Alexandria, VA: American Counseling Association.

CORMIER, W. H., & CORMIER, L. S. (1991). *Interviewing strategies for helpers* (3rd ed.). Pacific Grove, CA: Brooks/Cole.

CORSINI, R. J. (ED.). (1984). *Current psychotherapies* (3rd ed.). Itasca, IL: F. E. Peacock.

COUSINS, N. (1979). *Anatomy of an illness as perceived by the patient.* New York: Norton.

COUSINS, N. (1983). *The healing heart.* New York: Norton.

CUSHMAN, P. (1990). Why the self is empty. *American Psychologist, 45,* 599–611.

DAVIS, J. M. (1985). Minor tranquilizers, sedatives, and hypnotics. In H. I. Kaplan & B. J. Sadock

(Eds.), *Comprehensive textbook of psychiatry.* Baltimore: Williams & Wilkins.

DIXON, R. A., & LERNER, R. M. (1989). A history of systems in developmental psychology. In F. Masterpasqua, A competence paradigm for psychological practice. *American Psychologist, 44,* 1366–1371.

DOBSON, K. (ED.). (1988). *Handbook of cognitive-behavioral therapies.* New York: Guilford Press.

DOBSON, K., & BLOCK, L. (1988). Historical and philosophical bases of the cognitive-behavioral therapies. In K. Dobson (Ed.), *Handbook of cognitive-behavioral therapies.* New York: Guilford Press.

DOPPELT, G. (1983). Relativism in recent pragmatic conceptions of scientific rationality. In N. Rescher (Ed.), *Scientific explanation and understanding.* Lanham, MD: University Press of America.

DUSAY, J. M., & DUSAY, K. M. (1984). Transactional analysis. In R. J. Corsini (Ed.), *Current Psychotherapies* (3rd ed.). Itasca, IL: F. E. Peacock.

ECKMAN, P. (1984). Expression and the nature of emotions. In K. R. Scherer & P. Eckman (Eds.), *Approaches to emotion.* Hillsdale, NJ: Erlbaum.

EGAN, G. (1982). *The skilled helper* (2nd ed.). Pacific Grove, CA: Brooks/Cole.

ELLIOTT, F. A. (1988). In D. E. Papalia & S. Wendkos Olds, *Psychology.* New York: McGraw-Hill.

ELLIS, A. (1962). *Reason and emotion in psychotherapy.* New York: Lyle Stuart.

ELLIS, A. (1984). Rational-emotive therapy. In R. J. Corsini (Ed.), *Current psychotherapies* (3rd ed.). Itasca, IL: F. E. Peacock.

ERICKSON, E. (1968). *Identity, youth, and crisis.* New York: Norton.

ERON, L. D. (1988). In D. E. Papalia & S. Wendkos Olds, *Psychology.* New York: McGraw-Hill.

EVERLY, G. (1989). *Clinical guide to treatment of human stress response.* New York: Plenum.

EYSENCK, H. J. (1947). *Dimensions of personality.* London: Routledge & Kegan Paul.

EYSENCK, H. J., & EYSENCK, M. W. (1985). *Personality and individual differences.* New York: Plenum.

FITZGERALD, L. F., & OSIPOW, S. H. (1986). An occupational analysis of counseling psychology: How special is the specialty? *American Psychologist, 41,* 535–544.

FOLEY, V. D. (1984). Family therapy. In R. J. Corsini (Ed.), *Current psychotherapies* (3rd ed.). Itasca, IL: F. E. Peacock.

GALTON, F. (1883). *Inquiries into human faculty and development.* London: Macmillan.

GATZ, M. (1990). Interpreting behavioral genetic results: Suggestions for counselors and clients. *Journal of Counseling and Development, 68,* 601–605.

GELSO, C. J., & FRETZ, B. R. (1992). *Counseling psychology.* New York: Harcourt Brace Jovanovich.

GLASSER, W. (1984). Reality therapy. In R. J. Corsini (Ed.), *Current psychotherapies* (3rd ed.). Itasca, IL: F. E. Peacock.

GLOSOFF, H. L. (1992). Accrediting and certifying professional counselors. *Guideposts,* May 1992.

GREENBERG, L. S., & SAFRAN, J. D. (1987). *Emotion in psychotherapy.* New York: Guilford Press.

GREENWOOD, E. (1962). Attributes of a profession. In S. Nosow & W. Form (Eds.), *Man, work, and society.* New York: Basic Books.

GROVES, P. M., & REBEC, G. V. (1988). *Introduction to biological psychology.* Dubuque, IA: William C. Brown.

GUIDANO, V. (1988). A systems process-oriented approach to cognitive therapy. In K. Dobson (Ed.), *Handbook of cognitive-behavioral therapies.* New York: Guilford Press.

GUILFORD, J. (1959). Three faces of intellect. *American Psychologist, 14,* 469–479.

GUYTON, A. C. (1986). *Textbook of medical physiology* (7th ed.). Philadelphia: Saunders.

HAHN, M. E. (1980). Counseling psychology–2000 A.D. In J. Whiteley & B. Fretz (Eds.), *The present and future of counseling psychology.* Pacific Grove, CA: Brooks/Cole.

HALL, S. S. (1990). Biologists zero in on life's very essence. *Smithsonian, 20*(11), 40–51.

HELLMANS, A., & BUNCH, B. (1988). *The timetables of science.* New York: Simon & Schuster.

HERR, E. L., & CRAMER, S. H. (1992). *Career guidance and counseling through the lifespan: Systematic approaches* (4th ed.). New York: Harper & Row.

HILL, C. E. (1993). Editorial. *Journal of Counseling Psychology, 40,* 252–256.

HOLLAND, J. (1966). *The psychology of vocational choice.* Waltham, MA: Blaisdell Publishing Co.

HOLLAND, J. L. (1985). *Making vocational choices: A theory of vocational personalities and work environments* (2nd ed.). Englewood Cliffs, NJ: Prentice-Hall.

HOLLAND, J. L., WHITNEY, D. R., COLE, N. S., & RICHARDS, J. M., JR. (1969). *An empirical occupational classification derived from a theory of personality and intended for practice and research.* Iowa City: American College Testing.

HOOD, A. B., & JOHNSON, R. W. (1991). *Assessment in counseling.* Alexandria, VA: American Counseling Association.

IVEY, A. E. (1980). *Counseling and psychotherapy.* Englewood Cliffs, NJ: Prentice-Hall.

IZARD, C. E., KAGAN, J., & ZAJONC, R. (EDS.). (1984). *Emotions, cognition, and behavior.* New York: Cambridge University Press.

JORDAAN, J. P., MEYERS, R. A., LAYTON, W. L., & MORGAN, H. H. (1980). The counseling psychologist: A definition in 1968. In J. M. Whiteley (Ed.), *The history of counseling psychology.* Pacific Grove, CA: Brooks/Cole.

KAGAN, J. (1989). Temperamental contributions to social behavior. *American Psychologist, 44,* 668–674.

KAGAN, N., ARMSWORTH, M., ALTMAIER, E. M., DOWD, E. T., HANSEN, J.-I. C., SCHLOSSBERG, N., SPRINTHALL, N. A., TANNEY, M. F., & VASQUEZ, M. J. (1988). Professional practice of counseling psychology in various settings. *The Counseling Psychologist, 16*(3), 347–384.

KAHN, W. J. (1988). Cognitive-behavioral group counseling: An introduction. *The School Counselor, 35,* 343–351.

KAPES, J. T., & MASTIE, M. M. (1988). *A counselor's guide to career assessment instruments.* Alexandria, VA: American Counseling Association.

KAPLAN, H. I., & SADOCK, B. J. (EDS.). (1985). *Comprehensive textbook of psychiatry.* Baltimore: Williams & Wilkins.

KAUFMANN, Y. (1984). Analytical psychotherapy. In R. J. Corsini (Ed.), *Current psychotherapies* (3rd ed.). Itasca, IL: F. E. Peacock.

KAZDIN, A. E., & WILSON, G. T. (1978). *Evaluation of behavior therapy.* Cambridge, MA: Ballinger.

KEEN, S. (1990). *Fire in the belly.* New York: Bantam Books.

KEGAN, R. (1982). *The evolving self.* Cambridge, MA: Harvard University Press.

KING, P., KITCHENER, K. S., DAVIDSON, M. L., PARKER, C. A., & WOOD, P. K. (1983). A longitudinal study of reflective judgment and verbal aptitude in young adults. *Human Development, 26,* 106–116.

KNEFELKAMP, L. L., & SLEPITZA, R. (1976). A cognitive-developmental model of career development—An adaptation of the Perry scheme. *The Counseling Psychologist, 6*(3) 53–58.

KOHLBERG, L. (1976). *Collected papers on moral development and moral education.* Cambridge, MA: Center for Moral Development, Harvard University.

KRUMBOLTZ, J. (1991). Brilliant insights—platitudes that bear repeating. *The Counseling Psychologist, 19*(2), 298–315.

KRUMBOLTZ, J. (1993). Career Beliefs Inventory. Counseling Psychologists Press.

KRUMBOLTZ, J. D., & MENEFEE, M. (1980). Reflections on chronic health, self-control, and human ethology. In J. Whiteley & B. Fretz (Eds.), *The present and future of counseling psychology.* Pacific Grove, CA: Brooks/Cole.

KUHN, T. S. (1970). *The structure of scientific revolutions.* Chicago: University of Chicago Press.

KUKLA, A. (1989). Nonempirical issues in psychology. *American Psychologist, 44,* 789–794.

LAMB, R. R., & PREDIGER, D. J. (1981). *Technical report for the unisex edition of the ACT Interest Inventory.* Iowa City: American College Testing.

LAZARUS, A. A. (1984). Multimodal therapy. In R. J. Corsini (Ed.), *Current psychotherapies* (3rd ed.). Itasca, IL: F. E. Peacock.

LAZARUS, R. S. (1991a). Cognition and motivation in emotion. *American Psychologist, 46,* 352–367.

LAZARUS, R. S. (1991b). Progress on a cognitive-motivational relational theory of emotion. *American Psychologist, 46,* 819–834.

LEA, H. D., & LEIBOWITZ, Z. B. (1992). *Adult career development: Concepts, issues, and practices* (2nd ed.). Alexandria, VA: American Counseling Association.

LEVINSON, D. J. (1978). *The seasons of a man's life.* New York: Ballantine.

LEVY, L. H. (1984). The metamorphosis of clinical psychology: Toward a new charter as developmental psychology. *American Psychologist, 39,* 486–494.

LEWIN, K. (1963). *Field theory in social sciences: Selected theoretical papers.* London: Tavistock.

LINN, L. (1985). Clinical manifestations of psychiatric disorders. In H. I. Kaplan & B. J. Sadock (Eds.), *Comprehensive textbook of psychiatry.* Baltimore: Williams & Wilkins.

LYDDON, W. (1990). First- and second-order change: Implications for rationalist and constructivist cognitive therapies. *Journal of Counseling and Development, 69,* 122–127.

LYDDON, W. (1992). A rejoinder to Ellis: What is and what is not RET? *Journal of Counseling and Development, 70,* 452–454.

MAHONEY, M. (1988). The cognitive sciences and psychotherapy: Patterns in a developing relationship. In K. Dobson (Ed.), *Handbook of cognitive-behavioral therapies.* New York: Guilford Press.

MAHONEY, M. J., & ARNKOFF, D. B. (1978). Cognitive and self control therapies. In S. L. Garfield & A. E. Bergin (Eds.), *Handbook of psychotherapy and behavior change.* New York: Wiley.

MANICAS, P., & SECORD, P. (1983). Implications for psychology of the new philosophy of science. *American Psychologist, 38,* 399–414.

MANUELE-ADKINS, C. (1992). Career counseling is personal counseling. *Career Development Quarterly, 40*(4), 313–323.

MASTERPASQUA, F. (1989). A competence paradigm for psychological practice. *American Psychologist, 44,* 1366–1371.

MATARAZZO, J. (1987). There is only one psychology, no specialties, but many applications. *American Psychologist, 44,* 893–903.

MEYER, J. (1985). Normal human sexuality and psychosexual disorders. In H. I. Kaplan & B. J. Sadock (Eds.), *Comprehensive textbook of psychiatry.* Baltimore: Williams & Wilkins.

MITCHELL, J. V. JR. (ED.) (1985). *The ninth mental measurements yearbook.* Lincoln, NE: Buros Institute of Mental Measurement.

MORRIS, W. N. (1989). *Mood—the frame of mind.* New York: Springer-Verlag.

MORRISON P., & MORRISON, P. (1987). *The ring of truth.* New York: Random House.

MOSAK, H. (1984). Adlerian psychotherapy. In R. J. Corsini (Ed.), *Current psychotherapies* (3rd ed.). Itasca, IL: F. E. Peacock.

NEIMEYER, R. (1990). Personal construct therapy. In J. Zelig & W. Munion (Eds.), *What is psychotherapy?* San Francisco: Jossey-Bass.

NEMEROFF, S., & KAROLY, P. (1991). Operant methods. In F. Kanfer & A. Goldstein (Eds.), *Helping people change.* Elmsford, NY: Pergamon Press.

O'LEARY, S., & O'LEARY, K. (1976). Behavior modification in the school. In H. Leitenberg (Ed.), *Handbook of behavior modification and behavior therapy.* Englewood Cliffs, NJ: Prentice-Hall.

OSIPOW, S. (1980). Toward counseling psychology in the year 2000. In J. Whiteley & B. Fretz (Eds.), *The present and future of counseling psychology.* Pacific Grove, CA: Brooks/Cole.

PALLONE, N. J. (1980). Counseling psychology: Toward an empirical definition. In J. Whiteley & B. Fretz (Eds.), *The present and future of counseling psychology.* Pacific Grove, CA: Brooks/Cole.

PAPALIA, D. E., & WENDKOS OLDS, S. (1988). *Psychology.* New York: McGraw-Hill.

PARSONS, F. (1909). *Choosing a vocation.* Boston: Houghton Mifflin.

PATE, R. H., JR. (1992). Student suicide: Are you liable? *American Counselor, 1*(3).

PATTERSON, C. H. (1980). *Theories of counseling and psychotherapy* (3rd ed.). New York: Harper & Row.

PAVLOV, I. P. (1927). *Conditioned reflexes.* London: Oxford University Press.

PERRY, W., JR. (1970). *Intellectual and ethical development in college years.* New York: Holt, Rinehart & Winston.

PIAGET, J. (1952). *The origins of intelligence in children.* New York: International Universities Press.

PLUTCHICK, R. (1984). Emotions: A general psychoevolutionary theory. In C. E. Izard, J. Kagan, & R. Zajonc (Eds.), *Emotions, cognition, and behavior.* New York: Cambridge University Press.

POPE, K. S., & VETTER, V. A. (1992). Ethical dilemmas encountered by members of the American Psychological Association: A national survey. *American Psychologist, 47,* 397–411.

POPPER, K. (1962). *Conjectures and refutations.* New York: Harper & Row.

PREDIGER, D., SWANEY, K., & MAU, W.-C. (1993). Extending Holland's hexagon: Procedures, counseling applications, and research. *Journal of Counseling and Development, 71,* 422–428.

PRIBRAM, K. H. (1985). "Holism" could close cognition era. *APA Monitor, 16*(9).

PRIBRAM, K. H. (1986). The cognitive revolution and mind/brain issues. *American Psychologist, 41,* 507–520.

RAINE, A., & DUNKIN, J. J. (1990). The genetic and psychophysiological basis of antisocial behavior. *Journal of Counseling and Development, 68,* 637–644.

REHM, L. P., & ROKKE, P. (1988). Self-management therapies. In K. S. Dobson (Ed.), *Handbook of cognitive-behavioral therapies.* New York: Guilford Press.

REISER, L. W., & REISER, M. F. (1985). Endocrine disorders. In H. T. Sadock & B. J. Sadock (Eds.), *Textbook of psychiatry IV.* Baltimore: Williams & Wilkins.

RESTAK, R. M. (1988). *The mind.* New York: Bantam Books.

ROBINSON, F. P. (1950). *Principles and procedures in student counseling.* New York: Harper & Row.

ROGERS, C. (1942). *Counseling and psychotherapy.* Boston: Houghton Mifflin.

ROGERS, C. R. (1951). *Client-centered therapy.* Boston: Houghton Mifflin.

ROGERS, C., & SANFORD, R. (1985). Client-centered psychotherapy. In H. I. Kaplan & B. J. Sadock (Eds.), *Comprehensive textbook of psychiatry.* Baltimore: Williams & Wilkins.

ROSENBERG, A. (1983). Human science and biological science: Defects and prospects. In N. Rescher (Ed.), *Scientific explanation and understanding.* Lanham, MD: University Press of America.

ROSSI, E. (1986). *The psychobiology of mind-body healing.* New York: Norton.

ROWE, D. C. (1990). As the twig is bent? The myth of child-rearing influences on personality development. *Journal of Counseling and Development, 68,* 606–611.

RUBIN, S. E., & ROESSLER, R. T. (1987). *Foundations of the vocational rehabilitation process* (3rd ed.). Austin, TX: Pro Ed.

SAMSON, E. E. (1988). The debate on individualism: Indigenous psychologies of the individual and their role in personal and societal functioning. *American Psychologist, 43,* 1522.

SCHLOSSBERG, N. K. (1984). *Counseling adults in transition.* New York: Springer.

SCOTT, C. W. (1980). History of the division of counseling psychology: 1945–1963. In J. Whiteley (Ed.), *The history of counseling psychology.* Pacific Grove, CA: Brooks/Cole.

SEEMAN, J. (1989). Toward a model of positive health. *American Psychologist, 44,* 1099–1109.

SEGAL, N. L. (1990). The importance of twin studies for individual differences research. *Journal of Counseling and Development, 68,* 6, 612–622.

SHERMAN, P. R. (1992). *What do you want to be when you grow up? The ideology of vocational choice.* Paper delivered to the annual convention of the American Psychological Association.

SIEGEL, B. (1986). *Love, medicine, and miracles.* New York: Harper & Row.

SIMKIN, J. S., & YONTEF, G. M. (1984). Gestalt therapy. In R. J. Corsini (Ed.), *Current psychotherapies* (3rd ed.). Itasca, IL: F. E. Peacock.

SKINNER, B. F. (1953). *Science and human behavior.* New York: Macmillan.

SKOVHOLT, T. M. (1990). Counseling implications of genetic research. *Journal of Counseling and Development, 68,* 633–636.

SPEARMAN, C. (1904). General intelligence objectively determined and measured. *American Journal of Psychology, 15,* 201–293.

SPRINTHALL, N. A. (1990). Counseling psychology from Greystone to Atlanta: On the road to Armageddon? *The Counseling Psychologist, 18*(3), 455–463.

STEENBARGER, B. N. (1990). Toward a developmental understanding of the counseling specialty. *Journal of Counseling and Development, 68,* 434–437.

STERNBERG, R. J. (1985). *Beyond IQ.* Cambridge, England: Cambridge University Press.

STILES, W. B., SHAPIRO, D. A., & ELLIOT, R. (1986). Are all psychotherapies equivalent? *American Psychologist, 41,* 165–180.

STONE, G. L., & ARCHER, J. A., JR. (1990). College and university counseling centers in the 1990s. *The Counseling Psychologist, 18*(4), 539–607.

SUPER, D. (1957). *The psychology of careers.* New York: Harper & Row.

SUPER, D. (1980a). The identity crises of counseling psychologists. In J. Whiteley & B. Fretz (Eds.), *The present and future of counseling psychology.* Pacific Grove, CA: Brooks/Cole.

SUPER, D. (1980b). The year 2000 and all that. In J. Whiteley & B. Fretz (Eds.), *The present and future of counseling psychology.* Pacific Grove, CA: Brooks/Cole.

SWEENEY, T. J. (1992). CACREP: Precursors, promises, and prospects. *Journal of Counseling and Development, 70,* 667–672.

THOMPSON, J. G. (1988). The *psychobiology of emotions.* New York: Plenum.

THORESON, C. (1973). Behavioral humanism. In C. Thoreson (Ed.), *Behavioral modification in education,* Part 1, 72nd Yearbook. Chicago: National Society for the Study of Education.

THURSTONE, L. L. (1938). *Primary mental abilities.* Chicago: University of Chicago Press.

TOMPKINS, S. S. (1984). Affect theory. In K. R. Scherer & P. Eckman (Eds.), *Approaches to emotion.* Hillsdale, NJ: Erlbaum.

U. S. DEPARTMENT OF LABOR (1982). *Dictionary of occupational titles* (4th ed.) Washington, DC: U. S. Government Printing Office.

U. S. DEPARTMENT OF LABOR (1986). *Dictionary of occupational titles* (4th ed. suppl.). Washington, DC: U. S. Government Printing Office.

VANDENBERG, B. (1991). Is epistemology enough? An existential consideration of development. *American Psychologist, 46,* 1278–1286.

VON GLASERFELD, E. (1984). Introduction to radical constructivism. In P. Watzlanick (Ed.), *The invented reality.* New York: Norton.

WATKINS, C. E., JR., LOPEZ, F. G., CAMPBELL, V. L., & HIMMEL, C. D. (1986). Counseling psychology and clinical psychology: Some preliminary comparative data. *American Psychologist, 41,* 581–582.

WATSON, J. B., & RAYNER, P. (1920). Conditioned emotional reactions. *Journal of Experimental Psychology,* (3)1, 1–14.

WESCHLER, L. (1990). Profiles, *The New Yorker,* October 8th.

WHITELEY, J. M. (1980). *The history of counseling psychology.* Pacific Grove, CA: Brooks/Cole.

WHYBROW, P. (1984). Contributions from neuroendocrinology. In K. R. Scherer & P. Eckman (Eds.), *Approaches to emotion.* Hillsdale, NJ: Erlbaum.

WILLIAMSON, E. G. (1939). *How to counsel students; a manual of techniques for clinical counselors.* New York: McGraw-Hill.

WILLIAMSON, E. G. (1950). *Counseling adolescents.* New York: McGraw-Hill.

WILLIAMSON, E. G. (1965). *Vocational counseling.* New York: McGraw-Hill.

WILSON, G. T. (1984). Behavior therapy. In R. J. Corsini (Ed.), *Current psychotherapies* (3rd ed.). Itasca, IL: F. E. Peacock.

WINNICOTT, D. W. (1986). *Home is where we start from.* New York: Penguin.

WOLF, T. (1966, October 9). Oh rotten Gotham—sliding down the behavioral sink. New York: *World Journal Tribune.*

ZUNKER, V. G. (1990). *Career counseling: Applied concepts of life planning.* Pacific Grove, CA: Brooks/Cole.

# Index

TO THE OWNER OF THIS BOOK

We hope that you have found *Becoming a Master Counselor* useful. So that this book can be improved in a future edition, would you take the time to complete this sheet and return it? Thank you.

School and address: _____

Department: _____

Instructor's name: _____

1. What I like most about this book is: _____

_____

_____

2. What I like least about this book is: _____

_____

_____

3. My general reaction to this book is: _____

_____

4. The name of the course in which I used this book is: _____

_____

5. Were all of the chapters of the book assigned for you to read? _____

   If not, which ones weren't? _____

6. In the space below, or on a separate sheet of paper, please write specific suggestions  for improving this book and anything else you'd care to share about your experience in using the book.

_____

_____

_____

_____

_____

OPTIONAL

Your name: _____ Date: _____

May Brooks/Cole quote you, either in promotion for *Becoming a Master Counselor* or in future publishing ventures?

Yes: _____ No: _____

Sincerely,

*Richard Hill Byrne*

Brooks/Cole is dedicated to publishing quality books for the helping professions. If you would like to learn more about our publications, please use this mailer to request our catalogue.

Name: _____

Street Address: _____

City/State/Zip code: _____

FOLD HERE

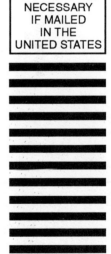

FOLD HERE